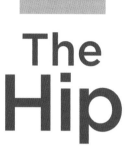

The
Hip

AANA Advanced Arthroscopic
Surgical Techniques

AANA Advanced Arthroscopic Surgical Techniques
SERIES

SERIES EDITORS, RICHARD K. N. RYU, MD
AND JEFFREY S. ABRAMS, MD

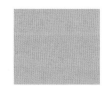

The
Hip

AANA Advanced Arthroscopic
Surgical Techniques

EDITED BY

J. W. THOMAS BYRD, MD
*Founder, Nashville Sports Medicine & Orthopaedic Center
and Nashville Sports Medicine Foundation
Clinical Professor, Department of Orthopaedics and Rehabilitation
Vanderbilt University
Nashville, Tennessee*

ASHEESH BEDI, MD
*Harold and Helen W. Gehring Professor
Chief, Sports Medicine
Department of Orthopaedic Surgery
University of Michigan Hospitals
Ann Arbor, Michigan*

ALLSTON J. STUBBS, MD
*Medical Director Hip Arthroscopy, Division of Sports Medicine
Associate Professor, Department of Orthopaedic Surgery
Wake Forest School of Medicine
Wake Forest Baptist Health
Winston-Salem, North Carolina*

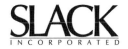

www.healio.com/books

ISBN: 978-1-63091-000-6

Published by: SLACK Incorporated
                  6900 Grove Road
                  Thorofare, NJ 08086 USA
                  Telephone: 856-848-1000
                  Fax: 856-848-6091
                  www.Healio.com/books

Contact SLACK Incorporated for more information about other books in this field or about the availability of our books from distributors outside the United States.

Library of Congress Cataloging-in-Publication Data

Names: Byrd, J. W. Thomas (John Wilson Thomas), 1957- , editor. | Bedi,
    Asheesh, 1978- , editor. | Stubbs, Allston J., editor. | Arthroscopy
    Association of North America.
Title: AANA advanced arthroscopic surgical techniques. Hip / [edited by] J.
    W. Thomas Byrd, Asheesh Bedi, Allston J. Stubbs.
Other titles: Advanced arthroscopic surgical techniques | Hip
Description: Thorofare, NJ : SLACK Incorporated, [2016] | Preceded by: AANA
    advanced arthroscopy. The hip / [edited by] J.W. Thomas Byrd, Carlos A.
    Guanche. Philadelphia : Saunders/Elsevier, c2010. | Includes
    bibliographical references and index.
Identifiers: LCCN 2015032288 | ISBN 9781630910006 (alk. paper)
Subjects: | MESH: Hip Joint--surgery. | Arthroscopy--methods.
Classification: LCC RD686 | NLM WE 860 | DDC 617.4/720597--dc23 LC record available at http://lccn.loc.gov/2015032288

Printed in the United States of America.

Last digit is print number: 10 9 8 7 6 5 4 3 2 1

DEDICATION

None of the innovations contained within the pages of this text would be possible without the support of our industry partners. Thus, I dedicate my efforts to an industry icon, Lisa Donnelly, who set the bar on industry commitment to the field of hip arthroscopy.

J. W. Thomas Byrd, MD

I dedicate this textbook to my family, whose countless sacrifices make my every endeavor possible, and also to my colleagues in hip preservation, who continue to enlighten me with insights that help me to be a more astute clinician and surgeon every day.

Asheesh Bedi, MD

To my wonderful children, Jack, Olivia, and Ava; your spirits make the world go round. Thank you for your love and support in this project and all orthopedic-related endeavors.

Allston J. Stubbs, MD

CONTENTS

ACKNOWLEDGMENTS

It is important to acknowledge the efforts of Sharon Simmons and Kay Jones and the entire Nashville Sports Medicine staff who tirelessly dedicate themselves to the patients who honor us by entrusting themselves to our care. Equally important is the ongoing commitment of this small village in disseminating our experiences to others who have taken on the responsibility of caring for those with complex hip disorders.

Lastly, I acknowledge the loving support of my family: Donna, Allison, and Ellen, who have graciously afforded me the luxury of being able to follow this trail.

J. W. Thomas Byrd, MD

I would like to acknowledge my colleagues and the thought leaders in hip preservation, many of whom are authors of this text, who continue to educate and enlighten me to make me a better clinician. It is the collective effort of these phenomenal individuals that make it a very exciting opportunity to be a hip preservation surgeon.

Asheesh Bedi, MD

In appreciation for their efforts on this project and in hip preservation, I would like to thank Angie Holland, Dana Lang, Brooke Miller, Tammy Olive, Kathy Prescott, Hope Touchtone, and Terri Windham.

Allston J. Stubbs, MD

ABOUT THE EDITORS

J. W. Thomas Byrd, MD is the founder of Nashville Sports Medicine & Orthopaedic Center, as well as the Nashville Sports Medicine Foundation, a nonprofit entity dedicated to research and education with a principal interest in hip disorders and arthroscopy. He is the third generation of physicians in his family to serve the Nashville community. He is team physician for the Tennessee Titans, has served as physician for the US Olympic team, and is a consulting orthopedic surgeon for numerous professional sports franchises from the National Football League, National Hockey League, National Basketball Association, Women's National Basketball Association, Major League Baseball, and Major League Soccer, as well as players from the Professional Golfers' Association, Ladies Professional Golf Association, and Association of Tennis Professionals. He is a Clinical Professor in Vanderbilt University's Department of Orthopaedic Surgery and Rehabilitation and serves on the Advisory Board for the Titleist Performance Institute.

Dr. Byrd is President of the International Society for Hip Arthroscopy and Immediate Past President of the Arthroscopy Association of North America. He is a member of the International Hip Society, Herodicus Society, Twentieth Century Orthopaedic Association, American Orthopaedic Society for Sports Medicine, International Society of Arthroscopy, Knee Surgery and Orthopaedic Sports Medicine, and Hip Society.

Dr. Byrd pioneered many of the techniques popular in hip arthroscopy today and designed many of the instruments commonly used for performing the procedure. He has authored 3 textbooks on hip arthroscopy, edited numerous other texts and journals, and published over 100 scientific papers, technical and review articles, and book chapters. He has been one of the leaders in defining and developing the role of less-invasive arthroscopic techniques in and around the hip.

Asheesh Bedi, MD is the Harold and Helen W. Gehring Professor of Orthopaedic Surgery and Chief of Sports Medicine and Shoulder Surgery at the University of Michigan and MedSport Program. He is also an Adjunct Assistant Professor at the Hospital for Special Surgery/Weill Cornell Medical College. He is a team physician for the University of Michigan, Eastern Michigan University, and Detroit Lions and a consultant for the National Football League and National Hockey League Players Association. Dr. Bedi specializes in both arthroscopic and open surgery for athletic injuries of the shoulder, elbow, hip, and knee. He is a Taubman Emerging Scholar and recognized clinician-scientist at the University of Michigan.

Dr. Bedi completed his undergraduate training at Northwestern University, where he graduated Summa Cum Laude. He graduated from the University of Michigan Medical School with AOA recognition and remained in Ann Arbor to pursue residency training in orthopedic surgery at the University of Michigan. After completing his training, Dr. Bedi completed a 2-year fellowship in sports medicine and shoulder surgery at the Hospital for Special Surgery and Weill Cornell Medical College in New York. He has also pursued additional dedicated training with Dr. Bryan Kelly in arthroscopic hip surgery for young athletes.

Dr. Bedi has also been recognized with the Leonard Marmor Outstanding Orthopaedic Resident Award and the Hospital for Special Surgery Philip D. Wilson Award for Excellence in both 2008 and 2009 for his efforts in orthopedic research and tendon-bone healing studies with Dr. Scott Rodeo. He is the winner of the 2010 Neer Award of the American Shoulder and Elbow Surgeons and a recipient of the 2010 Cabaud Award from the American Orthopedic Society for Sports Medicine. He has authored over 300 articles, chapters, and peer-reviewed publications on shoulder, elbow, knee, and hip injuries in athletes.

Allston J. Stubbs, MD is an Associate Professor of Orthopaedic Surgery at the Wake Forest School of Medicine in Winston-Salem, North Carolina. He specializes in orthopedic sports medicine and hip joint restoration. He serves as Medical Director of Hip Arthroscopy for Wake Forest Baptist Health. He is Board certified by the American Board of Orthopaedic Surgery and holds Subspecialty Certification in Sports Medicine. He is an active member of several orthopedic societies, serving on editorial and leadership boards. In the field of hip arthroscopy, he has authored research journal articles, created orthopedic instructional videos, and instructed at national and international orthopedic surgery conferences.

CONTRIBUTING AUTHORS

Geoffrey D. Abrams, MD (Chapter 8)
Assistant Professor
Department of Orthopedic Surgery
Stanford University School of Medicine
Redwood City, California
Veterans Administration
Palo Alto, California

William Brian Acker II, MD (Chapter 3)
Resident Surgeon
Department of Orthopaedic Surgery
University of Michigan
Ann Arbor, Michigan

Eduardo Acosta-Rodriguez, MD (Chapter 17)
Attendant Physician
Adult Joint Reconstruction Department
National Rehabilitation Institute of Mexico
Mexico City, Mexico

Marco Acuna-Tovar, MD (Chapter 17)
Clinical and Research Fellow
Adult Joint Reconstruction Department
National Rehabilitation Institute of Mexico
Mexico City, Mexico

Emily Cha, MD (Chapter 19)
Orthopedic Surgeon
Department of Orthopedics
Indiana University School of Medicine
Indianapolis, Indiana

John J. Christoforetti, MD (Chapter 5)
Director
Center for Athletic Hip Injury
Allegheny Health Network
Pittsburgh, Pennsylvania
Assistant Professor
Department of Orthopaedics
Drexel University School of Medicine
Philadelphia, Pennsylvania

Ryan M. Degen, MD (Chapter 14)
Sports Medicine Fellow
Hospital for Special Surgery
New York, New York

Michael Dienst, MD (Chapter 9)
Orthopedic Surgeon
Orthopädische Chirurgie München
Munich, Germany

Benjamin G. Domb, MD (Chapter 23)
Orthopaedic Surgeon
Hinsdale Orthopaedics
Medical Director
American Hip Institute
Westmont, Illinois

Michael B. Gerhardt, MD (Chapter 15)
Santa Monica Orthopaedic and Sports
    Medicine Group
Institute for Sports Science at Cedars-Sinai
FIFA Medical Center of Excellence
US Olympic Committee Sports Medicine
    Center
Team Physician, US Soccer and Major
    League Soccer
Santa Monica, California

Jonathan A. Godin, MD, MBA (Chapter 1)
Orthopedic Surgery Resident
Duke University Medical Center
Durham, North Carolina

Carlos A. Guanche, MD (Chapter 21)
Southern California Orthopedic Institute
Van Nuys, California

Joshua D. Harris, MD (Chapter 8)
Department of Orthopedics & Sports Medicine
Houston Methodist Hospital
Assistant Professor
Institute of Academic Medicine
Houston Methodist Research Institute
Houston, Texas

Munif Ahmad Hatem, MD (Chapter 20)
Hip Surgeon
Universidade Federal do Paraná and Hospital
  Pequeno Príncipe
Curitiba, Paraná, Brazil

Elizabeth A. Howse, MD (Chapters 2, 16)
Associate Physician
Department of Emergency Medicine
Kaiser Permanente Walnut Creek Medical
  Center
Walnut Creek, California

Víctor M. Ilizaliturri Jr, MD (Chapter 17)
Chief of Adult Joint Reconstruction
National Rehabilitation Institute of Mexico
Mexico City, Mexico

Pedro Joachin-Hernandez, MD (Chapter 17)
Clinical and Research Fellow
Adult Joint Reconstruction Service
National Rehabilitation Institute of Mexico
Mexico City, Mexico

Brandon Johnson, MD (Chapter 15)
Orthopedic Surgeon
Oklahoma Sports Science and Orthopedics
Oklahoma City, Oklahoma

Nicholas Johnson, MD (Chapter 15)
Medical Student
University of Oklahoma College of Medicine
Oklahoma City, Oklahoma

Michael R. Karns, MD (Chapter 4)
Department of Orthopaedic Surgery
University Hospitals Case Medical Center
Cleveland, Ohio

Bryan T. Kelly, MD (Chapters 14, 26)
Chief of Sports Medicine and Shoulder Service
Hospital for Special Surgery
New York, New York

Scott R. Kling, MD (Chapter 4)
Riverside Orthopedics Specialties
Newport News, Virginia

Andrew W. Kuhn, BA (Chapter 25)
George Wade Research Fellow
Department of Orthopaedic Surgery
University of Michigan Medical School
Ann Arbor, Michigan

Matthias Kusma, MD (Chapter 9)
Orthopedic Surgeon
Orthopädie an den Planken
Mannheim, Germany

Christopher M. Larson, MD (Chapters 3, 7, 10)
Program Director
MOSMI/Fairview Orthopedic Sports
  Medicine Fellowship Program
Minnesota Orthopedic Sports Medicine Center
Twin Cities Orthopedics
Edina, Minnesota

G. Peter Maiers II, MD (Chapter 19)
Methodist Sports Medicine
Assistant Professor
Indiana University
Indianapolis, Indiana

Matthew Mantell, MD (Chapter 11)
Chief Resident in Orthopedic Surgery
Department of Orthopaedics
George Washington University Hospital
Washington, DC

Hal D. Martin, DO (Chapter 20)
Medical and Research Director
Hip Preservation Center
Baylor University Medical Center at Dallas
Dallas, Texas

Richard C. Mather III, MD, MBA (Chapter 1)
Assistant Professor of Orthopedic Surgery
Duke University Medical Center
Durham, North Carolina

Lance Maynard, DO, MS (Chapter 5)
Orthopedic Surgeon
SportsMedicine Grant & Orthopaedic
  Associates
Columbus, Ohio

Jeffrey J. Nepple, MD (Chapter 10)
Assistant Professor
Washington University Orthopaedics
St. Louis, Missouri

Shane J. Nho, MD, MS (Chapter 12)
Assistant Professor
Hip Preservation Center, Division of Sports
    Medicine
Department of Orthopaedic Surgery
Rush University Medical Center
Chicago, Illinois

*Eilish O'Sullivan, PT, DPT, OCS, SCS
    (Chapters 14, 26)*
Clinical Care Coordinator
Center for Hip Preservation
Hospital for Special Surgery
New York, New York

Ian J. Palmer, PhD (Chapter 20)
Research and Education
Hip Preservation Center
Baylor University Medical Center at Dallas
Dallas, Texas

Sunny H. Patel, MD (Chapter 4)
Department of Orthopaedic Surgery
University Hospitals Case Medical Center
Cleveland, Ohio

Marc J. Philippon, MD (Chapter 13)
Managing Partner
The Steadman Clinic
Co-Chairman of the Board
Steadman Philippon Research Institute
Vail, Colorado

James R. Ross, MD (Chapters 3, 25)
Associate Professor and Orthopedic Surgeon
BocaCare Orthopedics—Boca Raton Regional
    Hospital
Florida Atlantic University, College of
    Medicine
Boca Raton, Florida

Marc R. Safran, MD (Chapter 8)
Professor
Department of Orthopedic Surgery
Stanford University School of Medicine
Redwood City, California

Michael J. Salata, MD (Chapter 4)
Assistant Professor, Orthopaedics
CWRU School of Medicine
Department of Orthopaedic Surgery
University Hospitals Case Medical Center
Cleveland, Ohio

John P. Salvo, MD (Chapter 22)
Rothman Institute
Clinical Associate Professor, Orthopaedic
    Surgery
Thomas Jefferson University Hospital
Philadelphia, Pennsylvania

Joshua D. Sampson, MD (Chapter 6)
Resident Physician
St. Joseph Mercy Livingston
Family Medicine Residency Program
Novi, Michigan

Thomas G. Sampson, MD (Chapter 6)
Medical Director of Hip Arthroscopy
Post Street Surgery Center
Orthopedic Surgeon and Consultant
Veterans Administration
Clinical Associate Orthopaedic Faculty
University of California, San Francisco
San Francisco, California

Chris Stake, DHA (Chapter 23)
Director of Research
American Hip Institute
Westmont, Illinois

Rebecca M. Stone, MS, ATC (Chapter 7)
Research and Education Supervisor
Twin Cities Orthopedics
Edina, Minnesota

Eric P. Tannenbaum, MD (Chapter 25)
Orthopaedic Surgery Resident
Department of Orthopaedic Surgery
University of Michigan Medical School
Ann Arbor, Michigan

Fotios Paul Tjoumakaris, MD (Chapter 22)
Associate Professor, Orthopaedic Surgery
Associate Director, Sports Medicine Research
Sidney Kimmel College of Medicine, Thomas
    Jefferson University
Sports Medicine, Rothman Institute
Egg Harbor Township, New Jersey

Christiano A. C. Trindade, MD (Chapter 13)
Research Scholar
Steadman Philippon Research Institute
Vail, Colorado

William Kelton Vasileff, MD (Chapter 4)
Assistant Professor
Department of Orthopaedics
The Ohio State University Wexner Medical
    Center
Columbus, Ohio

Patrick Vavken, MD, MSc (Chapter 24)
Alpha Clinic Zurich
Zurich, Switzerland

Andrew B. Wolff, MD (Chapter 11)
Hip Preservation and Sports Medicine
Washington Orthopaedics & Sports Medicine
Washington, DC

Thomas H. Wuerz, MD, MSc (Chapter 12)
Division of Sports Medicine
Department of Orthopedic Surgery
New England Baptist Hospital
Boston, Massachusetts

Yi-Meng Yen, MD, PhD (Chapter 24)
Assistant Professor
Department of Orthopaedics
Boston Children's Hospital
Harvard Medical School
Boston, Massachusetts

FOREWORD

Today, the arthroscope is an important tool in the diagnosis and treatment of hip conditions. It wasn't always that way, and it is still not being used as routinely as it is in other joints because the hip joint is difficult to reach due to its deep position within the pelvis. In order for surgeons to be adept at this difficult surgical procedure, they must perform it frequently. Because of the relative small number of indications for hip arthroscopy, it is almost impossible for surgeons who do not specialize in it to perfect the technique. They will often abandon the procedure or refer it to someone who has more experience performing it.

Unlike the knee, the hip joint is made up of 2 opposing joint surfaces. It is a well-contained and stable joint, so it is protected from trauma. Therefore, many of the problems that occur in the hip joint are chronic and result in conditions that are difficult to diagnose and treat. Although the arthroscope is invasive, it has a low potential for complications, and its low morbidity makes it useful for these chronic hip conditions. For instance, there is no better way to remove a symptomatic loose body from the hip than with the assistance of the arthroscope. The alternative method would involve a large incision and dislocation of the hip.

I first performed hip arthroscopy in 1977 to evaluate a painful hip that had been nailed for a subtrochanteric fracture. Radiographs and laboratory studies were normal. I suspected that the problem was due to arthritis. At that time, I was using the arthroscope in other joints mainly as a diagnostic tool, so I thought why not use if for the hip as well? Because at the time there were no procedural publications on the subject, I performed a technique that a colleague described to me. The procedure was performed with the patient supine on a fracture table. I visualized the hip through an anterior portal and found arthritis. A hip replacement was carried out shortly thereafter.

Between 1977 and 1984, I performed a total of 10 cases using the supine position. The patients were relatively young. Most of the cases were for diagnostic purposes. In one case, a synovial biopsy was performed and a diagnosis of rheumatoid arthritis was made. On occasion, it was difficult to enter the hip joint with this method, especially in obese individuals because the instruments that were available then were the same short instruments that were used in the knee. In the fall of 1983, I was unsuccessful in the removal of loose bodies from the hip of an obese woman placed in the supine position. Following the case, I discussed the problem with one of my colleagues who specialized in joint replacements and came to the conclusion that because the lateral approach (the approach he used for hip replacements) permits the fat to drop downward and away from the operative sight, better access to the hip joint would be achieved. To distract the hip, traction was applied through skin traction straps applied below the knee, which were connected to overhead weights by a rope placed through pulleys hung from the ceiling. After performing the procedure successfully in several patients placed on their sides, including a 5-ft-5-in, 270-lb patient, I contacted the woman who had loose bodies that I earlier failed to remove using the supine approach and scheduled her for another surgery, during which I successfully extracted 5 loose bodies using the lateral approach.

After using the overhead traction device in a dozen patients, I found that more distraction was needed to adequately examine the joint and keep from damaging the joint surfaces with the arthroscopic instruments. The distraction necessary to achieve this could not be obtained with overhead traction. I then used a fracture table with the attachments adjusted for patients placed on their sides. Satisfactory distraction was achieved in every case with this device. However, there were drawbacks, including difficulty in rearranging the table for the lateral approach, the inability to adjust the perineal post to prevent excessive pressure on the pudendal nerve, and the absence of a device to measure the amount of traction for safety reasons. In patients with stiff joints or hip contractures, a large amount of traction may be necessary to adequately distract the hip. In this situation, surgeons must be aware that a dangerous amount of pressure could be placed on the nerves of the limb and the perineum that could cause paralysis.

Once publications on the subject began to appear in the literature, more surgeons began to perform the procedure. Finally, specific instruments and traction devices were developed that made the procedure easier and safer. A few of the authors of this book led this early charge and were instrumental in refining the procedure so that it became more feasible. Instruments exclusive for the hip were developed, including longer arthroscopes and instruments that were essential to maintain the portals and reach the depths of the joint and curved instruments that helped in reaching the corners of the joint and made it possible to operate on the curved acetabulum. Several authors of this book developed techniques for viewing and operating on the extracapsular structures of the hip and repairing the intra-articular structures that were initially excised. These authors also developed ways of viewing and repairing damaged parts surrounding the hip joint, such as the structures around the greater and lesser trochanters. Despite these advancements, the procedure gained a fraction of the popularity that arthroscopy of the other joints had gained. The reasons at that time appeared to be a lack of indications and poor outcomes due to the association of degeneration in many cases. In the meantime, the few of us who were performing the procedure gained more experience.

In 2003, the condition of hip impingement brought new light to the cause of degeneration in the hip joint. The procedure to correct this was found to be adaptable to arthroscopy. Hip surgeons took notice and found arthroscopy to be beneficial in their practices, and they began to perform the procedure, increasing the number of surgeons who used it. As more hip arthroscopies were carried out, more refinements were made, more information about the anatomy of the hip was attained, and the outcomes of the procedure improved. Today, hip arthroscopy has become an integral part of the diagnosis and treatment of hip problems. As discussed in this book, more advances will come in the future, including imaging advances, new protocols for evaluating patients for this procedure, and developments in the correlation of 3-dimensional anatomy and computer modeling with navigation for streamlining the procedure. Furthermore, we can expect to see resurfacing techniques that could substitute for hip replacements. Already there have been trial studies using polymers for resurfacing knee joints in patients and hip joints in cadaver specimens.

The hip is the largest joint in the body and is the site of major diseases in patients of all ages, from children to the elderly. Therefore, it is imperative for surgeons who treat the hip to know the best treatment options available, which today most definitely includes hip arthroscopy. The significant features of arthroscopic surgery are not only that it uses minimal incisions and reduces morbidity, but also that it is designed to preserve the joint as much as possible. This book is invaluable because it discusses all of the current techniques necessary to diagnose and treat hip conditions. It will help surgeons in their endeavor to learn the principles of arthroscopy and hone the skills that will be essential for them to diagnose and treat the various hip diseases that they will encounter in their careers.

James M. Glick, MD
Clinical Professor
Orthopedic Department
University of California, San Francisco
San Francisco, California

INTRODUCTION

The *AANA Advanced Arthroscopic Surgical Techniques Series* represents the very best that AANA has to offer the practicing orthopedic surgeon. With premier arthroscopic surgeons taking the lead, each book in the series presents the latest diagnostic, therapeutic, and reconstructive techniques available in arthroscopic surgery today.

Each technique-based chapter is consistently organized with a user-friendly interface allowing for a quick reference or for prolonged study. Bulleted lists of easily accessed, high-yield information, including preoperative planning, patient selection, equipment checklists, step-by-step descriptions of procedures, and essential technical pearls, in addition to indications, contraindications, postoperative protocols, and potential complications, make this an invaluable resource for surgeons who want to improve not only their skill level, but also their mastery of the fundamentals that define arthroscopic surgery. Well-edited videos, accompanied by narration, further serve to support the materials systematically outlined in each chapter for each volume.

Education and innovation continue to be the top priority for AANA and its leadership. As such, all proceeds from this Series will be donated to the AANA Education Foundation, which, among other endeavors, helps support resident education at the Orthopedic Learning Center, The Traveling Fellowship, the Society of Military Orthopedic Surgeons (SOMOS)–AANA collaboration, resident scholarships to the Annual Meeting, as well as numerous research grants and awards. With the purchase of this book, AANA will also provide free electronic access to the text and videos from the same book in their initial series, AANA Advanced Arthroscopy (2010).

We believe that this 5-volume series is a must-have resource for those who rely on their arthroscopic skills and knowledge to improve patient outcomes. Concise, current, and cogent help describe the impact that these textbooks will have on your practice and in your clinical successes. AANA is delighted to have again taken on this critical leadership position in surgeon education, and is proud of the quality and immediacy of these 5 outstanding volumes.

Richard K. N. Ryu, MD
Jeffrey S. Abrams, MD
Series Co-Editors

SECTION I

Introduction

A Layered Approach to Patient Evaluation With Prearthritic Hip Pain

History and Physical Examination

Jonathan A. Godin, MD, MBA and Richard C. Mather III, MD, MBA

INTRODUCTION

Due to the myriad etiologies of prearthritic hip pain, the history may be equally varied in regard to symptom onset, duration, and severity. In general, a history of a significant traumatic event is a good prognostic indicator of a potentially correctable problem, whereas insidious onset of symptoms can suggest highly correctable pathology or can be a poor prognostic indicator, suggesting underlying degenerative disease or predisposition to injury.[1] The location, quality, radiation, severity, and timing of symptoms are essential information to obtain. With any hip joint problem, the clinician must look closely for predisposing and palliative factors. For example, femoroacetabular impingement (FAI) is a recognized cause of joint breakdown in young adults.[1] Often, the cause may be multifactorial, including age, activity level, and joint morphology. Perhaps not all factors can be identified or corrected, but the evaluation must be thorough.

The clinician must evaluate for the presence of mechanical symptoms, such as locking, catching, popping, or sharp stabbing.[2] This finding may indicate an unstable lesion inside the joint. However, painful intra-articular problems may never demonstrate this finding, and mechanical symptoms can occur due to many extra-articular causes, most of which are normal.[3] Audible popping is a common complaint and is often painless; this is typically psoas snapping and can be accentuated by intra-articular hip pathology, such as a joint effusion or large cam lesion. Mechanical symptoms that are sudden and painful, almost taking the breath away from the patient, are more likely to be an unstable labral and cartilage tear or intra-articular loose body.

With mechanical hip pathologies, the pain is worse with activities, although the degree is variable. Straight plane activities are often tolerated, whereas twisting maneuvers, such as cutting to change direction, may produce sharp pain.[4] This is especially true with any maneuver that places the affected hip in internal rotation. For example, right-handed golfers will complain of left hip pain on the follow-through. Sitting is frequently uncomfortable, especially if the hip is

Byrd JWT, Bedi A, Stubbs AJ, eds. *The Hip: AANA Advanced Arthroscopic Surgical Techniques* (pp 3-15). © 2016 AANA.

placed in excessive flexion.[2] Moreover, rising from a seated position is especially painful, and the patient may recount mechanical symptoms with this motion. Symptoms are usually described as worse with ascending or descending stairs or other inclines. Many patients with intra-articular hip symptoms will have some level of degeneration, and determining whether the pain is due to arthritis, FAI, or an unstable labral tear is critical to reaching the appropriate treatment decision. Positional pain as described previously without pain with standing might indicate the pain is more directly due to FAI than joint degeneration.

Typically, patients with intra-articular pathology will describe groin pain, but assuming all intra-articular hip pain is felt in the groin is a common cause for misdiagnosis. Byrd[5] described the "C" sign, in which patients cup their hands around the greater trochanter to describe deep hip pain. A variation of the "C" sign occurs when patients highlight several areas of pain independently, and the sum of the areas outlines the "C" distribution. Lastly, intra-articular hip pain is nearly always described as deep, and the patient often points to multiple areas in an attempt to reach the pain. Some patients will report gluteal or trochanteric pain, most commonly as a result of the aberrant gait mechanics secondary to abnormal hip morphology.[6] This is particularly common in collegiate or professional athletes who often have access to frequent therapy that allows them to avoid the acutely painful synovitis often accompanied by intra-articular hip pathology. However, these high-activity patients may be at highest risk of cartilage injury with continued at-risk sports, such as hockey, soccer, and dance. However, gluteal pain can also be a sign of posterior acetabular impingement or posterior cartilage degeneration.[6] With impingement or chondral injury, the gluteal pain will come about at night, as opposed to secondary pain brought about by poor biomechanics while walking.

Pain around the greater trochanter associated with mechanical snapping can be external snapping hip syndrome. This is common in young women and is often accompanied by hip abductor weakness. Rarely, this weakness is driven by intra-articular pathology and should be considered in refractory lateral hip pain or external snapping hip. Pain located in the lower abdomen and/or at the adductor tubercle can indicate athletic pubalgia. Pain located in the thigh, buttocks, or radiating below the knee is likely to originate from the lumbar spine or proximal thigh musculature.[7] Back pain and associated radiation down one or both legs, weakness, numbness, bowel or bladder symptoms, and exacerbation of symptoms with coughing or sneezing may indicate thoracolumbar pathology.[8] Radicular symptoms without low back pain that originate in the buttock might raise suspicion for deep gluteal space syndrome. Dyspareunia is often an issue due to hip joint pain and is commonly a problem among females, but it may be a difficulty for males as well.[1]

In addition, patients will complain of problems performing activities of daily living that rely on normal hip range of motion (ROM), such as shoe tying. These complaints suggest decreased ROM, which is commonly seen. The presence or absence of any medical or surgical history should be elucidated. Nonsurgical treatment efforts, including activity modification, medications, physical therapy, intra- or extra-articular injections, and assistive devices, should be noted.[3] In particular, the specific response to an intra-articular injection is arguably the most important piece of diagnostic information available.

The information obtained in the history should allow the clinician to draft a differential diagnosis. The history is vital to assisting the examiner in performing a directed physical examination.

PHYSICAL EXAMINATION

Unlike other joints, there is no systematic protocol for evaluating the hip. A number of tests have been developed, but there are limited data to support their effectiveness. Some authors have described a layered approach to categorize etiologies for pain around the hip.[2-4] The 4 layers are the osteochondral, intra-articular, muscular, and neural layers.[2,4]

The osteochondral layer includes the femur, pelvis, and acetabulum, which provide joint congruence and kinematics. Abnormalities within this layer can lead to static overload, dynamic impingement, and dynamic instability.[2,4] Anatomic variations resulting in static overload include lateral or anterior acetabular undercoverage or dysplasia, femoral anteversion, and femoral valgus that lead to abnormal stress across the femoral head and acetabulum in the axially loaded position.[2,4] Dynamic factors may lead to pain because abnormal stress and contact between the femoral head and acetabular rim occur with hip motion. When the functional ROM is greater than the amount of physiological motion allowed by the hip, forceful anterior contact occurring at the end range of internal rotation may lead to dynamic instability in the form of subtle posterior hip subluxation, which occurs as the femoral head levers out of the hip socket.[2,4] Altogether, these mechanical stresses lead to asymmetric wear of the chondral surfaces of the acetabulum and femoral head with or without associated instability of the hip.

Therefore, the osteochondral layer has a direct effect on the intra-articular layer, which comprises the labrum, joint capsule, ligamentous complex, and ligamentum teres, all of which contribute to the stability of the hip joint.[2,4] Injuries to this layer include labral injuries, ligamentum teres tears, capsular instability, and various ligament tears. The muscular layer includes all of the surrounding musculature, including the lumbosacral and pelvic floor muscles, that provides dynamic stability and muscular balance to the hip, pelvis, and trunk.[2,4] Abnormal mechanics within the osteochondral layer can lead to increased stresses of the sacroiliac (SI) joint, pubic symphysis, and ischium, as well as increases in the strains imparted to the muscles that attach to these pelvic structures.[2,4] Similarly, core muscle dysfunction can affect any of the muscles crossing the hip joint. Lastly, the neural layer includes the thoracolumbosacral plexus, lumbopelvic tissue, and lower extremity structures.[2,4] Compensatory injuries within this layer include nerve compression and pain syndromes, neuromuscular dysfunction, and spine referral patterns.[2,4] Commonly involved nerves include the ilioinguinal, iliohypogastric, genitofemoral, and pudendal nerves.

Inspection

The hip physical examination should begin with inspection (seated and standing) with a focus on limb-length discrepancy (LLD), pelvic obliquity, muscle contracture, atrophy, and scoliosis. Patients with unequal leg lengths can have symptoms related to FAI on the ipsilateral short side because of relative anterior overcoverage of the acetabulum created by anterior hemipelvic tilt.[6] Leg length is determined by measuring the distance measured between the anterior superior iliac spine and the distal aspect of the ipsilateral medial malleolus.[9] A true LLD is present when the bony structures are of different proportions. Meanwhile, a functional LLD is present when the leg lengths are equal in the presence of pelvic obliquity. Scoliosis, muscle spasms, contractures of the hip joint, or deformities of the pelvis have been implicated as a frequent cause of functional LLD.[6]

Stance/Gait

Arguably the most important aspect of inspection is evaluating a patient's gait and stance. Any splinting or protective maneuvers used to alleviate stresses on the hip joint are noted. While standing, a slightly flexed position of the involved hip, and concomitantly the ipsilateral knee, is common. In the seated position, slouching or listing to the uninvolved side avoids extremes of flexion. An antalgic gait is often present. Typically, the stance phase is shortened, and hip flexion appears accentuated as extension is avoided during this phase.[7] The antalgic gait pattern should be differentiated from the Trendelenburg gait (seen in patients with hip dysplasia who have weak abductors).[6] Varying degrees of abductor lurch may be present as the patient attempts to place the center of gravity over the hip, thereby reducing the forces on the joint. The foot progression angle should be assessed. Asymmetric external rotation of the legs may indicate acetabular retroversion, femoral retroversion, or femoral head-neck abnormalities.[10]

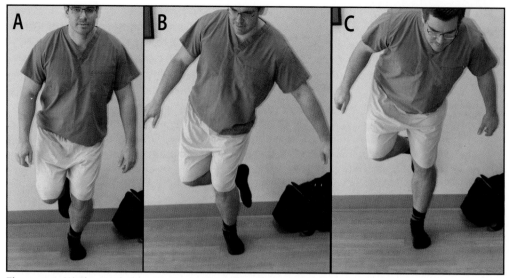

Figure 1-1. (A) The single-leg squat test allows the examiner to assess a patient's hip and trunk muscu-lature. Ask the patient to stand on one leg while the other leg is lifted off the ground. The hip is flexed to approximately 45 degrees, and the knee is flexed to approximately 90 degrees. This image depicts a normal test. (B) Weak trunk and hip stabilizers can lead to imbalance and trunk or pelvic shifting. (C) Leaning forward is a sign of tight hip flexors.

A single-leg stance phase stance is similar to the Trendelenburg test and is helpful in identify-ing a patient with weakened abductor muscles. It should be performed on both legs for compari-son. It is performed by having the patient standing with the feet shoulder width apart and then lifting the unaffected leg forward to 45 degrees of hip flexion and 45 degrees of knee flexion and holding this position for 6 seconds. A positive test is a pelvic shift or a decrease of more than 2 cm (Figure 1-1).[11]

Palpation

Palpation should be performed to localize any tenderness and identify any gross muscular atrophy. It is important to be systematic, palpating the lumbar spine, SI joints, ischium, iliac crest, lateral aspect of the greater trochanter and trochanteric bursa, muscle bellies, and pubic sym-physis, each of which may elicit information regarding a potential source of hip symptoms.[1] The examiner should palpate for fascial hernias by having the patient contract the rectus abdominus and obliques. The resisted sit-up test is helpful in diagnosing a sports hernia. The region of the ilioinguinal ligament should be evaluated, and the presence or absence of a Tinel's sign at this level indicative of femoral nerve pathology should be recorded.[3] Tenderness and swelling at the iliac crest following direct trauma are caused by hematoma formation and are commonly known as a hip pointer.

Apophyseal avulsion fractures or injury to the sartorius and rectus femoris off the anterior superior iliac spine and anterior inferior iliac spine (AIIS), respectively, are common in adoles-cents.[12] Moreover, heterotopic bone formation and chronic AIIS avulsions can lead to AIIS/subspine impingement.[13] Compression of the lateral femoral cutaneous nerve under the inguinal ligament (meralgia parasthetica) may produce dysesthesias over the proximal anterolateral thigh. Tenderness at the pubic symphysis or ramus may occur as the result of recurrent stress created by the hip adductors and rectus abdominus. Tenderness just superior to the greater trochanter is indicative of gluteus medius tendonitis. Tenderness over the greater trochanter is consistent with trochanteric bursitis, whereas tenderness posterior to the greater trochanter is suggestive of piriformis tendonitis or deep gluteal syndrome.[3] Hamstring avulsion injuries are associated with acute tenderness at the ischial tuberosity. Ischiogluteal bursitis, or weaver's bottom, is frequently found in seated athletes, such as bikers, rowers, and equestrian athletes.[14] Pain medial to the hamstring origin is concerning for pudendal nerve compression.

Range of Motion

Active and passive ROM should be assessed with the patient lying supine with the hips flexed, noting any asymmetry of motion. Care must be taken to stabilize the pelvis by extending the contralateral leg, with the pelvis level to the examination table.[15] This is important to avoid an overestimation of primary hip motion secondary to rotation of the hemipelvis or lumbosacral spine. Those with FAI will have limited internal rotation and asymmetric external rotation with the hips.[2,16] Excessive internal rotation (beyond 30 degrees) or excessive combined internal and external rotation should raise suspicion for dysplasia or ligamentous laxity as the primary cause of intra-articular pathology.

Neurovascular Examination

A thorough neurological and vascular evaluation should be performed in all patients. Motor strength should be assessed in muscles supplied by the femoral, obturator, superior gluteal, and sciatic nerves. The sensory assessment includes evaluation of the sensory nerves originating from the L2 through S1 levels.[3] Pain originating from neuralgia (ie, from the lateral femoral cutaneous nerve) should be ruled out.[17] Neurologic function can be further assessed by evaluation of deep tendon reflexes. If injury to a specific muscle group is suspected, resisted contraction should reproduce localized symptoms. The vascular assessment includes palpating the pulses of the dorsalis pedis and posterior tibial arteries. Moreover, skin color and warmth is assessed and compared between the extremities.

Special Tests

A systematic approach to special tests for the hip physical examination is based on the patient's position. The various tests are based on supine, lateral, and prone examinations.

Supine Assessment

The examiner should assess the resting position of the foot in the supine position. Moreover, the relative tightness of the hip joint compared with the contralateral side can be assessed (Figure 1-2). A quick, specific test for hip pain is log rolling of the hip back and forth. Log rolling moves only the femoral head in relation to the acetabulum and the surrounding capsule. Absence of a positive log roll test does not preclude the hip as a source of symptoms, but its presence greatly raises the suspicion and suggests the presence of degenerative disease or severe synovitis.[5] The Thomas test can help determine the presence of hip flexion contracture by eliminating lumbar lordosis on the perceived hip extension. By having the patient in the supine position and the contralateral hip flexed, the painful hip can be flexed and extended to assess for snapping.[2]

The most sensitive test for intra-articular pathology is the anterior impingement (flexion adduction internal rotation [FADIR]) test. This test requires the physician to flex the hip to 90 degrees, adduct, and internally rotate the hip. Patients with labral lesions or FAI will complain of deep anterior groin pain with decreased motion due to impingement of the anterior and anterolateral part of the femoral neck against the superior and anterior acetabular rim (Figure 1-3).[16,18] The subspine impingement test is performed in the supine position with passive movement of the thigh into maximum flexion, neutral adduction, and internal rotation (IR). Reproduction of anterior pain indicates impingement of the distal (anterolateral) and medial part of the femoral neck against the AIIS.[3] Meanwhile, the superolateral impingement test is performed with passive

Figure 1-2. The examiner should assess the resting position of the foot while the patient lies supine. Tightness can present with relative internal rotation compared with the contralateral side. The examiner should press on the foot, thereby creating an external rotation force, to further test hip tightness. Pain with this test is suggestive of synovitis.

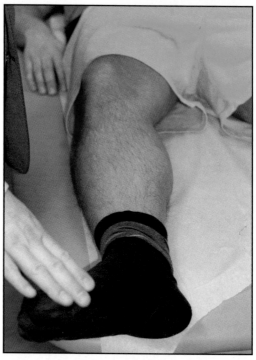

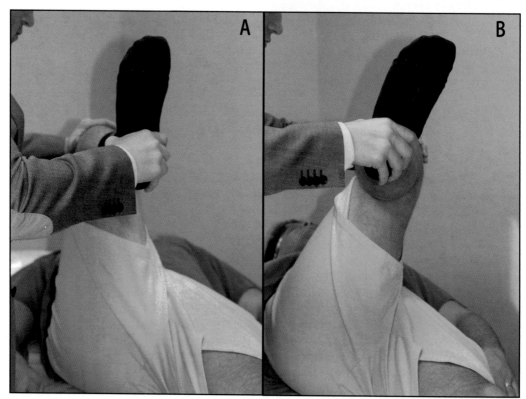

Figure 1-3. (A) To perform the flexion adduction internal rotation (FADIR) test, begin by flexing the hip and knee to 90 degrees. (B) Next, adduct and internally rotate the hip. Patients with labral lesions or FAI will complain of deep anterior groin pain with decreased motion due to impingement of the anterior and anterolateral part of the femoral neck against the superior and anterior acetabular rim.

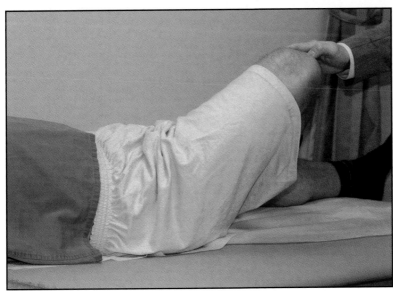

Figure 1-4. The FABER test places the affected limb in the figure-4 position with the ankle resting on the contralateral leg. This places the anterosuperior rim of the femoral neck against the 12-o'clock position of the acetabular rim. The examiner then presses down on the affected leg, with pain being an indicator of a positive test result.

movement of the thigh into flexion and external rotation (ER). Re-creation of anterolateral pain indicates impingement of the superior and superolateral part of the head-neck junction against the superior or acetabular rim.[3]

The dynamic external rotatory impingement test and the dynamic internal rotatory impingement test are performed with the contralateral leg maximally flexed to eliminate lumbar lordosis, and the affected hip is brought to 90 degrees of flexion. In the dynamic external rotatory impingement test, the hip is passively ranged through a wide arc of abduction and ER. In the dynamic internal rotatory impingement test, the hip is passively ranged through a wide arc of adduction and IR. For both maneuvers, the reproduction of the patient's pain in a specific position will correlate with the site of bony impingement in a clockwise fashion.[3,19] Similarly, the McCarthy hip extension test is used to assess for an anterior labral tear. The affected hip is rolled in arcs of IR and ER while the hip is brought from flexion to extension.[20,21] The test finding is positive when the patient's pain is recreated when the hip is extended in ER and then in IR.[20,21]

The Patrick—or flexion, abduction, and external rotation (FABER)—test can be useful, but noting the location of the pain is critical to correct interpretation of a positive test. The FABER test places the affected limb in the figure-4 position with the ankle resting on the contralateral leg. This places the anterosuperior rim of the femoral neck against the 12-o'clock position of the acetabular rim. The examiner then presses down on the affected leg, with pain being an indicator of a positive test result. Groin pain can indicate an iliopsoas strain or iliopsoas impingement on the labrum, posterior hip discomfort implies SI joint disorders, and lateral hip pain can suggest peritrochanteric space syndrome (Figure 1-4).[2] The posterior impingement test can assess posterior impingement lesions or cartilage degeneration. The patient lies supine with the contralateral hip flexed and held in position with his or her hands while the affected limb is extended and externally rotated. The test is considered positive if buttock pain results from the femoral head contacting the posterior acetabular cartilage and rim (Figure 1-5).[3,22-24]

Meanwhile, the lateral rim impingement test is performed by abducting the affected leg while in neutral rotation. Re-creation of lateral pain indicates impingement of the superolateral part of the femoral neck against the superoposterior acetabular rim. The ischiofemoral impingement sign is due to narrowing of the ischiofemoral and quadratus femoris spaces. The quadratus femoris muscle may be compressed directly between the lesser trochanter and the ischium. Clinically, this presents with pain in the groin and/or buttock that may radiate distally and can be reproduced by a combination of hip extension, adduction, and ER.[25]

Figure 1-5. The posterior impingement test can assess posterior impingement lesions or cartilage degeneration. The patient lies supine with the contralateral hip flexed and held in position with his or her hands, while the affected limb is extended and externally rotated. The test is considered positive if buttock pain results from the femoral head contacting the posterior acetabular cartilage and rim.

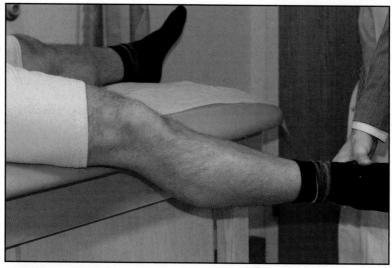

The straight-leg raise test is performed with the patient lying supine and the leg straight off the table. If the patient experiences a recurrence of radiating pain along a dermatomal distribution at an angle of 30 to 70 degrees, then the test finding is positive, and a herniated disk is likely the cause of the pain (Figure 1-6).[26] Mechanical symptoms can also be elicited by performing a resisted leg raise in the supine position (Stinchfield test) as the leg is raised to 45 degrees with the examiner placing downward force with the hand just proximal to the knee. The test is considered positive with weakness or reproduction of groin pain. This test assesses psoas strength, but pain is nonspecific because it can indicate an intra-articular problem or psoas tendinitis.[2,3]

Lateral Assessment

The gluteus medius and minimus muscles can be isolated in the lateral decubitus position. First, the examiner often must place one hand along the iliac crest to maintain the patient in a fully lateral decubitus position. A patient with abductor dysfunction will often roll toward supine as the leg is abducted to recruit the rectus. First, the leg is tested with the knee extended and then with the knee flexed (which lessens tension of the iliotibial band) to better isolate the gluteus medius and minimus function. Lastly, with the knee flexed and hip abducted, the examiner can test the ability of the patient to initiate abduction, which is another method of isolating gluteus medius and minimus function (Figure 1-7).

The Ober test examines the patient in the lateral position, and the examiner places a stabilizing hand on the patient's hip and lifts the affected leg straight up while extending the hip. Once the supportive hand of the examiner is removed, the affected leg should be able to adduct. A test result is determined to be positive when the leg stays abducted and is not able to passively adduct past the midline of the body, thus signifying iliotibial band or fascia lata tightness (Figure 1-8).[2,3,5] The flexion adduction IR and the lateral FABER tests can be performed in the lateral position to confirm intra-articular and peritrochanteric pathology. To perform the lateral FABER test, the examiner passively brings the affected hip through a wide arc from flexion to extension in continuous abduction. The lateral position is used to test the normal dynamic pelvic inclination because the supine position with the contralateral leg flexed eliminates lumbar lordosis. Pelvic inclination may influence physical examination findings, and both positions are valuable in assessment.[3] The anterior apprehension test assesses anterior instability using the same principles as in the shoulder. The leg is brought into adduction, ER, and extension. Pain and apprehension about instability and contraction of gluteal muscles to stabilize the hip suggest instability. Relocating the hip by

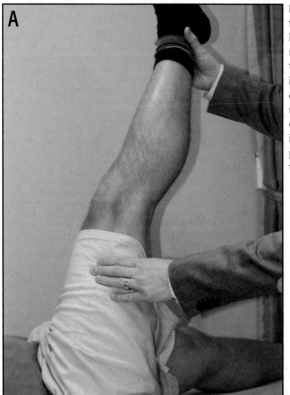

Figure 1-6. (A) The straight-leg raise test is performed with the patient lying supine and the leg straight off the table. A passive straight-leg raise is performed with the examiner assisting the patient in flexing the hip while maintaining full knee extension. Recreation of pain in a dermatomal manner suggests nerve impingement or herniated nucleus pulposus as the cause of pain. (B) A resisted straight-leg raise involves resistance from the examiner as the patient actively flexes at the hip while maintaining full knee extension.

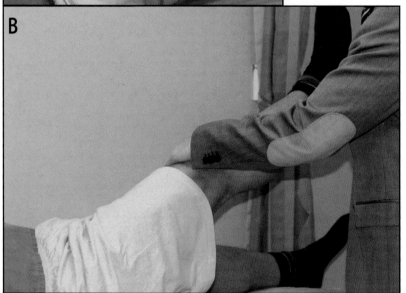

applying a posterior-directed force to the femoral head further supports the suggestion of instability (Figure 1-9).

Prone Assessment

In a prone patient, the Ely test has the patient flex the affected knee to bring the foot toward the buttocks (Figure 1-10). A positive test result suggesting rectus femoris contracture occurs

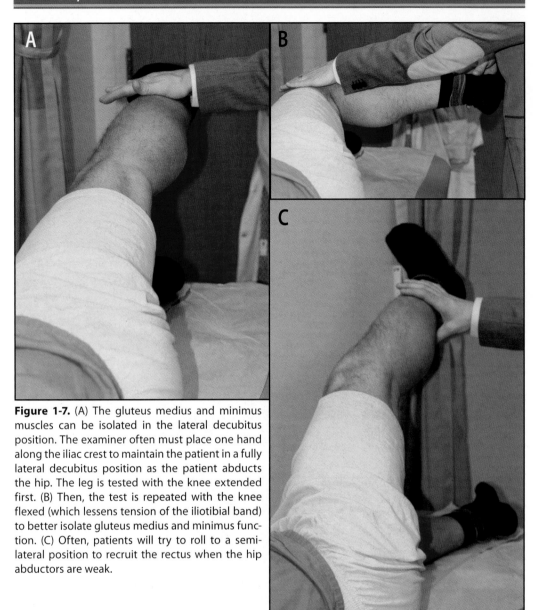

Figure 1-7. (A) The gluteus medius and minimus muscles can be isolated in the lateral decubitus position. The examiner often must place one hand along the iliac crest to maintain the patient in a fully lateral decubitus position as the patient abducts the hip. The leg is tested with the knee extended first. (B) Then, the test is repeated with the knee flexed (which lessens tension of the iliotibial band) to better isolate gluteus medius and minimus function. (C) Often, patients will try to roll to a semi-lateral position to recruit the rectus when the hip abductors are weak.

when knee flexion causes the pelvis to tilt and raise the buttocks from the table.[15] To perform the Phelps test, with the knees fully extended, passively abduct the hips as much as possible. Next, repeat with the knee flexed. Increased abduction is suggestive of a tight gracilis.[15]

Conclusion

In the past, hip joint problems were often neglected and went undetected due to poor assessment skills and, without interventional methods to address these problems, lack of incentive to pursue an investigation. However, advances in hip arthroscopy have defined numerous hip pathologies that previously went undiagnosed and untreated. These treatment advances have served

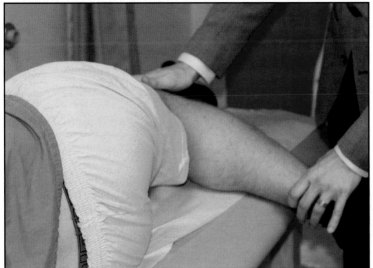

Figure 1-8. The Ober test examines the patient in the lateral position, and the examiner places a stabilizing hand on the patient's hip and lifts the affected leg straight up while extending the hip. Once the supportive hand of the examiner is removed, the affected leg should be able to adduct. The test is positive when the leg stays abducted and is not able to passively adduct past the midline of the body, thus signifying iliotibial band or fascia lata tightness.

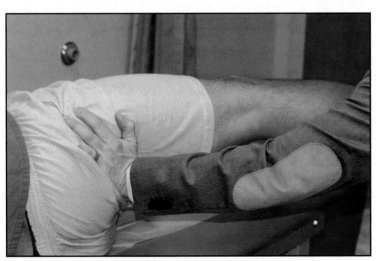

Figure 1-9. The anterior apprehension test assesses anterior instability using the same principles as in the shoulder. The leg is brought into adduction, external rotation, and extension. Pain and apprehension about instability, as well as contraction of gluteal muscles to stabilize the hip, suggest instability.

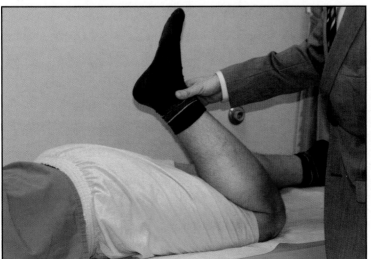

Figure 1-10. In a prone patient, the Ely test has the patient flex the affected knee to bring the foot toward the buttocks. A positive test result suggesting rectus femoris contracture occurs when knee flexion causes the pelvis to tilt and raise the buttocks from the table.

to enhance clinical assessment skills.[27] Using a thoughtful approach and thorough, systematic examination techniques, most hip joint problems can be detected and an appropriate treatment course established in a timely fashion.

References

1. Byrd JW. Evaluation of the hip: history and physical examination. *N Am J Sports Phys Ther.* 2007;2(4):231-240.
2. Lynch TS, Terry MA, Bedi A, Kelly BT. Hip arthroscopic surgery: patient evaluation, current indications, and outcomes. *Am J Sports Med.* 2013;41(5):1174-1189.
3. Poultsides LA, Bedi A, Kelly BT. An algorithmic approach to mechanical hip pain. *HSS J.* 2012;8(3):213-224.
4. Draovitch P, Edelstein J, Kelly BT. The layer concept: utilization in determining the pain generators, pathology and how structure determines treatment. *Curr Rev Musculoskelet Med.* 2012;5(1):1-8.
5. Byrd JW. Hip arthroscopy. *J Am Acad Orthop Surg.* 2006;14(7):433-444.
6. Sierra RJ, Trousdale RT, Ganz R, Leunig M. Hip disease in the young, active patient: evaluation and nonarthroplasty surgical options. *J Am Acad Orthop Surg.* 2008;16(12):689-703.
7. DeAngelis NA, Busconi BD. Assessment and differential diagnosis of the painful hip. *Clin Orthop Relat Res.* 2003;(406):11-18.
8. Martin HD, Shears SA, Palmer IJ. Evaluation of the hip. *Sports Med Arthrosc Rev.* 2010;18(2):63-75.
9. Harvey WF, Yang M, Cooke TD, et al. Association of leg-length inequality with knee osteoarthritis: a cohort study. *Ann Intern Med.* 2010;152(5):287-295.
10. Siebenrock KA, Schoeniger R, Ganz R. Anterior femoro-acetabular impingement due to acetabular retroversion. Treatment with periacetabular osteotomy. *J Bone Joint Surg Am.* 2003;85(2):278-286.
11. Martin HD, Kelly BT, Leunig M, et al. The pattern and technique in the clinical evaluation of the adult hip: the common physical examination tests of hip specialists. *Arthroscopy.* 2010;26(2):161-172.
12. Waters PM, Millis MB. Hip and pelvic injuries in the young athlete. *Clin Sports Med.* 1988;7(3):513-526.
13. McKinney BI, Nelson C, Carrion W. Apophyseal avulsion fractures of the hip and pelvis. *Orthopedics.* 2009;32(1):42.
14. Cho KH, Lee SM, Lee YH, et al. Non-infectious ischiogluteal bursitis: MRI findings. *Korean J Radiol.* 2004;5(4):280-286.
15. Plante M, Wallace R, Busconi BD. Clinical diagnosis of hip pain. *Clin Sports Med.* 2011;30(2):225-238.
16. Klaue K, Durnin CW, Ganz R. The acetabular rim syndrome: a clinical presentation of dysplasia of the hip. *J Bone Joint Surg Br.* 1991;73(3):423-429.
17. Braly BA, Beall DP, Martin HD. Clinical examination of the athletic hip. *Clin Sports Med.* 2006;25(2):199-210.
18. Philippon MJ, Stubbs AJ, Schenker ML, Maxwell RB, Ganz R, Leunig M. Arthroscopic management of femoroacetabular impingement: osteoplasty technique and literature review. *Am J Sports Med.* 2007;35(9):1571-1580.
19. McCarthy J, Noble P, Aluisio FV, Schuck M, Wright J, Lee JA. Anatomy, pathologic features, and treatment of acetabular labral tears. *Clin Orthop Relat Res.* 2003;(406):38-47.
20. McCarthy JC, Lee JA. Arthroscopic intervention in early hip disease. *Clin Orthop Relat Res.* 2004;(429):157-162.
21. McCarthy JC, Lee JA. Hip arthroscopy: indications, outcomes, and complications. *Instr Course Lect.* 2006;55:301-308.
22. Philippon MJ, Schenker ML. Arthroscopy for the treatment of femoroacetabular impingement in the athlete. *Clin Sports Med.* 2006;25(2):299-308.
23. Kelly BT, Williams RJ III, Philippon MJ. Hip arthroscopy: current indications, treatment options, and management issues. *Am J Sports Med.* 2003;31(6):1020-1037.
24. Shindle MK, Ranawat AS, Kelly BT. Diagnosis and management of traumatic and atraumatic hip instability in the athletic patient. *Clin Sports Med.* 2006;25(2):309-326.
25. Bano A, Karantanas A, Pasku D, Datseris G, Tzanakakis G, Katonis P. Persistent sciatica induced by quadratus femoris muscle tear and treated by surgical decompression: a case report. *J Med Case Reps.* 2010;4:236.

26. Scaia V, Baxter D, Cook C. The pain provocation-based straight leg raise test for diagnosis of lumbar disc herniation, lumbar radiculopathy, and/or sciatica: a systematic review of clinical utility. *J Back Musculoskelet Rehabil.* 2012;25(4):215-223.

27. Byrd JW, Jones KS. Diagnostic accuracy of clinical assessment, magnetic resonance imaging, magnetic resonance arthrography, and intra-articular injection in hip arthroscopy patients. *Am J Sports Med.* 2004;32(7):1668-1674.

Please see videos on the accompanying website at

www.ArthroscopicTechniques.com

2

Imaging in
Hip Preservation Surgery

Plain X-Rays, Computed Tomography, and Magnetic Resonance Imaging

Elizabeth A. Howse, MD and Allston J. Stubbs, MD, MBA

INTRODUCTION

Imaging of the hip serves as an adjunct to the history and physical examination in the evaluation of patients presenting with hip pain. The hip preservationist should develop a systematic method for evaluating each patient's imaging to develop a full picture of the cause of pain and determine an operative plan. This evaluation begins with a plain film assessment of the patient's hip. Plain x-rays will determine if the patient is eligible for arthroscopic surgery by displaying the extent of osteoarthritis, acetabular metrics, and morphology of the acetabulum and proximal femur. The surgeon may then use computed tomography (CT) and/or magnetic resonance imaging (MRI) to gain further perspective of pathology not evident on plain films.

PERTINENT IMAGING

Plain X-Rays

Primary imaging for the assessment of a patient with hip pain is plain radiography. The authors' standard plain radiographic assessment of the hip includes the following 4 views: a supine antero-posterior (AP) pelvic view (Figure 2-1), cross-table lateral view (Figure 2-2), Dunn (45-degree) or frog-leg lateral view (Figure 2-3), and a false-profile view (Figure 2-4). The AP pelvis, cross-table lateral, and Dunn views are nonweight bearing. The false-profile view is weight bearing. These plain films provide insight into the obvious and subtle forms of hip pathology that may be causing the patient's hip pain (Table 2-1). When evaluating plain x-rays for hip pathology, the surgeon should also evaluate patient position and radiographic angle to ensure accurate assessment. The degree of

Byrd JWT, Bedi A, Stubbs AJ, eds. *The Hip:*
AANA Advanced Arthroscopic Surgical Techniques (pp 17-34).
© 2016 AANA.

Figure 2-1. Centered AP pelvis x-ray with the tip of the coccyx approximately 15 mm above the symphysis pubis. The AP pelvis view is used to assess for bony morphology and metrics, degree of osteoarthritis, and additional pathology about the pelvis and lumbosacral junction.

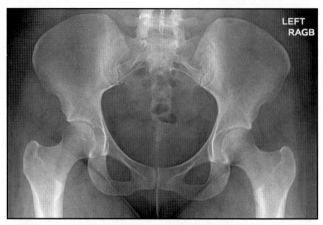

Figure 2-2. Cross-table lateral view of the hip demonstrating concentric joint space in a nonarthritic hip and evaluation of the anterior femoral head-neck junction.

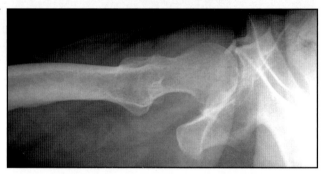

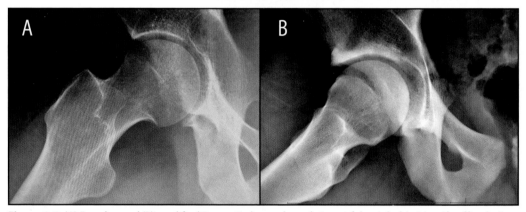

Figure 2-3. (A) Frog-leg and (B) modified Dunn 45-degree lateral views of the right hip identify offset lesions of the anterosuperior femoral head-neck junction. Compared with the modified Dunn 45-degree view, the relative increased abduction of the frog-leg lateral view may improve visualization of the femoral neck.

pelvic inclination on an AP pelvis, for example, affects the outcomes of calculated metrics and radiographic signs, such as the presence or absence of a posterior wall or crossover sign.[1]

X-Ray Views

- ▶ AP pelvic
- ▶ Cross-table lateral
- ▶ Dunn (45 or 90 degrees)

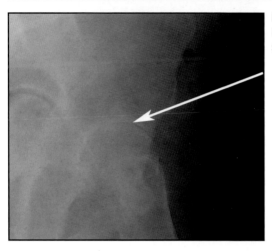

Figure 2-4. False-profile view of the left hip showing Tönnis grade 3 with significant loss of joint space.

Table 2-1. Recommended Radiographic Views and Observations

RADIOGRAPHIC VIEW	RADIOGRAPHIC OBSERVATIONS
AP pelvis	Saber tooth sign, coxa protrusio, coxa profunda, coxa magna, LCE, posterior wall sign, Tönnis classification, femoral head sphericity
Cross-table lateral	Cam, alpha angle, posterior joint space
Dunn (45 or 90 degrees) Frog-leg lateral	Cam, alpha angle
False-profile	ACE, AIIS morphology, joint space

ACE = anterior center-edge; AIIS = anterior inferior iliac spine; AP = anteroposterior; LCE = lateral center-edge.

- ► Frog-leg lateral
- ► False profile
- ► Deep-centered pelvis
- ► Functional abduction/adduction

Osteoarthritic Changes

- ► Tönnis classification
- ► Saber tooth sign
- ► Seagull sign
- ► Hammock sign
- ► Osteophytic changes
- ► Inferior femoral neck remodeling

Osteoarthritis Assessment

Femoroacetabular impingement (FAI) has been associated with the development of hip osteoarthritis.[2] The severity of osteoarthritis may negatively affect the outcome of hip arthroscopy.[2,3]

Table 2-2. Tönnis Classification of Osteoarthritis by Radiographic Changes

Grade	Description
0	No signs of osteoarthritis
1	Mild: Increased sclerosis, slight narrowing of the joint space, no or slight loss of head sphericity
2	Moderate: Small cysts, moderate narrowing of joint space, moderate loss of head sphericity
3	Severe: Large cysts, severe narrowing of obliteration of the joint space, severe deformity of the head
Reprinted with permission from Tönnis D, Heinecke A. Acetabular and femoral anteversion: relationship with osteoarthritis of the hip. *J Bone Joint Surg Am.* 1999;81(12):1747-1770.	

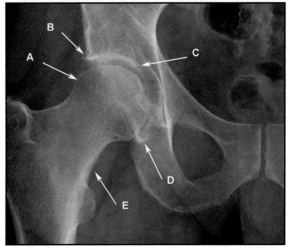

Figure 2-5. The 5 signs of osteoarthritis in a right hip. (A) Posterosuperior femoral head-neck junction remodeling sign. (B) Seagull sign. (C) Saber tooth sign. (D) Hammock sign. (E) Inferior femoral neck remodeling sign.

The authors' practice assesses the degree of osteoarthritis of the hip joint using the Tönnis radiological classification (Table 2-2) and other signs of degeneration, including a central acetabular cotyloid osteophyte (the saber tooth sign) best visualized on the AP view (Figure 2-5),[3] remodeling of the superolateral acetabulum (the seagull sign), sclerosis of the inferior acetabulum (the hammock sign), remodeling of the inferior femoral neck, and osteophytic changes of the femoral head fovea and posterosuperior femoral head-neck junction.

The Tönnis radiological classification evaluates degenerative arthritis of the high-pressure (weight-bearing) aspects of the hip, which manifests as destruction of the chondral surface and subchondral erosion (narrowing of the joint space, sclerosis, and loss of sphericity of the femoral head).[3-5] In the central acetabulum (nonweight-bearing) aspect of the hip joint, osteoarthritis presents as the saber tooth sign (osteophytosis).[3,5] In severe cases of osteoarthritis, the osteophytosis may result in lateralization of the femoral head due to the size of the osteophyte (ie, saber tooth) occluding the cotyloid fossa.[3,5] The authors' experience suggests articular cartilage loss is associated with acetabular radiographic findings, such as the saber tooth, seagull, and hammock signs, as well as femoral radiographic findings, such as osteophyte changes along the femoral head fovea, posterosuperior femoral head-neck junction, and inferior femoral neck.

Table 2-3. Radiographic Angles: Normal and Pathologic Measurements

RADIOGRAPHIC ANGLE	NORMAL	ABNORMAL
LCE of Wiberg	22 to 42	Less than 26 ~ dysplasia
Sharp	33 to 38	< 32: insignificant
		39 to 42: borderline
		> 42: dysplastic
ACE	> 20	
Neck-shaft	125 to 140	> 140: coxa valga
		< 125: coxa vara
MPFA		< 80: coxa vara
Tönnis	- 10 to 10	< -10: pincer
		> 10: dysplastic
Alpha	< 50.5	> 50.5: cam deformity

ACE = anterior center-edge; LCE = lateral center-edge; MPFA = medial proximal femoral angle.

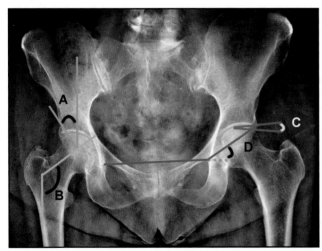

Figure 2-6. Plain film acetabular metrics depicted on an AP pelvis view. (A) LCE angle of Wiberg. (B) Neck-shaft angle. (C) Tönnis angle. (D) Sharp angle.

Acetabular and Femoral Metrics and Morphology

Acetabular metrics determine undercoverage (dysplasia) and overcoverage of the acetabulum on the femoral head (pincer-type FAI; Table 2-3). The authors routinely measure the lateral center-edge (LCE) angle of Wiberg, Sharp angle, and anterior center-edge angle (ACE; Figure 2-6). Other angles that may be measured include the femoral neck-shaft angle, Tönnis angle, and medial proximal femoral angle (MPFA).

Lateral Center-Edge Angle of Wiberg

The degree of acetabular coverage over the femoral head is evaluated by the LCE angle. The LCE is determined by the intersection of a line parallel to the longitudinal pelvic axis and a line between the center of the femoral head to the lateral edge of the acetabulum (Figure 2-7).[6] An

Figure 2-7. (A) Coxa profunda identified by the center of rotation of the femoral head medial to the posterior wall of the acetabulum, (B) Wiberg angle > 35 degrees, and the base of the acetabulum medial to the (C) ilioischial line.

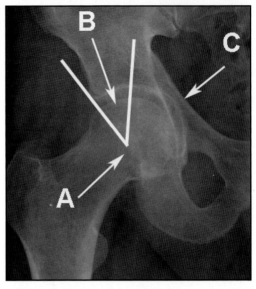

LCE angle of less than 26 degrees may be indicative of a borderline (18 to 23 degrees) or dysplastic hip (less than 20 degrees); however, normal values in adults may range from 22 to 42 degrees.[6]

Sharp Angle

The Sharp angle, or acetabular angle, was first proposed by Sharp[7] in 1961 as a simple method to measure the degree of acetabular development in the adult pelvis. He hypothesized that an underdeveloped acetabular roof leads to a rise in pressure over a proportionately smaller surface and thereby predisposes the hip to the development of osteoarthritis.[7] This angle is measured by drawing a horizontal line between the inferior end projections of the floor of the acetabular fossa of each hip (teardrops) and then an additional line to the lateral edge of the acetabular roof (see Figure 2-6).[7] Sharp[7] argued that although the acetabular angle does not measure the depth of the acetabulum, the angle of the slope is fairly consistent with the degree of acetabular development. In a normal hip, the acetabular angle is between 33 and 38 degrees. Angles less than 32 degrees were found to be clinically insignificant, angles of 39 to 42 degrees were borderline, and angles greater than 42 degrees were consistent with a dysplastic hip.[7]

Agus et al[8] later proposed a modified acetabular angle, stating that when used on hips with a defective acetabular roof, the traditional acetabular angle was difficult to measure and overestimated the acetabular slope due to the resultant teardrop deformity (Figure 2-8). In the modified version of the acetabular angle, the second line is drawn connecting the inferior tip of the teardrop to the sourcil of the acetabular roof (the most lateral point of subchondral bone condensation) instead of the lateral acetabular roof.[8]

Anterior Center-Edge Angle

The examiner evaluates the anterior coverage of the femoral head with the ACE (also known as the vertical-center-anterior margin) on the false-profile view of the hip. The ACE angle is traditionally measured by drawing a vertical line through the center of the femoral head and a second line to the most anterior aspect of the acetabulum.[9-11] Chosa and Tajima[12] proposed that the angle should instead be calculated with the second line slightly posterior traversing the dense shadow of the subchondral bone (Figure 2-9).[10] Comparison between these 2 methods by Sakai et al[10] revealed that the results of both techniques are similar in normal hips, with a value of greater than 20 degrees. In dysplastic hips, the traditional angle should be interpreted with caution, however, because the anterior acetabular coverage may be overestimated.[10] Furthermore, in this projection,

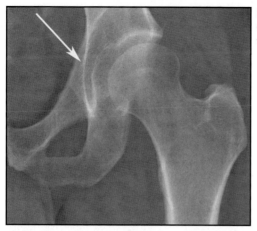

Figure 2-8. AP pelvis x-ray (cropped to show detail) depicting a V-shaped teardrop deformity associated with acetabular dysplasia of the left hip.

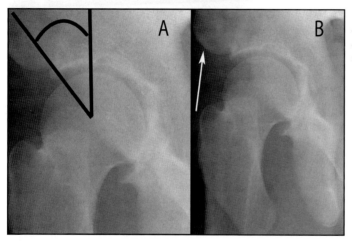

Figure 2-9. False-profile view of a hip demonstrating (A) an ACE angle and (B) anterior inferior iliac spine impingement.

visualization of the true lateral view of the proximal end of the femur is seen, as well as a profile of the acetabulum's anterosuperomedial edge.[13]

Lequesne and Laredo[13] demonstrated that subtle signs of degenerative joint disease could be appreciated in the false-profile view due to joint loading, which may be missed on supine projections. The false-profile view allows for comparison between the anterosuperior and posterosuperior joint space. In the normal hip, the anterosuperior joint space is wider than the posteroinferior joint space. Therefore, subtle anterior subluxation of the femoral head should be suspected when these measurements are equal. Narrowing of the anterosuperior joint space is a sign of osteoarthritis. Additional signs of osteoarthritis that may be appreciated on this view include osteophytosis of the posterior acetabular horn, localization of subchondral bone cysts, minimal concentric joint space narrowing, and subchondral sclerosis.[13] Furthermore, in the authors' experience, inflammatory joint disease will compromise the central joint space on false-profile views.

Medial Proximal Femoral Angle

The MPFA is measured by drawing a line from the shaft of the femur to the tip of the greater trochanter to the center of the femoral head (Figure 2-10). Bardakos and Villar[2] found that the MPFA had the highest predictive value regarding the development of osteoarthritis in patients with FAI. They theorized that a reduced MPFA (less than 80 degrees) results from an isolated overgrowth of the greater trochanter or a varus deformity of the proximal femur, thereby resulting in abductor dysfunction by distorting the position of the greater trochanter in relation to the

Figure 2-10. AP pelvis x-ray (cropped to show detail) demonstrating measurement of a medial proximal femoral angle of the left hip.

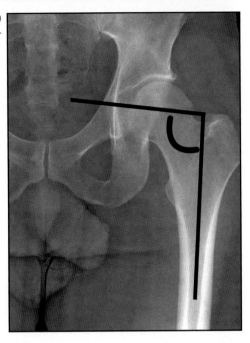

femoral head. Bardakos and Villar[2] postulated that the resulting abductor pathology from the distorted position of the greater trochanter ultimately results in a biomechanical imbalance and osteoarthritis progression.

Neck-Shaft Angle

The neck-shaft angle is measured from the shaft of the femur through the center of the femoral head along the axis of the femoral neck. An angle less than 125 degrees may signify coxa vara, and an angle greater than 145 degrees may signify coxa valga. Both extremes may be associated with abnormal hip development and biomechanics.

Coxa Profunda and Coxa Protrusio

A deep acetabular socket is known as coxa profunda and is identified by the center of rotation of the femoral head lying medial to the posterior wall of the acetabulum. In coxa profunda, the floor of the acetabular fossa touches or is medial to the ilioischial line (see Figure 2-7), whereas in coxa protrusio (Figure 2-11), the femoral head projects medial to the ilioischial line. Coxa profunda and coxa protrusio are evaluated on AP pelvic x-rays.

Femoroacetabular Impingement: Cam/Pincer

FAI of the hip is a form of abnormal bony morphology in which the proximal femur contacts the acetabulum, thereby restricting the range of motion. FAI has become an increasingly recognized cause of hip pathology, and continued FAI results in cartilage degeneration and labral tears. FAI is classified as the following 3 types: cam impingement in which the abnormal contact is due to an aspherical femoral head, pincer impingement from acetabular overcoverage or retroversion, and combined impingement, which has elements of pincer and cam (Figure 2-12).[14] Pincer impingement compresses the labrum as the femoral neck abuts with the acetabulum. This contact may lead to ossification of the labrum and further restrict hip range of motion (Figure 2-13).[14] Although cam-type FAI is most commonly recognized on plain films in lateral-type projections, MRI is often useful for evaluation of the secondary concomitant pathology, such as chondral damage, labral injury, and associated cystic changes of the acetabulum and femoral head-neck junction.

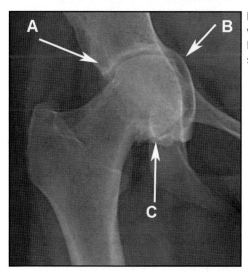

Figure 2-11. Coxa protrusio of the right hip in a patient with Marfan syndrome. (A) Acetabular overcoverage. (B) Pseudocortex of the medial acetabulum. (C) Inferior joint space narrowing.

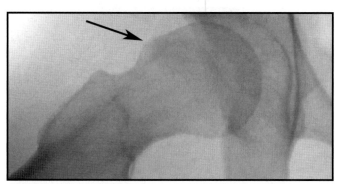

Figure 2-12. Intraoperative fluoroscopic image showing cam lesion across anterosuperior head-neck junction. Fluoroscopy allows dynamic radiographic assessment.

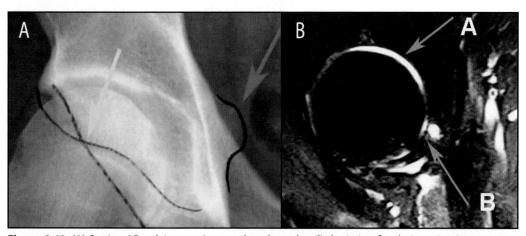

Figure 2-13. (A) Supine AP pelvis x-ray (cropped to show detail) depicting focal pincer impingement as cephalad acetabular retroversion with a crossover sign (yellow arrow) and ischial spine sign (red arrow). (B) Pincer contracoup lesion visualized on T2-weighted sagittal MRI showing asymmetric joint space (A) and posteroinferior chondral loss with a subchondral cyst (B).

Figure 2-14. AP pelvis x-ray (cropped to show detail) with anterior inferior iliac spine impingement and a pseudo-crossover sign (blue arrow) of the right hip.

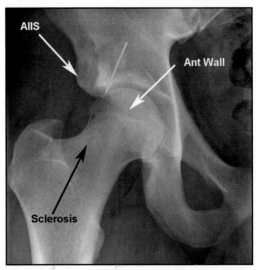

Figure 2-15. AP pelvis x-ray (cropped to show detail) depicting the posterior wall sign. The posterior wall (black arrow) is medial to the center of rotation (white arrow).

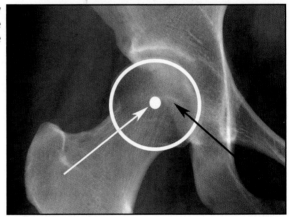

Acetabular Retroversion: Crossover Sign, Ischial Spine Sign, and Posterior Wall Sign

Acetabular retroversion may also result in hip impingement of the anterosuperior femoral neck and is defined as an LCE angle less than 35 degrees with a positive crossover sign (Figure 2-14).[1,15] The crossover sign is defined by the convergence of the anterior and posterior acetabular walls caudally to the lateral edge. The ischial spine sign is where the ischial spine projects medial to the inner wall of the pelvis or quadrilateral plate (see Figure 2-13). The posterior wall sign (ie, a shallow posterior wall) is a subtle sign of acetabular dysplasia and is also associated with acetabular retroversion. The posterior wall sign is defined as the posterior wall of the acetabulum lying medial to the center of rotation, therefore providing undercoverage of the femoral head (Figure 2-15). The posterior wall of the acetabulum will intersect with the center of the femoral head in normal hips.

Tönnis Angle

The Tönnis angle is referenced from a line drawn from teardrop to teardrop to a tangential line to the acetabular sourcil (see Figure 2-6). An angle less than -10 degrees may signify a pincer-type morphology, and an angle greater than 10 degrees may signify a dysplastic morphology. Research by Stubbs et al[16] suggests that the Tönnis angle is the most representative of the actual acetabular volume and femoral head coverage.

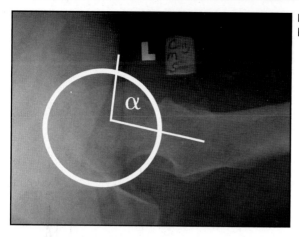

Figure 2-16. Cross-table lateral x-ray of the left hip demonstrating alpha angle measurement.

Alpha Angle

The contour of the femoral head-neck is best evaluated on the Dunn view. The degree of cam-type FAI anterior deformity may be quantified by the alpha angle, with an angle of greater than 50.5 degrees signifying a cam deformity.[17] The alpha angle is obtained by drawing a line between the center of the narrowest point of the femoral neck to the center of the best-fit circle and a second line anteriorly from the center of the best-fit circle to the point where the anterior femoral head cortex extends beyond the circle (Figure 2-16).[17] Greater alpha angles have been associated with greater acetabular articular surface damage.[18] The same measurement can be performed along the posterior femoral head cortex and is referred to as the beta angle.

Coxa Magna and Coxa Breva

Asymmetrical enlargement of the femoral head is known as coxa magna and was first described by Ferguson and Howorth in 1935.[19] Coxa magna is hypothesized to be a sequela from hyperplasia and hypertrophy of the cartilage due to a reactive hyperemia from a pathology that ultimately results in the enlargement of the femoral head and neck.[19] Legg-Calvé-Perthes disease, juvenile rheumatoid arthritis, transient synovitis, septic arthritis, osteomyelitis, congenital hip dislocation, and trauma have all been implicated as inciting pathologies.[19,20] Coxa breva, also associated with Legg-Calvé-Perthes disease, is when the hip has an abnormally shortened femoral neck. The clinical significance of coxa magna remains disputed.[19]

Computed Tomography

Computed Tomography Protocol

► Pritchard O'Donnell view

► Portable intraoperative CT (O-Arm, Medtronic)

► Tera 3-dimensional reconstruction (TeraRecon Systems)

► Dyonics PLAN 4-dimensional reconstruction (Smith & Nephew)

Additional bony detail can be identified with CT scans. CT scans, in particular fine-cut CT scans, are recommended for hip joint evaluation. The most common use for CT scanning is the evaluation of FAI morphology. Acetabular morphology can be assessed with measurements of acetabular version. Femoral morphology can be assessed with measurements of alpha angle, proximal femoral torsion, and neck-shaft angle. Early use of CT scans for FAI included the Pritchard O'Donnell view, in which the patient was scanned in a position of hip impingement, as well as the use of portable intraoperative CT scanning (O-Arm).[21,22] More recently, software programs

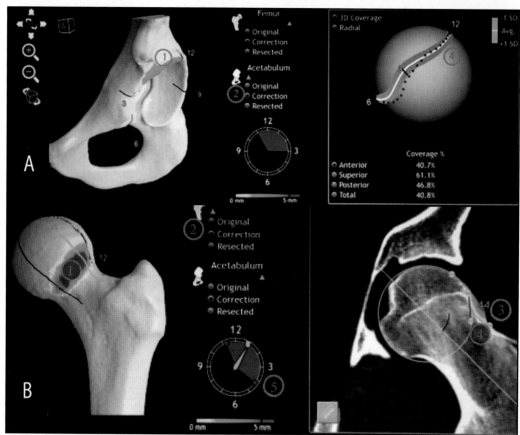

Figure 2-17. Four-dimensional analysis and templating with proprietary software. (A) Left acetabular analysis demonstrating anterosuperior overcoverage. (B) Left femoral analysis demonstrating anterior head-neck junction asphericity. Each demonstrates a 3-dimensional topographic map and analysis for correction.

are available to reconstruct the 2-dimensional CT images into 3-dimensional models (TeraRecon Systems) and 4-dimensional models (Dyonics PLAN; Figure 2-17).

CT scanning has had the benefit of providing detailed modeling of the hip joint prior to surgical exploration. However, risks of CT evaluation include the radiation of a reproductive pelvis, static assessment of a dynamic joint, and the inability to differentiate between morphology and pathology. Newer CT scanning protocols may reduce the radiation exposure of traditional CT imaging.

Magnetic Resonance Imaging

Magnetic Resonance Imaging Protocol

- ▶ T1- and T2-weighted orthogonal views of hip, including T2-weighted fat-suppressed body sagittal view
- ▶ T2-weighted fat-suppressed axial pelvis
- ▶ MR arthrography (MRA) of the hip
- ▶ Delayed gadolinium-enhanced MRI of the hip

MRI evaluation of the hip joint provides the hip arthroscopist with additional information regarding the extra-articular soft tissue that surrounds the hip joint, as well as further intra-articular information. MRI is most helpful at eliminating the following causes of hip pain: avascular necrosis,

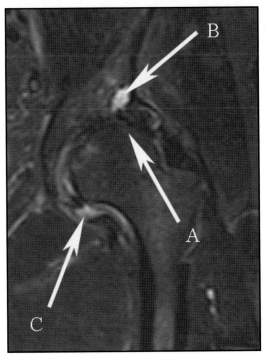

Figure 2-18. MRI of the left hip depicting Tönnis grade 3 with (A) significant joint space narrowing, (B) subchondral edema with cystic formation, and (C) mild to moderate joint effusion.

stress fracture, and neoplasm. Furthermore, pathology of muscles and tendons that may be clinically suspected but are not able to be visualized on plain x-rays can be evaluated with this modality (Figure 2-18). MRI of the hip is less standardized than plain film or CT evaluation; as such, the surgeon should be proactive in communicating with the radiologist regarding the protocol of the hip.

The first decision when ordering an MRI is to determine whether it should include gadolinium. MRA involves the injection of contrast and potentially anesthetic into the hip joint. The injection of contrast into the joint prior to imaging results in a displacement of the capsule and therefore improves the imaging of intra-articular pathology. The addition of an anesthetic may help predict the success of arthroscopy. Byrd and Jones[23] found anesthetic injection to be 90% accurate in diagnosing intra-articular pathology. The examiner must be aware that although there are benefits to MRA, the injection of the contrast may conceal some pathology along the insertion tract and mislead the interpreter with abnormal pooling of contrast, such as the keyhole complex or pinhole sign. Intravenous contrast may be used in the setting of delayed gadolinium-enhanced MRI scanning to assess the charge differentials across articular cartilage.[24] The charge patterns are indicative of an articular index, which is correlated with outcomes following periacetabular osteotomy.

Although contrasted MRI scanning has some benefits, it is associated with increased pain, cost, and contrast artifact along the track of injection. As such, the authors typically do not order contrasted MRI scans of the hip but recommend higher-quality scans of 1.5 T or greater with at least 3 fields of view with T1 and T2 sequencing. The authors have found the body sagittal T2-weighted fat-suppressed sequence to be the most sensitive at detecting anterosuperior joint damage, as well as more subtle posteroinferior contracoup lesions (see Figure 2-12).

MRI is ideal for intra-articular assessment to detect labral tears and paralabral cysts of the acetabulum, as well as chondromalacia and subchondral cysts of the acetabulum and femoral head (Figure 2-19). Furthermore, MRI may help to determine additional extra-articular pathologies that may be treated with hip endoscopy. Tears of the gluteal muscle insertion and ischiofemoral impingement are readily identifiable on MRI (Figure 2-20). Ischiofemoral impingement, first recognized by Johnson[25] in 1977 in patients who had previously undergone total hip arthroplasty or proximal femoral osteotomy, has become an increasingly recognized source of groin and atypical

Figure 2-19. (A) Axial MRA depicting anterosuperior chondral abnormality and (B) body sagittal MRA showing an anterosuperior labral tear.

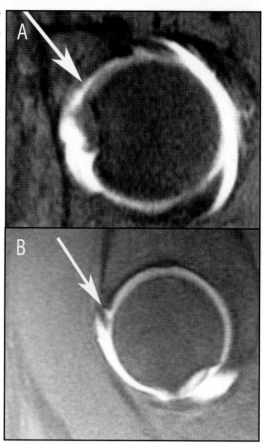

hip pain in the native hip over the past few years.[26] On plain x-rays, a narrowing (13±5 mm; approximately 20 mm is considered normal) of the space between the lesser trochanter of the femur and the ischial tuberosity can be determined.[26] In addition to measuring the ischiofemoral space on MRI, volume loss, inflammation, and fatty replacement of the quadratus femoris muscle are clearly displayed on MRI.[26]

MRI has also identified other anatomic findings that are physiologically normal in the prearthritic hip. The keyhole complex is a fluid-filled defect noticed on MRI first described by Byrd.[27] A supramedial acetabular recess of the bone, the keyhole complex, is filled with amorphous fibrous tissue and may have bands that extend down to the formal acetabular fossa. When directly visualized through an arthroscope, fibrotic bands in this recess resemble the shape of a keyhole (Figure 2-21). The pinhole sign is an additional variant the authors have found that has not previously been described. The pinhole sign is a physiologic defect of the physeal cleft due to contrast extravasation on MRA (Figure 2-22). This defect was initially interpreted as a posterior labral tear with an associated posterolateral paralabral cyst. In 2 patients, the radiologist missed the corresponding anterosuperior pathologic labral tear secondary to FAI due to this physeal defect.

CONCLUSION

Evaluation of the young adult hip is not complete without evaluation of hip imaging. A systematic approach for assessment of the images is necessary to obtain a complete picture of what is causing the patient's pain. Imaging of the symptomatic hip begins with plain x-rays to assess

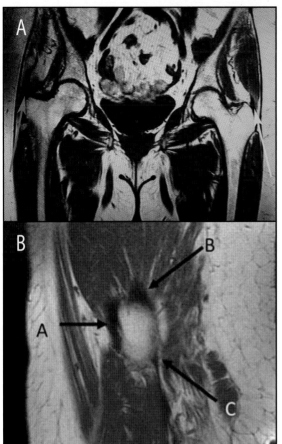

Figure 2-20. (A) T1-weighted coronal pelvis MRI depicting a right abductor muscle tear with a left intact abductor muscle. (B) T1-weighted sagittal MRI of the left hip demonstrating the gluteus minimus, medius, and maximus.

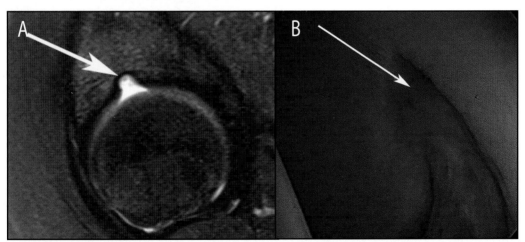

Figure 2-21. (A) Supra-acetabular fossa in a sagittal T2-weighted MRI of the right hip. (B) Arthroscopic view of the keyhole complex as viewed from the mid-anterior portal with a 70-degree arthroscope.

for gross pathology, osteoarthritis, and morphology. Advanced imaging comprising CT and MRI scanning may further elucidate bony and soft tissue pathology. Future dynamic imaging will better assist hip arthroscopists in modeling the prearthritic hip.

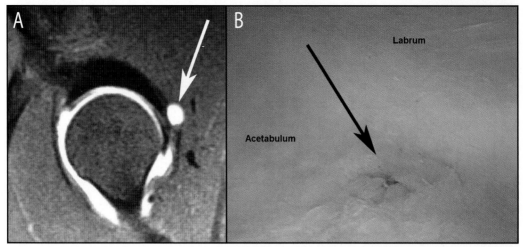

Figure 2-22. (A) T2-weighted sagittal MRI demonstrating the pinhole sign. (B) Arthroscopic visualization of the associated physeal defect (arrow) as viewed from the anterolateral portal with a 70-degree arthroscope.

TOP TECHNICAL PEARLS AND PITFALLS FOR THE PROCEDURE

Pearls

1. Obtain complete radiographic evaluation of the hip, including AP pelvis, cross-table lateral, false-profile, and frog-leg views.

2. Know the signs of early osteoarthritis on plain films and MRI.

3. Obtain femoral torsion analysis in cases of suspected femoral anteversion.

4. Use dynamic fluoroscopic or ultrasound testing when available.

Pitfalls

1. Inadequate radiographic assessment of the hip can be misleading because it does not provide the surgeon with a full picture of the patient's anatomy and subsequent pathology.

2. Not recognizing pseudoacetabular retroversion in cases of subspinous impingement.

3. Failure to recognize subtle anterior subluxation resulting in loss of anterosuperior joint space on the false-profile view.

4. Unstable acetabular dysplasia resulting in a break in Shenton's line.

REFERENCES

1. Siebenrock KA, Kalbermatten DF, Ganz R. Effect of pelvic tilt on acetabular retroversion: a study of pelves from cadavers. *Clin Orthop Relat Res.* 2003;(407):241-248.
2. Bardakos NV, Villar RN. Predictors of progression of osteoarthritis in femoroaceabular impingement: a radiological study with a minimum of ten years follow-up. *J Bone Joint Surg Br.* 2009;91(2):162-169.
3. Mofidi A, Shields JS, Stubbs AJ. Central acetabular osteophyte (saber tooth sign), one of the earliest signs of osteoarthritis of the hip joint. *Eur J Orthop Surg Traumatol.* 2011;21(2):71-74.
4. Altman RD, Gold GE. Atlas of individual radiographic features in osteoarthritis, revised. *Osteoarthr Cartilage.* 2007;15(suppl A):A1-A56.
5. Tönnis D, Heinecke A, Nienhaus R, Thiele J. Predetermination of arthrosis, pain and limitation of movement in congenital hip dysplasia [in German]. *Z Orthop Ihre Grenzgeb.* 1979;117(5):808-815.
6. Martin HD. Clinical examination and imaging of the hip. In: Byrd JWT, Guanche CA, eds. *AANA Advanced Arthroscopy: The Hip.* Philadelphia, PA: Elsevier; 2010:3-30.
7. Sharp IK. Acetabular dysplasia: the acetabular angle. *J Bone Joint Surg Br.* 1961;43(2):268-272.
8. Agus H, Biçmoglu A, Omeroglu H, Tümer Y. How should the acetabular angle of Sharp be measured on a pelvic radiograph? *J Ped Orthop.* 2002;22(2):228-231.
9. Crockarell JR Jr, Trousdale TR, Guyton JL. The anterior centre-edge angle. A cadaver study. *J Bone Joint Surg Br.* 2000;82(4):532-534.
10. Sakai T, Nishii T, Sugamoto K, Yoshikawa H, Sugano N. Is vertical-center-anterior angle equivalent to anterior coverage of the hip? *Clin Orthop Relat Res.* 2009;467(11):2865-2871.
11. Lequesne M, de Seze S. The false-profile view of the hip: new radiographic method of the hip evaluation and the utility for the diagnosis of the dysplasia and different coxopathy. *Rev Rhum.* 1961;28:643-652.
12. Chosa E, Tajima N. Anterior acetabular head index of the hip on false-profile views. New index of anterior acetabular cover. *J Bone Joint Surg Br.* 2003;85(6):826-829.
13. Lequesne MG, Laredo JD. The faux profil (oblique view) of the hip in the standing position. Contribution to the evaluation of osteoarthritis of the adult hip. *Ann Rheum Dis.* 1998;57(11):676-681.
14. Beck M, Kalhor M, Leunig M, Ganz R. Hip morphology influences the pattern of damage to the acetabular cartilage: femoroacetabular impingement as a cause of early osteoarthritis of the hip. *J Bone Joint Surg Br.* 2005;87(7):1012-1018.
15. Boone G, Pagnotto MR, Walker JA, Trousdale RT, Sierra RJ. Radiographic features associated with differing impinging hip surgeries with special attention to coxa profunda. *Clin Orthop Relat Res.* 2012;470(12):3368-3374.
16. Stubbs AJ, Anz AW, Frino J, Lang JE, Weaver AA, Stitzel JD. Classic measures of hip dysplasia do not correlate with three-dimensional computed tomographic measures and indices. *Hip Int.* 2011;21(5):549-558.
17. Nötzli HP, Wyss TF, Stoecklin CH, Schmid MR, Treiber K, Hodler J. The contour of the femoral head-neck junction as a predictor for the risk of anterior impingement. *J Bone Joint Surg Br.* 2002;84(4):556-560.
18. Johnston TL, Schenker ML, Briggs KK, Philippon MJ. The relationship between offset angle alpha and hip chondral injury in femoroacetabular impingement. *Arthroscopy.* 2008;24(6):669-675.
19. Young EY, Gebhart JJ, Bajwa N, Cooperman DR, Ahn NU. Femoral head asymmetry and coxa magna: anatomic study. *J Pediatr Orthop.* 2014;34(4):415-420.
20. Rowe SM, Moon ES, Song EK, Seol JY, Seon JK, Kim SS. The correlation between coxa magna and final outcome in Legg-Calve-Perthes disease. *J Pediatr Orthop.* 2005;25(1):22-27.
21. Grabinski R, Ou D, Saunder K, et al. Protocol for CT in the position of discomfort: preoperative assessment of femoroacetabular impingement—how we do it and what the surgeon wants to know. *J Med Imaging Radiat Oncol.* 2014;58(6):649-656.
22. Mofidi A, Shields JS, Tan JS, Poehling GG, Stubbs AJ. Use of intraoperative computed tomography scanning in determination of the magnitude of arthroscopic osteochondroplasty. *Arthroscopy.* 2011;27(7):1005-1013.
23. Byrd JW, Jones KS. Diagnostic accuracy of clinical assessment, magnetic resonance imaging, magnetic resonance arthrography, and intra-articular injection in hip arthroscopy patients. *Am J Sports Med.* 2004;32(7):1668-1674.

24. Kim YJ, Jaramillo D, Millis MB, Gray ML, Burstein D. Assessment of early osteoarthritis in hip dysplasia with delayed gadolinium-enhanced magnetic resonance imaging of cartilage. *J Bone Joint Surg Am.* 2003;85(10):1987-1992.

25. Johnson KA. Impingement of the lesser trochanter on the ischial ramus after total hip arthroplasty. Report of three cases. *J Bone Joint Surg Am.* 1977;59(2):268-269.

26. Howse EA, Mannava S, Tamam C, Martin HD, Bredella MA, Stubbs AJ. Ischiofemoral space decompression through posterolateral approach: cutting block technique. *Arthrosc Tech.* 2014;3(6):e661-e665.

27. Byrd JW. The supine position. In: Zini R, ed. *Hip Arthroscopy.* Urbino, Italy: Edizioni Argalìa Editore; 2010:55-70.

Indications for
Hip Arthroscopy

William Brian Acker II, MD; James R. Ross, MD;
Christopher M. Larson, MD; and Asheesh Bedi, MD

INTRODUCTION

Although initially described in 1931, hip arthroscopy has been gaining popularity in the medical field only since the 1980s.[1] The use of hip arthroscopy was initially limited due to the technical difficulties presented by the anatomy of the hip joint, which, compared with other joints, presents additional challenges due to the thick soft tissue envelope, the constrained bony anatomy, the proximity of neurovascular structures, and a lack of instrumentation capable of handling the depth of the joint. The development of specific instrumentation and improved techniques in exposure and patient positioning have allowed for greater accessibility to the joint and have expanded the indications for the procedure. Hip arthroscopy is a minimally invasive procedure that may offer decreased morbidity, diminished risk of neurovascular injury, and shorter recovery periods compared with traditional open exposures to the hip.[1]

INDICATIONS

Intra-articular

- ► Femoroacetabular impingement (FAI; cam and pincer type)
- ► Labral pathology
- ► Chondral lesions
- ► Ligamentum teres injuries
- ► Loose bodies/synovial chondromatosis
- ► Septic arthritis

Byrd JWT, Bedi A, Stubbs AJ, eds. *The Hip:*
AANA Advanced Arthroscopic Surgical Techniques (pp 35-42).
© 2016 AANA.

- Synovial-based diseases
- Adhesive capsulitis
- Capsular laxity and instability
- Staged interventions
- Adjunct to total hip arthroplasty

Periarticular

- Greater trochanteric pain syndrome
- Snapping hip syndromes
- Proximal hamstring repair
- Sciatic nerve entrapment
- FAI (ischiofemoral and anterior inferior iliac spine [AIIS]/subspine type)

Intra-articular (Central Compartment) Pathology

Femoroacetabular Impingement

FAI is a disorder of the hip joint that results from abnormal contact between the femoral head-neck junction and acetabulum that can lead to chondral and/or labral pathology. Recurrent impingement may result in pain and discomfort in patients and is one of the predominant causes of arthritis in the nondysplastic hip.

Leunig et al[2] pioneered the open surgical dislocation approach via a trochanteric osteotomy to surgically address FAI in symptomatic patients. Recent literature suggests that arthroscopy may provide equal or greater improvement in outcomes when compared with open surgical dislocation for the treatment of FAI, with a lower reoperation and complication rate.[3,4] Arthroscopy also minimizes trauma to the periarticular soft tissues without the need for trochanteric osteotomy, potentially reducing recovery time and morbidity related to abductor dysfunction.

Labral Pathology

The acetabular labrum is a ring of fibrocartilage that acts as a suction seal to ensure continuous lubrication of the hip joint and improve joint stability and kinematics by distributing contact forces and deepening the hip joint. Labral damage may result in painful clicking and locking, reduced range of motion (ROM), and interference with activities of daily living. Labral pathology most commonly occurs in the form of a tear and can be secondary to FAI, dysplasia, degeneration, or trauma. During surgical treatment of labral tears, the labrum is typically debrided or repaired based on tear pattern and healing potential.

Labral pathology most commonly occurs along the anterior and superior acetabular margins, but the location typically reflects the areas of mechanical conflict between femoral and acetabular pathomorphology.[5] Osseous pathomorphology must be addressed in addition to the labral damage to avoid recurrent injury. The objectives of labral preservation are to treat the resultant symptoms and restore the hip seal and stability. In addition, labral repair is performed with the goal of preventing the premature development of arthritis, which has been shown to correlate with labral tears.[6] Studies have demonstrated superior clinical outcomes among patients who underwent labral repair when compared with debridement and/or excision.[7] However, if repair is not possible, labral debridement also has good clinical outcomes.

Chondral Lesions

Insults to the chondral surfaces can occur traumatically, acutely, and chronically from cyclical impingement (ie, FAI), or as a result of a degenerative process, such as the static overload that occurs in dysplasia. Injury can occur on the articular surface of the femoral head (more common with acute trauma) or the chondral surface of the acetabulum, as is typical with FAI.

Chondral lesions of the acetabulum are commonly associated with intra-articular hip disorders and reflect a morphological incongruity between the femoral head-neck junction and the acetabulum. Loss of normal sphericity and offset at the head-neck junction can cause delamination of the acetabular chondral surface via cyclical wear, leading to pain and mechanical symptoms. Arthroscopy allows for identification of chondral lesions and debridement and/or marrow stimulation to treat these lesions. Chondral delamination in the presence of an intact labrochondral junction can be successfully managed with labral refixation, which indirectly stabilizes the chondral surface.

Chondral lesions of the femoral head are less common. The femoral head cartilage is thinner; thus, it is more difficult to prepare an adequate border for marrow stimulation. Mosaicplasty has been described on the femoral head via an open approach, but this treatment has yet to be described arthroscopically.[8]

Given the limited joint space for instrumentation during hip arthroscopy, the risk of iatrogenic chondral injury exists. Injuries to friable cartilage have been shown to heal poorly, and no perfect arthroscopic treatment for smaller defects has been reported.[9] Great caution should be exercised by hip arthroscopists during joint entry and surgical maneuvers to avoid iatrogenic chondral injury.

Ligamentum Teres Injuries

The ligamentum teres is a strong intra-articular ligament that is thought to be important for stabilization of the hip, particularly in adduction, flexion, and external rotation.[10] Lesions of the ligamentum teres include partial or complete traumatic tears, degenerative tears, and avulsion fractures at the foveal insertion. Traumatic hip subluxations or dislocations have a high incidence of ligamentum teres tears.

Ligamentum teres injuries are difficult to diagnose, and patients may present with mechanical hip pain and describe painful locking, clicking, or giving way. Arthroscopy is an effective technique that has greatly enhanced the diagnosis of such injuries and is nearly the only treatment modality used to resect or debride the ligament, although reconstruction techniques have been described despite limited evidence.[10] When significant tears in the ligamentum teres are encountered in the absence of degenerative change, traumatic (subluxation) and atraumatic (dysplasia/multidirectional instability) instability should be suspected. Botser et al[11] and Gray and Villar[12] proposed various classification systems based on arthroscopic findings for ligamentum teres injuries, with each class determined by the completeness and character of the tear.

Septic Arthritis

Septic arthritis is an infection of the hip joint, occurring most commonly in young children and in immunocompromised and elderly adults. It can cause acute chondrolysis and irreversible damage to joint articular surfaces, and, if left untreated, may lead to osteomyelitis, sepsis, and eventually osteoarthritis of the joint.

Open arthrotomy with adequate irrigation and debridement has been considered the standard form of treatment of patients with septic arthritis. Arthroscopic drainage of septic arthritis of the hip has been used as an alternative to an open arthrotomy based on its successful use in the knee. In a comparative study, El-Sayed[13] showed equal eradication of infection at greater than 12-month follow-up, with no recurrence or development of complications when comparing arthroscopic vs open treatment of septic arthritis. Arthroscopic drainage of septic arthritis of the hip appears to be a valid alternative to an open arthrotomy, especially in acute, promptly diagnosed cases and in the hands of experienced arthroscopists.

Loose Bodies/Synovial Chondromatosis

Loose bodies are small fragments of bone, cartilage, or diseased synovium that are typically mobile within the hip joint, typically causing mechanical symptoms, such as popping, catching, and locking. Due to the variable location and composition of loose bodies, physical examination and radiological imaging are unreliable. Hip arthroscopy has become a valuable tool allowing for direct visualization and minimally invasive treatment of loose bodies.[14]

A large number of small loose bodies may be the product of primary or secondary synovial chondromatosis/osteochondromatosis. Primary synovial chondromatosis is a proliferative disease affecting the joint synovium. Synovial membrane metaplasia enlarges, calcifies, and breaks away, becoming free in the joint to potentially cause pain and mechanical symptoms. Secondary synovial chondromatosis is more common and typically occurs secondary to trauma. Traumatic damage to articular cartilage can result in loose chondral fragments. Hip arthroscopy allows for identification and removal of these fragments that advanced imaging, such as computed tomography and magnetic resonance imaging, frequently fails to identify and also affords the opportunity for simultaneous treatment of the damaged chondral surface.

Synovial Diseases

The synovial membrane is a thin layer of soft tissue that lines the inner surface of the hip joint capsule and functions to maintain the volume of lubricating joint fluid needed for optimal joint function. The synovial lining can degenerate over time secondary to trauma, repetitive stress, and/ or a variety of inflammatory arthropathies, such as synovial chondromatosis, rheumatoid arthritis, and pigmented villonodular synovitis.

Arthroscopy in the setting of synovial disease allows for minimally invasive treatment and definitive diagnosis. Synovial biopsy via arthroscopy can confirm the diagnosis of inflammatory arthropathy and guide subsequent treatment with appropriate disease-modifying agents. Arthroscopic synovectomy has been shown to slow deterioration of the articular cartilage and preserve hip function; however, more diffuse disease extending outside the joint space into adjacent soft tissues may warrant more complete excision via surgical dislocation.[14]

Adhesive Capsulitis

Adhesive capsulitis of the hip, recognized since 1999, is a newer indication for hip arthroscopy.[15] It is similar to adhesive capsulitis of the shoulder but can be nonspecific in the presence of other hip pathologies that cause pain and a decreased passive ROM of the joint, such as FAI.

Adhesive capsulitis is likely underreported in the literature relative to shoulder adhesive capsulitis because decreased ROM of the more constrained hip is less functionally noticeable and limiting.[16] Arthroscopy can effectively treat patients with adhesive capsulitis of the hip in a minimally invasive fashion via capsulotomy or capsulectomy.

Capsular Laxity and Instability

Capsular laxity can be associated with hip pain and instability. The causes can be divided into traumatic and atraumatic etiologies. Traumatic injuries can result in capsular incompetence with or without labral damage. Atraumatic hip instability can be the consequence of repetitive external rotation with axial loading resulting in anterior subluxation. Other individuals may be predisposed to hip instability due to general ligamentous laxity, acetabular dysplasia, or connective tissue disorders.[16]

Arthroscopic capsular or labral repair or reconstruction may be beneficial for patients with recurrent hip instability, particularly in the setting of prior trauma. Recent case series have proposed that the structural abnormalities associated with FAI may predispose patients to traumatic posterior hip instability and subluxation events, with one series reporting favorable outcomes after arthroscopic osteoplasty and labral re-fixation.[17,18] However, these procedures should be approached with caution in atraumatic cases and should primarily be used in patients with normal bony morphology.

Staged Interventions

Acetabular dysplasia can lead to static overload and cartilage injury, hypertrophy and degeneration of the labrum, and hypertrophy and/or tearing of the ligamentum teres. Correction of a shallow acetabulum is most completely addressed with a periacetabular osteotomy (PAO), which, by reorienting the acetabulum, improves load-sharing and contact forces. Arthroscopy in conjunction with a PAO is increasingly used because it affords an opportunity for more precise diagnosis, classification, and treatment of associated intra-articular pathology. A recent study demonstrated that labral and chondral pathologies may be as high as 86% and 69%, respectively, and if left unaddressed could be a potential source of residual hip pain after PAO.[19]

Arthroscopy can be an effective adjunct to a more powerful extra-articular osteotomy; however, one should be cautious when using this as an isolated treatment of dysplasia. Isolated arthroscopy in the setting of acetabular dysplasia may result in iatrogenic instability with or without bony resections, labral debridements, and capsulotomies. Global acetabular deformities (eg, protrusio acetabula, acetabular retroversion) are currently better addressed via open approaches to allow for more comprehensive anatomic correction.

Total Hip Arthroplasty

Arthroscopy in the setting of a painful total hip arthroplasty may be used to evaluate the integrity of implants, assess component wear, remove loose acetabular screws, and perform debridements of soft tissue impingement or infection.

There have also been reports of psoas pain and impingement after hip arthroplasty with associated component malpositioning.[20] Definitive treatment with psoas tenotomy or component revision has proven successful, but revision arthroplasty is associated with a significant rate of complications. Psoas lengthening or release may be performed arthroscopically to reliably improve pain and function, with similar outcomes documented after revision hip arthroplasty and psoas tenotomy.[21]

Periarticular (Peripheral Compartment) Pathology

Greater Trochanteric Pain Syndrome

Greater trochanteric pain syndrome (GTPS) is an entity encompassing several pathologies causing chronic lateral hip pain around the greater trochanter. GTPS is relatively common, reportedly affecting up to 10% to 25% of the population.[22] Trochanteric bursitis is the most common form and involves inflammation of the bursa between the trochanteric facets and the gluteus medius, gluteus minimus, and the iliotibial band (ITB) caused by repetitive trauma. Tears in the abductor tendons and musculature can result and contribute to pain generation, analogous to rotator cuff tears in the shoulder. The gluteus medius, which inserts on the lateral and posterior facets of the greater trochanter, is usually torn along its articular side and, akin to the shoulder, can be partial, intrasubstance, or complete. GTPS can be effectively treated with arthroscopic bursectomy, ITB release, and/or tendon repair.

Snapping Hip Syndrome

Snapping hip syndrome is characterized by an audible or visible snapping of the hip when the joint is in motion and may be accompanied by pain. Sources of the snapping can include loose bodies in the joint and extra-articular causes, including a thickened ITB or gluteus maximus (external coxa saltans), which may visibly snap over the greater trochanter when the hip is flexed and then extended. Audible snapping may also result from the iliopsoas tendon (internal coxa saltans) displacing over the iliopectineal eminence, AIIS, acetabular rim, or femoral head. Friction from repetitive snapping leads to chronic inflammation and potential tendon tears. Arthroscopic procedures for recalcitrant symptoms are effective and include the removal of osseous impingements and/or the release or lengthening of the iliopsoas or ITB to alleviate symptoms.[23]

Extra-articular Femoroacetabular Impingement

Extra-articular hip impingement commonly results from ischiofemoral impingement, AIIS/subspine impingement, or both. Arthroscopic decompression of these structures can improve outcomes. Ischiofemoral impingement occurs between the lesser trochanter and ischium, which may result in quadratus femoris injury. Subspine impingement, however, is thought to result from osseous contact between a prominent AIIS and the femoral neck in flexion. Hetsroni et al[24] classified AIIS morphology, and one must be aware of the variations in the anatomy because a low-lying AIIS may be mistaken as a false-positive crossover sign on an anteroposterior pelvic x-ray.[25]

CONTRAINDICATIONS

A successful outcome from arthroscopy or endoscopy of the hip requires careful patient selection and recognition of technical factors that may preclude the procedure or compromise clinical outcomes.

Absolute Contraindications

► Advanced osteoarthritis
► Severe proximal femoral deformity (Legg-Calvé-Perthes disease, slipped capital femoral epiphysis) necessitating an osteotomy
► Ankylosis
► Dysplasia with femoral head migration
► Greater trochanteric impingement
► Severe acetabular retroversion

In cases of severe osteoarthritis with fully denuded articular cartilage, arthroscopy should not be performed because universally poor results have been reported.[26] There is also good evidence demonstrating inferior outcomes and a higher rate of conversion to total hip arthroplasty when radiographic joint space is less than 2 mm.[27] Arthroscopy should not be performed in septic arthritis that has migrated beyond the joint, and an open arthrotomy should be used if osteomyelitis is suspected.[28] Ankylosis of the joint is an important absolute contraindication because arthroscopic instruments cannot be safely used if the hip cannot be distracted or distended. Dysplastic features with femoral head migration (> 1 cm lateral or break in Shenton's line) indicate more global structural instability, and arthroscopic treatment alone should be avoided. Symptomatic greater trochanteric impingement is best treated via open approaches that include relative femoral neck lengthening and/or greater trochanter distalization. Finally, rim resection in the presence of severe acetabular retroversion can exacerbate instability from a posteriorly deficient acetabulum; thus, an anteverting PAO is indicated.

Relative Contraindications

► Moderate osteoarthritis
► Dysplasia

- ▶ Inflammatory arthritis
- ▶ Neurological injury
- ▶ Chronic proximal hamstring avulsions
- ▶ Chronic abductor avulsions with severe retraction and fatty atrophy
- ▶ Internal snapping hip with severe femoral neck anteversion

Obesity multiplies the technical challenges of hip arthroscopy and increases the risk of complications because current arthroscopic instrumentation may not have sufficient length to access the joint.[5] Obesity and deconditioning also make compliance with postoperative rehabilitation more difficult. Arthroscopic procedures have poor outcomes in the presence of mild to moderate osteoarthritis, dysplasia, and inflammatory arthritis.[26] As previously mentioned, arthroscopy may be a useful adjunct tool in the setting of acetabular dysplasia, but its corrective ability is limited and should typically be used in combination with a PAO. Arthroscopic procedures may also be contraindicated for patients with known neurological injury or disorders, such as pudendal neuralgia, because hip traction may risk further neurologic impairment. Finally, internal snapping hip caused by severe femoral neck anteversion may be more safely addressed with a derotational femoral osteotomy.

CONCLUSION

Until recently, hip arthroscopy was not widely endorsed due to the complexity of a deep joint with a thick surrounding tissue envelope and constrained alignment of the osseous structures. Currently, arthroscopic and endoscopic hip procedures are rapidly evolving and can be safely and effectively performed to address an increasing number of disorders involving the hip and pelvis, allowing for the precise diagnosis and treatment of an increasing number of hip injuries and pathologies. Indications and contraindications will continue to evolve as new technological advances and outcomes are reported. Adherence to evidence-based indications and contraindications will optimize patient outcomes from these procedures.

REFERENCES

1. Burman MS. Arthroscopy or the direct visualization of joints. *J Bone Joint Surg Am.* 1931;13(4):669-695.
2. Leunig M, Beaulé PE, Ganz R. The concept of femoroacetabular impingement: current status and future perspectives. *Clin Orthop Relat Res.* 2009;467(3):616-622.
3. Domb BG, Stake CE, Botser IB, Jackson TJ. Surgical dislocation of the hip versus arthroscopic treatment of femoroacetabular impingement: a prospective matched-pair study with average 2-year follow-up. *Arthroscopy.* 2013;29(9):1506-1513.
4. Harris JD, Erickson BJ, Bush-Joseph CA, Nho SJ. Treatment of femoroacetabular imgingement: a systematic review. *Curr Rev Musculoskelet Med.* 2013;6(3):207-218.
5. Khanduja V, Villar RN. Arthroscopic surgery of the hip: current concepts and recent advances. *J Bone Joint Surg Br.* 2006;88(12):1557-1566.
6. McCarthy JC, Noble PC, Schuck MR, Wright J, Lee J. The watershed labral lesion: its relationship on early arthritis of the hip. *J Arthroplasty.* 2001;16(8 suppl 1):81-87.
7. Larson CM, Giveans MR, Stone RM. Arthroscopic debridement versus refixation of the acetabular labrum associated with femoroacetabular impingement: mean 3.5-year follow-up. *Am J Sports Med.* 2012;40(5):1015-1021.
8. Hart R, Janecek M, Visna P, Bucek P, Kocis J. Mosaicplasty for the treatment of femoral head defect after incorrect resorbable screw insertion. *Arthroscopy.* 2003;19(10):E1-E5.
9. Jordan MA, Van Thiel GS, Chahal J, Nho SJ. Operative treatment of chondral defects in the hip joint: a systematic review. *Curr Rev Musculoskelet Med.* 2012;5(3):244-253.

10. Bardakos NV, Villar RN. The ligamentum teres of the adult hip. *J Bone Joint Surg Br.* 2009;91(1):8-15.
11. Botser IB, Martin DE, Stout CE, Domb BG. Tears of the ligamentum teres: prevalence in hip arthroscopy using 2 classification systems. *Am J Sports Med.* 2011;39 suppl:117S-125S.
12. Gray AJ, Villar RN. The ligamentum teres of the hip: an arthroscopic classification of its pathology. *Arthroscopy.* 1997;13(5):575-578.
13. El-Sayed AM. Treatment of early septic arthritis of the hip in children: comparison of results of open arthrotomy versus arthroscopic drainage. *J Child Orthop.* 2008;2(3):229-237.
14. Fu FH. *Master Techniques in Orthopaedic Surgery: Sports Medicine.* Philadelphia, PA: Wolters Kluwer Health/Lippincott Williams & Wilkins; 2010.
15. Byrd JW, Jones KS. Adhesive capsulitis of the hip. *Arthroscopy.* 2006;22(1):89-94.
16. Smith MV, Sekiya JK. Hip instability. *Sports Med Arthrosc.* 2010;18(2):108-112.
17. Berkes MB, Cross MB, Shindle MK, Bedi A, Kelly BT. Traumatic posterior hip instability and femoroacetabular impingement in athletes. *Am J Orthop (Belle Mead NJ).* 2012;41(4):166-171.
18. Krych AJ, Thompson M, Larson CM, Byrd JW, Kelly BT. Is posterior hip instability associated with cam and pincer deformity? *Clin Orthop Relat Res.* 2012;470(12):3390-3397.
19. Ross JR, Zaltz I, Nepple JJ, Schoenecker PL, Clohisy JC. Arthroscopic disease classification and interventions as an adjunct in the treatment of acetabular dysplasia. *Am J Sports Med.* 2011;39 suppl:72S-78S.
20. Lachiewicz PF, Kauk JR. Anterior iliopsoas impingement and tendinitis after total hip arthroplasty. *J Am Acad Orthop Surg.* 2009;17(6):337-344.
21. Van Riet A, De Schepper J, Delport HP. Arthroscopic psoas release for iliopsoas impingement after total hip replacement. *Acta Orthop Belg.* 2011;77(1):41-46.
22. Strauss EJ, Nho SJ, Kelly BT. Greater trochanteric pain syndrome. *Sports Med Arthrosc.* 2010;18(2):113-119.
23. Kelly BT, Williams RJ III, Philippon MJ. Hip arthroscopy: current indications, treatment options, and management issues. *Am J Sports Med.* 2003;31(6):1020-1037.
24. Hetsroni I, Poultsides L, Bedi A, Larson CM, Kelly BT. Anterior inferior iliac spine morphology correlates with hip range of motion: a classification system and dynamic model. *Clin Orthop Relat Res.* 2013;471(8):2497-2503.
25. Zaltz I, Kelly BT, Hetsroni I, Bedi A. The crossover sign overestimates acetabular retroversion. *Clin Orthop Relat Res.* 2013;471(8):2463-2470.
26. Larson CM, Giveans MR, Taylor M. Does arthroscopic FAI correction improve function with radiographic arthritis? *Clin Orthop Relat Res.* 2011;469(6):1667-1676.
27. Philippon MJ, Briggs KK, Carlisle JC, Patterson DC. Joint space predicts THA after hip arthroscopy in patients 50 years and older. *Clin Orthop Relat Res.* 2013;471(8):2492-2496.
28. Kamiński A, Muhr G, Kutscha-Lissberg F. Modified open arthroscopy in the treatment of septic arthritis of the hip. *Ortop Traumatol Rehabil.* 2007;9(6):599-603.

4

Arthroscopic and Open Anatomy of the Hip

Scott R. Kling, MD; Michael R. Karns, MD; Sunny H. Patel, MD; William Kelton Vasileff, MD; and Michael J. Salata, MD

INTRODUCTION

A thorough and comprehensive understanding of hip anatomy is essential to the safe and effective arthroscopic treatment of hip disorders. This chapter aims to highlight the anatomic considerations that will facilitate a safe and efficient hip arthroscopy. The authors begin with patient positioning and anatomic structures related to portal placement. They then examine in depth the arthroscopic anatomy of each hip compartment.

ANATOMIC CONSIDERATIONS DURING PATIENT POSITIONING AND TRACTION

One of the most important, but often overlooked, steps in a successful hip arthroscopy is proper patient positioning. Furthermore, the key to safely accessing the central compartment of the hip is distraction of the hip joint. Proper distraction allows safe clearance during introduction of the arthroscope and instruments. A fracture table, or hip arthroscopy–specific bed attachment, is typically used. The operative foot is placed in a well-padded boot, and distraction is accomplished through countertraction on a well-padded perineal post. Techniques of obtaining hip distraction without a perineal post,[1] or even through temporary spanning external fixation,[2] have also been described. Traction-related complications may occur from distraction itself or from compression via the perineal post. Traction-related neuropraxias have been reported and are fortunately almost exclusively transient.[3] The femoral and sciatic nerves are most at risk, and the hip should be positioned in slight flexion to minimize risk of these injuries.[4]

Byrd JWT, Bedi A, Stubbs AJ, eds. *The Hip:*
AANA Advanced Arthroscopic Surgical Techniques (pp 43-57).

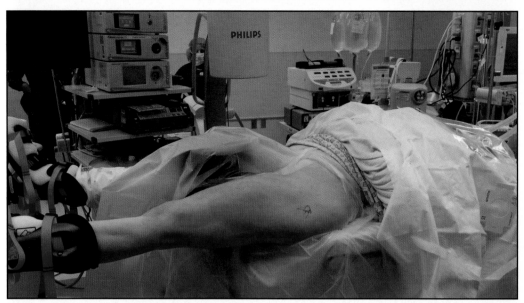

Figure 4-1. Traction setup for hip arthroscopy.

Compression-type injuries related to pressure induced by the perineal post include hematoma/necrosis of the perineal tissues and pudendal nerve injuries.[5] The incidence of pudendal nerve injury from traction varies from 1.9% to 27.6%[6] within the trauma literature but appears to be significantly lower during hip arthroscopy. In a systematic review, Harris et al[3] recently reported the overall incidence of nerve injury to be 1.4%, with pudendal nerve neuropraxias comprising 40% of these injuries. The injuries varied from parasthesias/dysesthesias to sexual dysfunction and were transient in all cases.[3] Brumback et al[7] looked specifically at pudendal nerve injuries with a perineal post and found an increased risk with greater overall force applied (73.3 vs 34.9 kg-hours). Adduction of the operative leg significantly increased the force generated. Duration of traction did not appear to increase risk of injury.[7] However, basic science literature suggests that tissue pressures of 70 mm Hg applied for 2 hours have been found to result in microscopic tissue damage.[8] Thus, traction time is thought of in a similar regard as tourniquet time and should be limited to 2 hours. The perineal post should be well padded, and the diameter of post is inversely related to the incidence of pudendal nerve injury.[6] A diameter greater than 10 cm significantly decreases perineal pressures.[5,8] There are several commercially available large-diameter posts. The post is placed eccentrically on the operative hip, which allows for distribution of force away from the perineum. This technique also yields a more colinear distraction vector referencing the femoral neck axis.

The authors' method for hip distraction uses a hip arthroscopy–specific traction device (Smith & Nephew Hip Positioning System). The feet are secured in well-padded traction boots, and a large (12-cm outer diameter) padded perineal post is place eccentrically on the side of the operative hip. The hip is then abducted and flexed approximately 20 degrees. Enough force is applied to snug the perineum to the post, and the slack is then taken out by applying traction to the contralateral leg. Traction is then placed on the operative hip via adduction to neutral in short increments until the suction seal is broken and hip distraction occurs (Figure 4-1). Often, an audible pop is heard when the suction seal is breached. Fluoroscopic imaging is then used to quantify distraction, and traction is lowered to the minimal amount, allowing access to the joint. In cases of difficult distraction, an air arthrogram can be performed to vent the joint. The air arthrogram technique has the added benefit of better defining the labrum to fluoroscopically guide needle and cannula passage between the labrum and chondral surfaces. Once adequate distraction is obtained, a traction start time is noted, and the leg is prepped and draped. An alarm is signaled routinely at the 1-hour mark of traction time, followed by alerts in 15-minute intervals. Traction time is limited to 2 hours, and a break of 20 minutes is given if additional traction time is required, although this is rarely the case.

ANATOMIC CONSIDERATIONS
PRIOR TO PORTAL PLACEMENT

An understanding of neurovascular anatomy is essential for safe arthroscopic portal placement. The neurovascular injury rate is 0.6% during hip arthroscopy.[9] The structure most susceptible to injury is the lateral femoral cutaneous nerve (LFCN). The LFCN travels approximately 1 cm medial to the anterior superior iliac spine (ASIS) and underneath the inguinal ligament. It courses over the sartorius muscle just below the epidermis. It then branches out in a fan-like distribution. The lateralmost branches are often in close proximity to the location of the traditional anterior portal. Injury can result in the patient experiencing localized parasthesias. The LFCN is most at risk while making the skin incision with a scalpel if the surgeon cuts too deep. Less commonly, LFCN injury can also be caused by blunt trauma during trocar insertion.

The femoral neurovascular bundle consists of the femoral nerve, artery, vein, and associated lymphatics. It crosses the hip joint anteromedially and lays only a few centimeters medial to the anterior portal. To avoid these structures, arthroscopic portals should remain lateral to the line in the body sagittal plane drawn distally from the ASIS toward the medial border of the patella.

The sciatic and superior gluteal nerves are most at risk while making the posterolateral portal. The sciatic nerve enters the gluteal region inferior to the piriformis from the greater sciatic foramen. It lies between the superficial and deep gluteal muscles along the posterior surface of the obturator internus and gemelli. It is normally located at the midpoint of the greater trochanter and ischial tuberosity deep to the gluteus maximus. The sciatic nerve then exits into the posterior thigh just inferior to the quadratus femoris. The superior gluteal nerve exits the sciatic notch and courses transversely in a posterior-to-anterior direction along the deep surface of the gluteus medius.

There has been a case report of significant morbidity due to inferior gluteal vessel injury that occurred with an accessory posterior portal.[10] The superior and inferior gluteal vessels are branches of the internal iliac artery. They exit through the sciatic notch, and the superior and inferior gluteal vessels emerge superior and inferior to the piriformis, respectively. A portal made more distal and with the same trajectory as the standard posterolateral portal has the potential to pass just inferior to the piriformis and into the area of the inferior gluteal artery exit from the sciatic notch.[10]

The medial femoral circumflex artery (MFCA) supplies the majority of the blood to the adult hip. It arises from the posteromedial aspect of the deep femoral artery and, less frequently, from the femoral artery. It travels into the femoral triangle and dives under the neck of the femur before continuing to the posterior thigh. Along the way, it reliably gives off the deep, trochanteric, posterior, anterior, and transverse branches. The deep branch lies in close proximity to the posterior portal. It runs posterior to the obturator externus and anterior to the obturator internus and the gemilli. The MFCA reaches the hip capsule by diving between the inferior gemellus and quadratus femoris. The retinacular branches ascend along the superior femoral neck and lie in close proximity to the tract created by the posterolateral portal.

The lateral femoral circumflex artery (LFCA) is the other major vessel supplying the hip. The LFCA arises from the deep femoral artery the majority of the time. It travels posterior to the sartorius and rectus femoris and divides into ascending, transverse, and descending limbs. The ascending branch of the LFCA is often at risk during anterior portal placement as it passes upward beneath the rectus femoris and tensor fascia lata (TFL).[6]

Figure 4-2. Arthroscopic view of the (A) modified mid-anterior portal and (B) a traditional anterior portal.

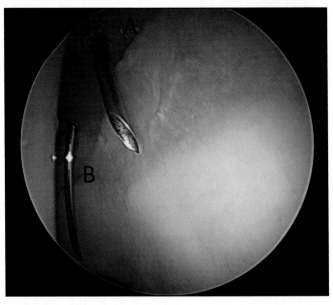

Understanding the bony anatomy of the hip joint is of utmost importance for successful portal placement. The femoral neck-shaft angle is 135 degrees on average. The center of the femoral head lies at the level of the tip of the greater trochanter. Femoral neck anteversion is generally 10 to 15 degrees, referenced off the posterior condylar axis of the distal femur. The normal bony acetabulum is slightly less than a hemisphere, although its functional dimensions are extended by the labrum. In the erect position (ASIS and pubic symphysis in the same plane), acetabular anteversion is 14 to 19 degrees on average, with women having a slightly higher angle. Acetabular coverage, as measured by the lateral center-edge angle on an anteroposterior x-ray, is typically 25 to 35 degrees. Angles less than 20 degrees and greater than 40 degrees are considered to meet the criteria for dysplasia and overcoverage, respectively.

ANATOMIC CONSIDERATIONS DURING ARTHROSCOPIC PORTAL PLACEMENT

The greater trochanter and the ASIS are outlined first. Next, intersecting vertical and horizontal lines are made from the superior tip of the greater trochanter and the inferior aspect of the ASIS. Traditional hip arthroscopy portals include the anterolateral, anterior, and posterolateral hip portals as described by Byrd et al.[11] The authors' preferred method consists of anterolateral, modified mid-anterior, and distal anterolateral accessory portals (Figure 4-2).

The anterolateral portal is generally the first portal established because it is considered the safest portal. It is also considered the most utilitarian portal because it allows for visualization of the central, peripheral, and peritrochanteric compartments. First, a superficial incision is made over the anterior and superior tip of the greater trochanter. A blunt trocar is used to reach the hip capsule. It is aimed approximately 15 degrees posterior and 15 degrees cephalad. There should be little resistance encountered as the trocar enters at the junction of the anterior gluteal fascia and posterior TFL and then passes just anterior to the gluteal musculature. The superior gluteal nerve lies between 4.4 to 6.4 cm away, and the sciatic nerve is 4.0 cm away.[12]

Next, the anterior or mid-anterior portal can be established. The anterior portals allow for visualization of the anterior femoral neck, ligamentum teres, transverse acetabular ligament, lateral aspect of the labrum, and superior retinacular folds. The anterior portal has been traditionally placed at the intersection of a line drawn distally from the ASIS and transversely from the superior tip of the greater trochanter. It is inserted at an angle of 35 degrees cephalad and 35 degrees posterior. This approach penetrates the sartorius and rectus femoris origin and may cause tendinopathy. Therefore, more recently, the anterior portal has been made 1 cm lateral to the traditional anterior portal. This location allows for the portal to pass through the TFL and then through the interval between the gluteus minimus and rectus femoris. The LFCN, especially its lateral branch, is most likely to be injured during anterior portal placement. It is approximately 1.5 cm away from the lateralized anterior portal. The femoral nerve is approximately 5.4 cm away at the level of the sartorius and is 3.5 cm away at the level of the hip capsule. In addition, the ascending branch of the LCFA is approximately 3.1 cm away, but there is frequently a small terminal branch that extends superiorly toward the anterior portal at a distance of approximately 1.5 cm from the portal.[12] The mid-anterior portal is formed distal and lateral to the anterior portal and forms an equilateral triangle with the anterior and anterolateral portals. The portal is aimed 35 degrees cephalad and 25 degrees posterior and, like the anterior portal, pierces the TFL and uses the interval between the gluteus medius and rectus femoris to reach the hip capsule. The LFCN and the femoral nerve are approximately 1 cm farther away using the mid-anterior portal compared with the anterior portal. However, the LFCA and its terminal branch are closer at 1.9 and 1.0 cm, respectively.[12] There have been no reports of iatrogenic injury to this branch, and because these vessels provide no significant contribution to femoral head vascularity, it is unlikely that injury would cause avascular necrosis. The traditional anterior and mid-anterior portals are typically made under direct visualization by viewing from the anterolateral portal. A spinal needle is directed through the capsule in the anterior triangle, which is bordered by the anterior labrum, femoral head, and edge of the arthroscope superiorly.

The posterolateral portal is rarely needed but can be used to examine the posterior aspect of the hip. The skin incision is placed 1 cm posterior and 1 cm superior to the tip of the greater trochanter. It is aimed 5 degrees cephalad and 5 degrees anteriorly to visualize the central compartment. It passes through the gluteus medius and minimus and courses superior and anterior to the piriformis before reaching the posterior hip capsule. The sciatic nerve and medial femoral circumflex artery are on average 2.2 cm[12] and 1.0 cm[13] away, respectively. Although the MFCA lies in close proximity, a bony ridge on the posterior aspect of the greater trochanter protects its branches from injury during posterolateral portal placement.[13]

The distal anterolateral accessory (DALA) portal is useful in the placement of anchors and for accessing the peripheral compartment. The portal is made 4 to 6 cm distal to and in line with the anterolateral portal. The path to the hip joint is made by aiming for the acetabular rim. This can be accomplished under direct visualization while using a needle. The DALA enters the peripheral compartment by piercing through the fascia located just anterior to the iliotibial band (ITB). The structure most at risk is the transverse branch of the LFCA, which is located approximately 2.3 cm medial to the portal. The sciatic nerve is located posterior and medial to the femoral insertion of the gluteus maximus and will be protected as long as the portal is established lateral to the femur and superior to the gluteus maximus tendon.[12]

ANATOMIC CONSIDERATIONS DURING COMPARTMENTAL HIP ARTHROSCOPY

When considering arthroscopic examination of the hip, surgeons typically separate the joint into the following 3 distinct compartments: the central compartment, the peripheral compartments, and the more recently described peritrochanteric compartment. A sound understanding of intra- and extracapsular anatomy is required to successfully and safely navigate the hip arthroscopically.

Figure 4-3. View of the intra-artic-ular hip capsule from the modified mid-anterior portal.

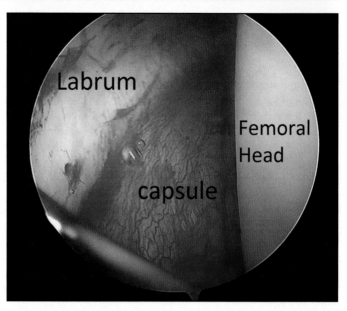

Central Compartment

Capsule

The hip capsule is a thick and fibrous structure that takes a spiraling course around the hip. In an anatomic sense, it is a coalescence of the following 3 distinct ligaments: the ischiofemoral, iliofemoral, and pubofemoral ligaments (Figure 4-3). Collectively, these ligaments function in a screw home mechanism to tighten in extension and impart stability to the joint. The ischiofemoral ligament courses from the ischium and inserts laterally along the femoral neck just medial to the base of the greater trochanter. Relative to the more anterior ligamentous structures, it is thin and generally does not pose a problem in accessing the joint during arthroscopy because most of the work is done anteriorly. It provides resistance to internal rotation in flexion and extension.[14] Distally, the fibers of the ischiofemoral ligament condense to a thick circular collar around the femoral neck dubbed the *zona orbicularis* (Figure 4-4). This circular leash tightens in extension and relaxes in flexion. Its primary function is not clearly delineated, but it has been shown to provide stability during hip distraction.[3] The pubofemoral ligament courses anteromedially from the pubic rami and anterior acetabulum distally to the anteromedial femoral neck and becomes confluent with fibers of the iliofemoral ligament. It helps provide control of external rotation in extension with contributions of the iliofemoral ligament, as well as resisting abduction.[14] Lastly, the ilio-femoral ligament, or Y ligament of Bigelow, courses from the AIIS in 2 distinct lateral and medial limbs to insert along the intertrochanteric line. It is the strongest ligament in the human body and can resist tensile loads upward of 350 N. It is taut in extension and prevents anterior subluxation of the femoral head, contributes to rotational stability, and limits adduction.[11,15]

Because the majority of work occurs anteriorly at the source of the pathoanatomy, the anterior capsular structures provide a barrier to accessing the joint. The strategies for managing the capsule vary from surgeon to surgeon, but in all circumstances, some degree of capsulotomy is used. A limited capsulotomy may be sufficient for accessing the central compartment only. However, if access is needed to the more peripheral areas (ie, femoral neck osteoplasty), then a more extensile capsulotomy is needed. Some authors advocate for a T capsulotomy to gain unobstructed access to the central and peripheral compartments. With certain techniques, however, adequate access can be had without the need for a T capsulotomy.

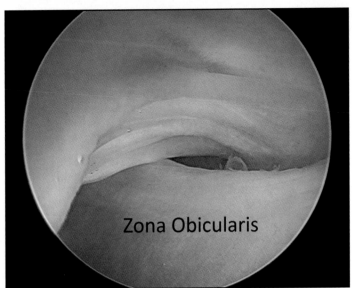

Figure 4-4. Zona orbicularis seen from the anterolateral portal.

Zona Obicularis

The authors prefer to perform an extensile capsulotomy from approximately 9 o'clock posterolaterally to 3 o'clock anteromedially and use a traction stitch to allow retraction of the capsule and provide access to the femoral neck. The authors first begin the capsulotomy with a beaver blade from the anterolateral portal. They then switch portals and connect their capsulotomy anteriorly via a modified mid-anterior portal. Once completed, the indirect head of the rectus femoris can be seen inserting at the 12 o'clock position on the acetabular rim. This serves as an important landmark for acetabular rim recession because the majority of pincer lesions occur in the 12-to-3-o'clock arc. The overlying iliocapsularis muscle can be visualized anteromedially. This is a lesser known capsular muscle originating from the AIIS and inserting distal to the lesser trochanter and assists in tightening the capsule.[16] The gluteus minimus can be visualized anterolaterally. An important plane exists between these 2 muscles and represents the division between the medial and lateral limbs of the iliofemoral ligament and is where the T capsulotomy is made. In addition, the iliopsoas tendon can be accessed if iliopsoas lengthening is needed. In order to provide adequate visualization in the peripheral compartment, a traction stitch is placed in the femoral capsular limb using a single cannula capsular repair device (CapsulePass, Pivot Medical, Stryker Sports Medicine) and brought out through a DALA portal where traction can be applied by an assistant as needed. This provides ample exposure of the femoral neck and allows for 180 degrees of femoral osteoplasty.

Management of the capsule at the completion of the case continues to be debated.[17] Traditionally, capsulotomy without repair, or even capsulectomy, was preferred and had favorable short-term results. There is a recent trend toward capsular closure because literature implicates the capsule as a source of potential instability and rare dislocation.[18] There is growing support for routine capsular closure.[17-19] The authors recommend routine capsular closure and use a single portal technique using a capsular repair device (CapsulePass) to perform the capsular repair through the modified mid-anterior portal. Alternating half hitches are tied beginning medial to lateral to facilitate visualization. In cases of generalized ligamentous laxity, a capsular plication is performed in an attempt to tighten the anterior capsular structures (Figure 4-5). In addition, some authors advocate thermal capsulorrhaphy in addressing capsular laxity, although long-term data are lacking.[20]

Figure 4-5. A capsular plication seen from the anterolateral portal in the peripheral compartment.

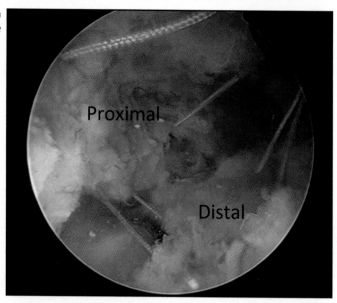

Figure 4-6. The cotyloid fossa (CF) seen arthroscopically. LT = ligamentum teres.

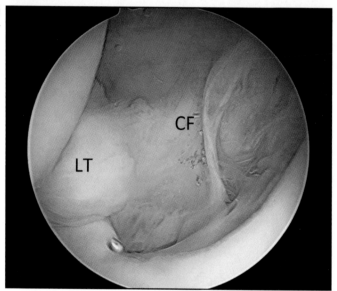

Femoral Head/Lunate Cartilage/Cotyloid Fossa

The distracted hip allows excellent visualization of the femoral head and lunate articular surfaces with the exception of the most posteromedial aspect. Nearly 80% of the femoral head surface may be visualized. This allows definitive diagnosis and management of articular cartilage lesions, including debridement and microfracture. Deep within the lunate cartilage lies the cotyloid fossa. The fossa does not participate in weight bearing because it is devoid of articular cartilage. It renders the articular surface of acetabulum a horseshoe geometry. This specific horseshoe, or lunate, morphology has been shown to contribute to a lower and more homogeneously distributed hip joint contact stress.[21] Within the cotyloid fossa exists the pulvinar, consisting of fibrofatty tissue and small synovial vessels.

The most significant structure within the fossa is the ligamentum teres (Figure 4-6). This synovial invested ligament has a broad origin, blending with the transverse acetabular ligament

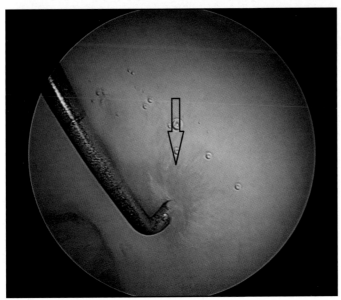

Figure 4-7. Stellate crease seen arthroscopically (should not be confused with a chondral defect).

and ischial and pubic sides of the notch, and inserts on the fovea capitis of the femoral head. Its biologic role has yet to be fully characterized, but it has been implicated in hip stability, nociception, and proprioception. It transmits the anterior branch of the posterior division of the obturator artery; it is negligible in adults but contributes to vascular supply of the femoral head in children. It has been implicated as a pain generator and is responsible for mechanical symptoms. It is most commonly treated with debridement/shrinkage.[22] The physeal scar may be seen as a linear structure that courses along the medial wall of the acetabulum, representing the fusion of the triradiate cartilage. The stellate crease, located directly superior to the cotyloid fossa, is a focal area of chondromalacia and a normal anatomic variant (Figure 4-7). It is the remnant of the supra-acetabular fossa, as seen in young adults.[23,24]

Labrum

The most commonly injured structure in the hip joint is the acetabular labrum (Figure 4-8). With the growth in hip arthroscopy research, understanding of labral pathology and management continues to evolve. The labrum is a semilunar structure along the bony acetabular rim and is continuous with the transverse acetabular ligament. The labrum is triangular in cross-section and gradually lessens in size when moving from posterosuperior to anteroinferior. A normal labral cleft may be visualized that separates the acetabular articular surface from the labrum and should not be misinterpreted as a traumatic detachment.[23] Histologically, the labrum differs in composition with the capsular side primarily composed of type I and III cartilage, and the articular surface is composed of fibrocartilage.[13] The acetabulum projects a wedged bony rim into the substance of the labrum circumferentially and attaches to the labrum via a tidemark of calcified cartilage on the articular side.[13] The blood supply to the labrum is derived mostly from an anastomotic capsular ring, with contributions from the superior gluteal vessels, the obturator artery, and one ascending branch of the medial femoral circumflex artery.[25] Interestingly, anatomic studies have demonstrated increased microvessel proliferation in the substance of a labral tear.[25] Moreover, histologic retrieval studies in patients undergoing conversion to total hip arthroplasty following labral repair with progression of preexisting chondral damage demonstrated histologic healing.[26] In stark contrast to the knee meniscus, the acetabular labrum has been shown to be well innervated with evidence of nociceptive and proprioceptive nerve end organs.[27,28]

Figure 4-8. Arthroscopic view of the acetabular labrum.

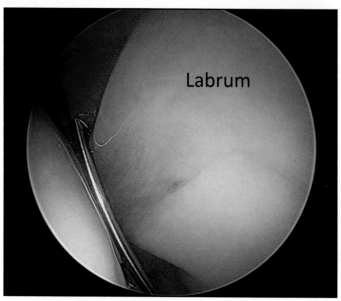

The function of the labrum is not completely understood. Anatomically, it increases the articular surface area by 22% and the acetabular volume by 33%. Although the significance of this is unknown, an important function that is becoming clear is its role in sealing the central and peripheral compartments. This suction seal is thought to have at least 2 important functions. First, by creating a negative intra-articular pressure, it is thought to provide some stability by resisting distraction.[25] Second, and likely most significant, is the resistance of fluid flow out of the central compartment and consequent decrease in articular contact stresses.[29] This latter function has been supported in cadaveric studies showing improved intra-articular fluid pressurization with labral repair and reconstruction and improved resistance to hip distraction when compared with a torn state or partial labral resection.[12,30] The management of labral tears varies by surgeon. A multitude of retrospective studies suggest improved outcomes with labral repair compared with labral debridement.[31] To the authors' knowledge, only one prospective, randomized trial exists comparing labral debridement vs repair. Krych et al[14] demonstrated significantly improved hip outcome scores with labral repair in a randomized trial of 36 patients. However, there is a paucity of Level I evidence supporting resection vs repair vs reconstruction. Given the biomechanical data supporting restoration of more normal labral function, the authors believe the labrum should be repaired if possible, and in the case of an irreparable tear, they advocate reconstruction.

Peripheral Compartment

The peripheral compartment is considered an intra-capsular extra-articular compartment. It contains the acetabular rim and the femoral neck and extends to the distal reaches of the capsular insertion. It is usually accessed after examination of the central compartment because traction is not needed to examine and work in this compartment. Often, a T capsulotomy is used to gain full exposure. Two critical structures to examine are the medial and lateral synovial folds. They serve as important anatomic landmarks with regard to the femoral neck. The medial synovial fold (ligament of Weitbrecht) is found at about the 6-o'clock position, and the lateral synovial fold is at the 12-o'clock position. This is important not only for orientation, but also because cam lesions generally are found within these boundaries and require recession depending on the functional arc of impingement (Figure 4-9).

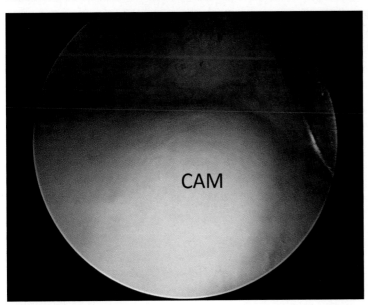

Figure 4-9. Arthroscopic view of a cam lesion in the peripheral compartment.

CAM

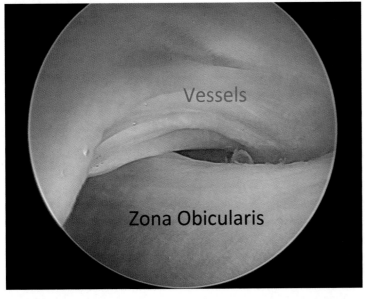

Figure 4-10. Lateral retinacular vessels observed from the peripheral compartment.

Vessels

Zona Obicularis

Most importantly is the lateral synovial fold as a landmark for MFCA and lateral retinacular vessels that are just posterior and the main vascular supply to the femoral head (Figure 4-10). Extreme caution must be observed when working in this area to avoid iatrogenic injury and the potential for avascular necrosis of the femoral head. The deep branch of the MFCA supplies the femoral head and runs just posterior to the lateral retinacular fold with a mean clock face position of 11:15.[32] An average of 4 retinacular vessels travel along the same orientation diving into the femoral head at the femoral neck/chondral junction, and 97% are posterior to the 12-o'clock position. Thus, a relative a safe zone is established from the 12- to 6-o'clock positions.[33]

Moving distally is the zona orbicularis, a thick capsular collar encompassing the femoral neck. Lying just cranial and in line with the medial synovial fold is the iliopsoas tendon. This tendon occasionally needs lengthening in the case of internal snapping hip and may be addressed from the central or peripheral compartment.[6] As seen from the central compartment, the iliopsoas tendon

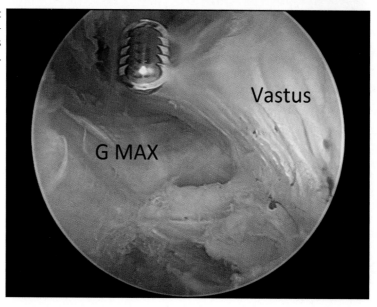

Figure 4-11. Arthroscopic view of the peritrochanteric space gluteus maximus insertion and vastus lateralis. G MAX = gluteus maximus.

creates a medial indentation in the anterior labrum defined as the psoas U. At this level, the iliopsoas is approximately 40% tendon and 60% muscle in cross-section.[34] MCFA anatomy is critical when considering the location of iliopsoas release. The safe zone for release is on either side of the middle-third of the capsule, thus maximizing distance from the MCFA.[33] A central compartment release is consequently fairly safe, whereas a peripheral compartment release places the MCFA at risk.

Peritrochanteric Compartment

More recently described is the peritrochanteric space, which is located between the ITB and the proximal femur. Disorders such as recalcitrant trochanteric bursitis, external snapping ITB, and gluteus medius/minimus tears are now being treated endoscopically via this compartment.[6,35] Access to the peritrochanteric space can be best achieved through the anterior portal. The cannula is directed into the space and then swept back and forth between the greater trochanter and ITB in a fashion analogous to establishing the subacromial space in the shoulder. A DALA portal may then be used as a working portal, and an anterolateral portal added if more proximal work is needed (gluteus minimus/medius repair). Voos et al[35] described a diagnostic examination that begins distally by visualizing the gluteus maximus as it inserts into the posterior border of the ITB (Figure 4-11). The arthroscope is then directed cephalad, and the proximal vastus lateralis can be identified and traced back to the vastus tubercle on the greater trochanter. Next, the abductor insertion should be assessed for tears. The gluteus minimus can be seen inserting relatively anteriorly on the trochanter. Conversely, the gluteus medius inserts more posterior, with 2 separate attachments (lateral and superoposterior facets) (Figure 4-12). Finally, the arthroscope can be directed laterally, and the ITB can be visualized after thorough debridement of the trochanteric bursa. Specific attention should be directed to the posterior third of the ITB because it is implicated in external coxa saltans and may be released.

CONCLUSION

Safe and successful hip arthroscopy hinges on a solid understanding of the anatomy of the hip and surrounding structures. Proper patient positioning and safe portal placement must closely

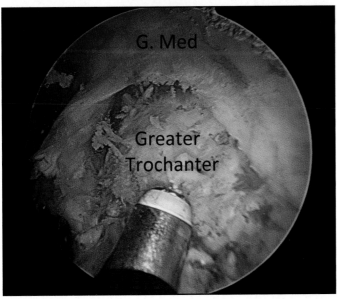

Figure 4-12. Arthroscopic view of a gluteus medius tear seen in the peritrochanteric space. G. Med = gluteus medius.

consider the local anatomy to avoid complications, such as nerve injury. An understanding of hip capsule anatomy and function aids in accessing the joint safely and can help guide its management during and at the completion of the case. Navigating and working within the 3 compartments of the hip is performed safely and effectively with a solid grasp of the intricate anatomic relationships around the hip. With safe access and mobility, surgeons are best prepared to address pathologies affecting the labrum, articular surface, and bony structures in nondegenerative hips.

Top Technical Pearls for the Procedure

1. Proper and careful patient positioning, usage of appropriate traction devices for hip joint distraction, and careful monitoring of the amount of force applied and length of time are important for successful hip arthroscopy and prevention of complications.

2. Thorough understanding of bony pelvic anatomy and the neurovascular structures and muscles crossing the hip joint is important for safe placement of arthroscopic portals that allow for effective surgical procedures.

3. Important structures to visualize during evaluation of the central compartment include the capsule, articular cartilage of the femoral head and acetabulum, cotyloid fossa and ligamentum teres, and labrum.

4. In the peripheral compartment of the hip, anatomic structures to visualize include the acetabular rim and femoral neck, iliopsoas, and zona orbicularis. Also, the medial and lateral retinacular folds can be appreciated, as well as their respective circumflex vessels.

5. Peritrochanteric space evaluation is a more recent development; here, the ITB, gluteus maximus tendon, and vastus lateralis fibers can be appreciated and associated with the trochanteric bursa. Deep to these structures lie the gluteus medius and minimus tendon insertions onto the greater trochanter.

REFERENCES

1. Mei-Dan O, McConkey MO, Young DA. Hip arthroscopy distraction without the use of a perineal post: prospective study. *Orthopedics*. 2013;36(1):e1-e5.
2. Sadri H. Complex therapeutic hip arthroscopy with the use of a femoral distractor. In: Sekiya JK, Safran MR, Ranawat AS, Leunig M, eds. *Techniques in Hip Arthroscopy and Joint Preservation Surgery*. Philadelphia, PA: Elsevier Saunders; 2011:113-120.
3. Harris JD, McCormick FM, Abrams GD, et al. Complications and reoperations during and after hip arthroscopy: a systematic review of 92 studies and more than 6,000 patients. *Arthroscopy*. 2013;29(3):589-595.
4. Papavasiliou AV Bardakos NV. Complications of arthroscopic surgery of the hip. *Bone Joint Res*. 2012;1(7):131-144.
5. Pailhé R, Chiron P, Reina N, Cavaignac E, Lafontan V, Laffosse JM. Pudendal nerve neuralgia after hip arthroscopy: retrospective study and literature review. *Orthop Traumatol Surg Res*. 2013;99(7):785-790.
6. Gerhardt MB, Logishetty K, Meftah M, Ranawat AS. Arthroscopic and open anatomy of the hip. In: Sekiya JK, Safran M, Ranawat AS, Leunig M, eds. *Techniques in Hip Arthroscopy and Joint Preservation Surgery*. Philadelphia, PA: Saunders; 2011:9-22.
7. Brumback RJ, Ellison TS, Molligan H, Molligan DJ, Mahaffey S, Schmidhauser C. Pudendal nerve palsy complicating intramedullary nailing of the femur. *J Bone Joint Surg Am*. 1992;74(10):1450-1455.
8. Topliss CJ, Webb JM. Interface pressure produced by the traction post on a standard orthopaedic table. *Injury*. 2001;32(9):689-691.
9. Clarke MT, Arora A, Villar RN. Hip arthroscopy: complications in 1054 cases. *Clin Orthop Relat Res*. 2003;(406):84-88.
10. Bruno M, Longhino V, Sansone V. A catastrophic complication of hip arthroscopy. *Arthroscopy*. 2011;27(8):1150-1152.
11. Byrd JW, Pappas JN, Pedley MJ. Hip arthroscopy: an anatomic study of portal placement and relationship to the extra-articular structures. *Arthroscopy*. 1995;11(4):418-423.
12. Philippon MJ, Nepple JJ, Campbell KJ, et al. The hip fluid seal—Part I: the effect of an acetabular labral tear, repair, resection, and reconstruction on hip fluid pressurization. *Knee Surg Sports Traumatol Arthrosc*. 2014;22(4):722-729.
13. Seldes RM, Tan V, Hunt J, Katz M, Winiarsky R, Fitzgerald RH Jr. Anatomy, histologic features, and vascularity of the adult acetabular labrum. *Clin Orthop Relat Res*. 2001;(382):232-240.
14. Krych AJ Thompson M, Knutson Z, Scoon J, Coleman SH. Arthroscopic labral repair versus selective labral debridement in female patients with femoroacetabular impingement: a prospective randomized study. *Arthroscopy*. 2013;29(1):46-53.
15. Flierl MA, Stahel PF, Hak DJ, Morgan SJ, Smith WR. Traction table-related complications in orthopaedic surgery. *J Am Acad Orthop Surg*. 2010;18(11):668-675.
16. Babst D, Steppacher SD, Ganz R, Siebenrock KA, Tannast M. The iliocapsularis muscle: an important stabilizer in the dysplastic hip. *Clin Orthop Relat Res*. 2011;469(6):1728-1734.
17. Domb BG, Philippon MJ, Giordano BD. Arthroscopic capsulotomy, capsular repair, and capsular plication of the hip: relation to atraumatic instability. *Arthroscopy*. 2013;29(1):162-173.
18. Harris JD, Slikker W III, Gupta AK, McCormick FM, Nho SJ. Routine complete capsular closure during hip arthroscopy. *Arthrosc Tech*. 2013;2(2):e89-e94.
19. Bedi A, Galano G, Walsh C, Kelly BT. Capsular management during hip arthroscopy: from femoroacetabular impingement to instability. *Arthroscopy*. 2011;27(12):1720-1731.
20. Philippon MJ. The role of arthroscopic thermal capsulorrhaphy in the hip. *Clin Sports Med*. 2001;20(4):817-829.
21. Daniel M, Iglic A, Kralj-Iglic V. The shape of acetabular cartilage optimizeship contact stress distribution. *J Anat*. 2005;207(1):85-91.
22. Bardakos NV, Villar RN. The ligamentum teres of the adult hip. *J Bone Joint Surg Br*. 2009;91(1):8-15.
23. Byrd JW. Hip arthroscopy, the supine approach: technique and anatomy of the intraarticular and peripheral compartments. *Tech Orthop*. 2005;20(1):17-31.
24. Keene GS, Villar RN. Arthroscopic anatomy of the hip: an in vivo study. *Arthroscopy*. 1994;10(4):392-399.
25. Safran MR. The acetabular labrum: anatomic and functional characteristics and rationale for surgical intervention. *Am Acad Orthop Surg*. 2010;18(6):338-345.

26. Audenaert EA, Dhollander AA, Forsyth RG, Corten K, Verbruggen G, Pattyn C. Histologic assessment of acetabular labrum healing. *Arthroscopy.* 2012;28(12):1784-1789.

27. Alzaharani A, Bali K, Gudena R, et al. The innervation of the human acetabular labrum and hip joint: an anatomic study. *BMC Musculoskelet Disord.* 2014;15:41.

28. Kim YT, Azuma H. The nerve endings of the acetabular labrum. *Clin Orthop Relat Res.* 1995;(320):176-181.

29. Ferguson SJ, Bryant JT, Ganz R, Ito K. An in vitro investigation of the acetabular labral seal in hip joint mechanics. *J Biomech.* 2003;36(2):171-178.

30. Nepple JJ, Philippon MJ, Campbell KJ, et al. The hip fluid seal—Part II: the effect of an acetabular labral tear, repair, resection, and reconstruction on hip stability to distraction. *Knee Surg Sports Traumatol Arthrosc.* 2014;22(4):730-736.

31. Haddad B, Konan S, Haddad FS. Debridement versus re-attachment of acetabular labral tears: a review of the literature and quantitative analysis. *Bone Joint J.* 2014;96(1):24-30.

32. Martin HD, Savage A, Braly BA, Palmer IJ, Beall DP, Kelly B. The function of the hip capsular ligaments: a quantitative report. *Arthroscopy.* 2008;24(2):188-195.

33. McCormick F, Kleweno CP, Kim YJ, Martin SD. Vascular safe zones in hip arthroscopy. *Am J Sports Med.* 2011;39 suppl:64S-71S.

34. Blomberg JR, Zellner BS, Keene JS. Cross-sectional analysis of iliopsoas muscle-tendon units at the sites of arthroscopic tenotomies: an anatomic study. *Am J Sports Med.* 2011;39 suppl:58S-63S.

35. Voos JE, Rudzki JR, Shindle MK, Martin H, Kelly BT. Arthroscopic anatomy and surgical techniques for peritrochanteric space disorders in the hip. *Arthroscopy.* 2007;23(11):1246.e1-1246.e5.

Please see videos on the accompanying website at

www.ArthroscopicTechniques.com

SECTION II

Operative Setup

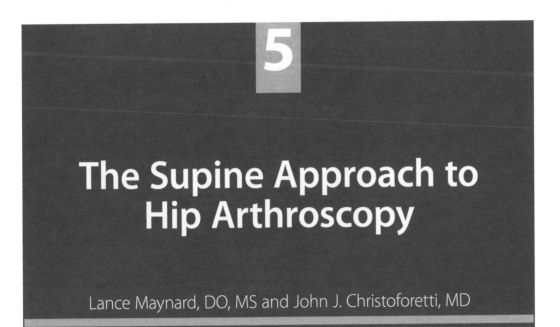

ANESTHESIA

The supine position for hip arthroscopy can be performed with any acceptable combination of general or regional anesthetic techniques deemed safe by the anesthesiology staff and orthopedic surgeon. The authors advocate preoperative clearance for general endotracheal anesthesia according to established facility guidelines. Although some authors have advocated for the use of regional techniques (lumbar plexus block) in combination with sedation or general anesthetic,[1] the current authors have typically relied on general anesthesia with complete neuromuscular blockade (during hip distraction). Their results for the safe outpatient discharge of supine hip arthroscopy using this technique have been presented. The most common complaints associated with this approach have been nausea and a requirement for narcotic pain control in the recovery room. No perineal or genital injury complications were reported.

Communication between the surgical and anesthesiology teams is important. Preoperative familiarization with the intended complexity of the case, including anticipation for bone resection, length of traction time anticipated, and clinical complaints leading to surgery, helps the anesthesia staff. Education for certified registered nurse anesthetists or resident anesthesiologists who are present or will substitute for relief coverage during the case is also required. Often, there can be gaps in this communication in the main operating room setting, and vigilance is required.

In addition to the typical expertise required to manage the operative patient, the anesthesiology team must be aware of specific needs and warning signs in hip arthroscopy. Preoperative placement of monitoring devices and intravenous access points should occur on the nonsurgical upper extremity. Positioning the patient against the traction post typically requires assistance from the anesthesiologist to transfer the patient safely into position. Upper extremity control for hip joint access and dynamic examination with attention to avoiding compressive injury to the upper extremities must be instructed. Intraoperative considerations include maintenance of paralysis during the traction

Byrd JWT, Bedi A, Stubbs AJ, eds. *The Hip:*
AANA Advanced Arthroscopic Surgical Techniques (pp 61-70).
© 2016 AANA.

Figure 5-1. The authors' preferred equipment and setup for supine operative hip arthroscopy.

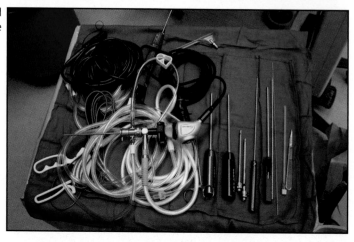

portions of the case, control of the mean arterial pressure (MAP) to close to 60 mm Hg, and continuous monitoring of core temperature for rapid hypothermia (a warning sign of abdominal extravasation of arthroscopy fluid). Gentle Trendelenburg positioning in the supine patient will allow for safer maintenance of low MAP and may also reduce traction force against the perineal post.[2]

Postoperatively, patients are placed in a hip brace, and continuous passive motion may be initiated in the early postoperative period. Postoperative pain control is typically managed in the recovery room by the anesthesiology staff. Intravenous ketorolac, opioid narcotic, and acetaminophen are frequently used for analgesia. Patients are mobilized immediately with assistance from nurses, family members, or physical therapists. There is little consensus concerning venous thromboembolic prevention strategies for hip arthroscopy.

ARTHROSCOPIC EQUIPMENT

Operative hip arthroscopy requires several instruments to make the procedure possible and improve patient and articular cartilage safety (Figure 5-1). These include access cannula systems, 30- and 70-degree lenses, arthroscopic knife, a standard set of hip-length arthroscopic tools, radiofrequency devices, arthroscopic shavers, burrs, and suture passing/shuttling devices. In general, the access systems will offer longer cannulas than standard knee or shoulder systems and typically come in standard and extended length for patients with a larger soft tissue envelope. The access cannula systems come equipped with spinal needles and nitinol wires for portal establishment via the Seldinger technique.

There are many different hip-length arthroscopic tools available. In addition to length, the tools are specially designed to navigate the constrained space of the hip with flexible designs and different angles in radiofrequency devices, shavers, burrs, and standard arthroscopic tools. It is not recommended to schedule operative hip arthroscopic procedures without the presence of hip-specific instrumentation.

An arthroscopy fluid delivery system (pump or gravity powered) that allows for monitoring of flow and pressure adds safety. The surgeon should be aware that the pressure display on most arthroscopy pump monitors may not reflect the exact conditions in the surgical environment. Manual palpation of the thigh and abdomen should occur at frequent intervals to assess for increased tension due to extravasation of arthroscopy fluid. The supine position allows for easy access to this safety-based maneuver. Reports of symptomatic intra-abdominal fluid extravasation have been linked to high pump pressure, iliopsoas tenotomy, and post-acetabular fracture.[3-6] Even with meticulous care, it is possible to encounter elevated abdominal or thigh compartment pressures. No evidence is available to support more advanced monitoring than the simple method described here.

TABLE OPTIONS

Operative tables that facilitate lower extremity distraction are essential to performing hip arthroscopy. Options include a standard fracture table or commercially available limb spar and post attachments designed for use with a standard operating room table. Key elements mandatory for comprehensive arthroscopy of the hip include radiolucent or open access to the pelvis and proximal femur to the level of the diaphysis; a large-circumference, well-padded perineal post; a secure, well-padded foot-to-table connection; gross and fine traction application ability; and a mobile table or detachable foot connection for sterile dynamic examination.

Unlike traditional fracture surgery–based requirements, distraction for hip arthroscopy requires a substantial traction force. Limiting the duration and force of distraction will reduce iatrogenic damage to the soft tissues and nervous structures of the groin and lower extremity. In addition because the point of contact for distal distraction is typically the foot and ankle, sufficient padding and protection must be provided to avoid injury to these structures during traction. A large-circumference, well-padded perineal post has been shown to decrease the likelihood of injury to the pudendal nerve or genitalia.[7-9] The large size of the post also provides a lateralizing vector of force in addition to the standard longitudinal force vector to aid in distraction and increase access to the central compartment of the hip joint. When using a standard fracture table, the authors have augmented the perineal post and foot attachments with commercially available post and boot disposables designed for arthroscopy.

Purchase of specialized arthroscopy table attachments is not required for the completion of hip arthroscopy. However, for advanced joint preservation surgery and increased ease of complete dynamic assessment, high-volume centers may benefit from the increased efficiency afforded by newer designs. Nonsterile assistant safety may also be improved with the newer designs vs the traditional fracture table.

Design features of specialized tables include independent limb spar attachments, specialized foot connections designed for ease and safety of traction and dynamic examination, "freeze and hold" positioning of spar and limb to achieve mobile examination, and removable perineal post designs. Regardless of the table selected, the authors recommend a full setup and nonsterile positioning with fluoroscopic examination prior to attempting supine arthroscopy in each case. This ensures that the patient-to-table contact points are adequately secured to achieve traction prior to risking contamination of the field or excessive distraction time due to sterile preparation, draping, or equipment passage.

OPERATING ROOM SETUP AND PATIENT POSITIONING

The general operating room setup should include an arthroscopic monitor at the head of the nonoperative side of the table for the surgeon and, if possible, an additional tower at the head of the operative side for the assistant. The arthroscopic pump and equipment are located on the nonoperative side. The C-arm should be located diagonally from the lower portion of the nonoperative side at an angle with the monitor directly at the foot of the table. A Mayo stand is positioned near the head of the operative side, with the side table and scrub assistant on the lateral aspect of the operative side (Figure 5-2).

After induction of general anesthesia, transfer the patient to the operative table. The authors suggest first performing an evaluation of the hip under anesthesia. Flex the hip to 90 degrees and internally and externally rotate the hip to assess rotational motion. Rotational limits are defined

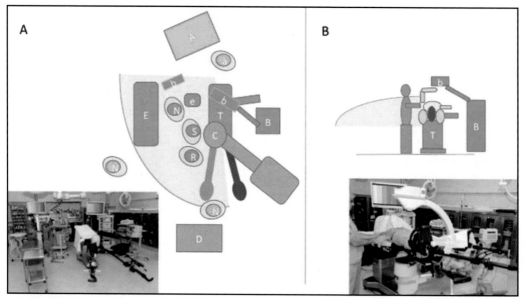

Figure 5-2. (A) Photograph and illustrated overhead view of the operative setup for hip arthroscopy showing the sterility zone in light green. A = anesthesia machine, a = anesthetist, T = table, B = arthroscopy tower, b = boom arm for display monitor, e = sterile Mayo stand, S = surgeon, N = sterile assistant, R = resident surgeon if present, E = sterile instrument table, N = nonsterile assistants, C = C-arm fluoroscopy, D = fluoroscopy monitor. (B) Photographic and illustrated side view from the vantage point of the nonsterile assistant showing the sterility zone in light green.

by the point where hip motion stops and pelvic motion begins. Next, check the stability of the hip by performing a hip distraction test. The examiner secures the limb and pelvis and applies a firm pull to the hip at 30 and 70 degrees of hip flexion. One should feel for subluxation indicating hip laxity. This provides clues to the amount of force that will be required for central compartment access and cautions excessive capsulotomy in cases of generalized ligamentous laxity.

The patient's feet are then snugly wrapped in foam boots, and preparations are made to slide the patient onto the post. The surgeon or circulating nurse should always perform a visual inspection of the genitalia prior to positioning on the post. Any vaginal tearing preoperatively or testicular abnormalities should be noted and placed in the operative chart. The team then transfers the patient's perineum onto the post, and the feet are locked into boots in the spars of the table. Care should be taken to ensure that the heel is placed firmly into the boot and that the foot is adequately locked into the boot to avoid loss of traction intraoperatively. Regardless of the foot-to-table connection mechanism, efforts should be made to maintain a 90-degree foot-to-shin dorsiflexion. Foot plantarflexion is a common cause of slippage at the foot-table interface and results in poor distraction or, in extreme cases, detachment of the foot from the table.

The nonoperative side arm is placed out to the side of the patient and is left open for vascular access, pulse oximetry, and blood pressure monitoring. The patient's chest is padded with blankets, and the operative side arm is draped across the chest with the shoulder and elbow bent at 90 degrees. Foam padding is then used to protect all bony prominences and the ulnar nerve and is secured in place with table belts or athletic tape, forming an X across the chest of the patient (Figure 5-3).

With the upper extremities secure, a time out is called prior to applying traction. The nonoperative leg is abducted, and slight countertraction of 10 to 20 lb is applied. The operative leg should be in approximately 10 degrees of flexion to relax the anterior capsule and neutral rotation. Manual traction is then applied to the operative hip in approximately 20 to 30 degrees of abduction, and the gross distraction mechanism is locked. The operative spar is then adducted to 0 degrees with

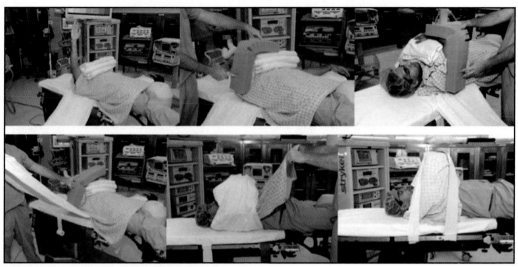

Figure 5-3. Patient arm positioning demonstrating safe and secure control of the operative side with maintenance of well-padded free access to the contralateral side.

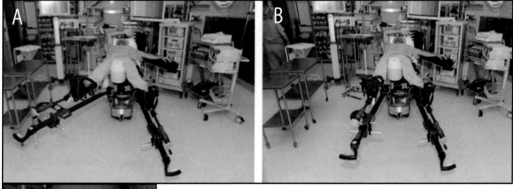

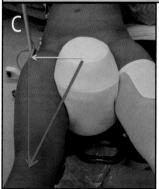

Figure 5-4. Position of the supine patient against the perineal post for hip distraction for right hip surgery. (A) Seating the pelvis safely against the post with limbs abducted. (B) Adduction of the operative limb to neutral. (C) Offset distraction vector clinical photograph showing the offset vector (yellow), traction vector (blue), and resultant vector (green).

the proximal medial thigh in contact with the oversized, padded perineal post. The oversized post in contact with the medial thigh provides a lateralizing force to the hip to aid in subluxation.[9,10] Fine traction is applied until at least 1 cm of distraction is obtained (Figure 5-4). The surgeon and staff should now inspect the operative positioning to ensure that it is appropriate for the case and that the foot is well secured prior to draping.

The operative hip is then prepped, and a spinal needle is used under fluoroscopic guidance to perform an air arthrogram (Figure 5-5). Once obtained, traction is added or decreased as

Figure 5-5. Fluoroscopic images obtained (A) before and (B) after air arthrogram using a spinal needle placed into the hip capsule.

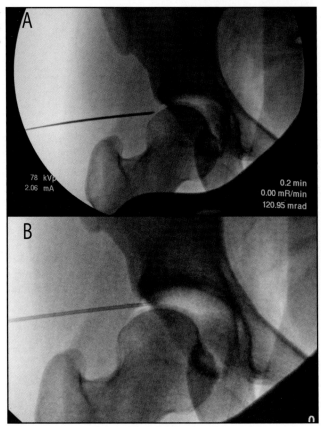

appropriate for the anticipated demands of the case. Traction is then released. The authors suggest routinely performing an air arthrogram to ensure that after breaking the suction seal of the hip, one is applying the least amount of distraction force to perform the case. Most patients may require up to 50 lb of traction, with instability patients requiring less and arthritic patients or patients with global overcoverage (profunda or protrusio deformity) requiring greater force.[9,10]

Perform the standard prepping and draping without traction to decrease the amount of time the patient is in distraction, allowing more time during pertinent portions of the case. Studies have shown that increased traction time and force correlate to the development of significant somatosensory-evoked potential waveform changes and neuropraxia.[11-13] The authors' draping system focuses on maintaining a sterile but moveable field given the importance of dynamic assessment during arthroscopy (Figure 5-6).

A standard shower curtain–style drape with central adhesive field is applied centered on the trochanter. The upper portion of the drape is laid across the patient rather than securing it with standard vertical shower curtain bar attachments. A sterile drape is then attached to the arm/padding construct using a nonpenetrating clamp. This allows for a secure point of attachment of the shower curtain drape and the accessory sterile drape, allowing for the creation of a sterile zone between the upper torso of the patient, the anesthesia team, and the operative field. The C-arm intensifier is draped sterilely to allow for image acquisition over the surgical field.

Traction is now applied to the operative extremity, and once adequate distraction is obtained, a spinal needle is inserted under fluoroscopic guidance to establish the anterolateral portal. Care must be taken to pierce the hip capsule without causing iatrogenic cartilage damage on the femoral head or within the labrum. Tactile feel is necessary during placement of the needle because significant resistance is likely the result of piercing the labrum. An important tip for success is to consider the

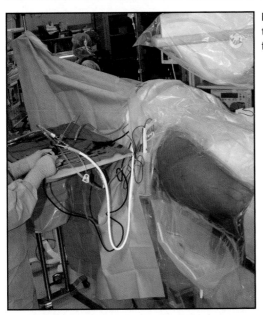

Figure 5-6. Draping of the hip using adhesive contact drapes ("shower curtain") and a limited sterile field opening for portal access.

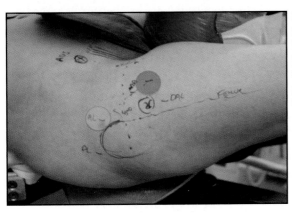

Figure 5-7. Clinical photograph of a supine patient with skin sites for portal placement. Portals marked include anterolateral (yellow), posterolateral, and mid-anterior (green). The anterolateral is the authors' preferred initial portal, and the mid-anterior is the preferred second portal.

acetabular morphology when selecting the skin and deep-entry position. Proximal femoral morphology can obscure the best approach for instrument access and require modification from traditional palpation-based portal start points. The authors use the anterolateral portal as described by Byrd[9,10] and the mid-anterior portal as their standard 2 portals (Figure 5-7). The mid-anterior portal is favored over a traditional anterior portal to increase the margin of safety from the lateral femoral cutaneous nerve and to improve the trajectory for acetabular instrumentation and labral anchor placement.

Once inside the joint, a nitinol wire is advanced gently until bony contact is made. Accurate placement of this portal will result in the nitinol wire contacting the ilioischial line on fluoroscopy. If the wire does not contact the ilioischial line, this could indicate inappropriate capsular entry of the portal. A Seldinger technique is used to widen the portal site, and the cannula and scope are placed at a point just entering the capsule.[14] The authors prefer to avoid initial use of fluid inflow to avoid the poor visualization that often results due to clotted blood from the lower joint prior to establishment of a second portal for outflow.

The authors' first arthroscopic assessment is to direct the camera posteriorly to confirm that the scope is not in the substance of the labrum and then angle the camera anteriorly to view the anterior triangle. This triangle is formed by the border of the femoral head, the labrum, and the edge of the arthroscopic image on the screen (Figure 5-8). This is the projected entry site for

Figure 5-8. Arthroscopic view from AL portal demonstrating the femoral head (asterisk), labrum (L), and capsule (green triangle). This view is termed the anterior triangle, and a spinal needle is shown as placed via the mid-anterior portal.

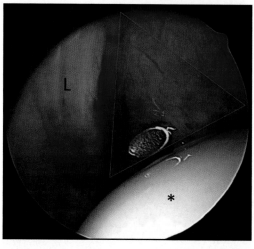

the mid-anterior working portal. A spinal needle is once again used to develop this portal with a Seldinger technique.[14] Once the portal is established, the camera is removed and placed in the mid-anterior working portal to view the blindly placed anterolateral portal to ensure it is not translabral. The camera is then placed back into the anterolateral portal, the flow is turned on, and diagnostic arthroscopy is performed in the central compartment.

HIP ARTHROSCOPY WITHOUT JOINT DISTRACTION

Once the central compartment work is completed, the surgeon must transition to the peripheral compartment. In the supine approach, all planes of hip motion may be examined without limitation beyond those created by the table itself. Traditional fracture tables require detachment of the spar-foot connection for comprehensive dynamic examination. Specialized distractors allow an easy transition and add the benefit of complete mobility of the hip to aid in access to areas of the peripheral compartment. Peripheral compartment work typically consists of management of the cam lesion, loose bodies, and synovial disorders, and some surgeons manage pincer and labral disorders without traction.

To first access the peripheral compartment, traction is released from the hip. The hip is then flexed to 30 degrees to relax the anterior capsule. The surgeon can then gain access to this compartment through their interportal capsulotomy or redirect a modified anterolateral portal into the peripheral compartment via a Seldinger technique as described by Dienst et al.[15] Unlocking the boot connection on specially developed tables allows an assistant to fully internally and externally rotate the hip while adding flexion or extension of the hip through the spar to aid in arthroscopic access of the peripheral compartment. Having an assistant slightly flex the hip aids in relaxing the anterior capsule and further increasing working space (Figure 5-9). Using these techniques, the surgeon should be able to work in the peripheral compartment from the lateral to the medial synovial fold. Although the completion of advanced hip preservation techniques is possible on any operative table, realistic assessment of the skill and availability of the surgical team and surgeon, as well as the equipment, must be considered in advance.

POTENTIAL COMPLICATIONS

The supine and lateral approaches share complications, such as genital injury, nerve palsy, and skin injury.[7,8,16,17] These complications result more from increased force and length of time

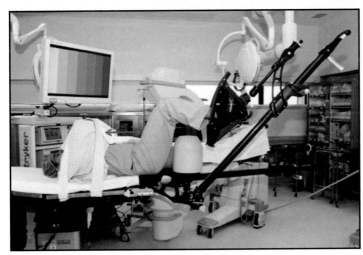

Figure 5-9. Photograph showing the working room for instruments during dynamic examination with the hip joint reduced.

associated with traction as opposed to surgical approach. The authors' rule of thumb is to have the circulating nurse call out every 10 minutes while in traction to keep the surgeon aware. The authors suggest limiting traction to no longer than 1 continuous hour and no longer than 2 hours per case to limit these issues.[7,10]

BENEFITS AND DISADVANTAGES OF THE SUPINE APPROACH

The supine approach provides easier patient positioning and anesthesia access than the lateral approach.[9,10] Use and interpretation of C-arm fluoroscopy during the case is straightforward in the supine position. Although many specialized tables and table attachments exist to aid in the supine approach, the procedure can easily be accomplished with the use of a standard fracture table. This aids in decreasing the cost of incorporating hip arthroscopy into one's practice because most centers have a standard fracture table.

One could make the argument that the lateral position could have an easier learning curve for surgeons who have extensive experience in laterally based positioning for hip replacement surgery; however, the setup is extensive. There is also the benefit in obese patients that the adipose tissue falls away from the operative field, aiding in identifying anatomic landmarks, and the arthroscope passes through less tissue.[18]

CONCLUSION

The supine approach to hip arthroscopy provides easier patient positioning, use of a commercially available specialized or standard fracture table, and straightforward use of C-arm fluoroscopy intraoperatively. This is a team approach, and all staff should be educated as to their role to facilitate timely patient positioning and completion of the operative goal. Strict care should be taken when positioning the patient against the perineal post, as well as with the force and duration of traction time, to avoid potential complications.

TOP TECHNICAL PEARLS FOR THE PROCEDURE

1. Reduce neuropraxia through the use of a large, padded perineal post; limiting traction time and force to a minimum; adding gentle Trendelenburg to the operating room table; and obtaining an air arthrogram prior to joint distraction.

2. When placing portals, consider the required approach to the acetabulum along with standard surface references to the femoral trochanter.

3. Ensure that the foot is properly secured to the table and boot prior to sterile preparation to avoid loss of traction intraoperatively.

4. If patient health allows, maintain MAP close to 60 mm Hg for adequate visualization.

5. Educate staff members as to their roles in the procedure to enhance efficiency.

REFERENCES

1. Ward JP, Albert DB, Altman R, Goldstein RY, Cuff G, Youm T. Are femoral nerve blocks effective for early postoperative pain management after hip arthroscopy? *Arthroscopy.* 2012;28(8):1064-1069.
2. Mei-Dan O, McConkey MO, Young DA. Hip arthroscopy distraction without the use of a perineal post: prospective study. *Orthopedics.* 2013;36(1):e1-e5.
3. Kocher MS, Frank JS, Nasreddine AY, et al. Intra-abdominal fluid extravasation during hip arthroscopy: a survey of the MAHORN group. *Arthroscopy.* 2012;28(11):1654.e2-1660.e2.
4. Bartlett CS, Difelice GS, Buly RL, Quinn TJ, Green DST, Helfet DL. Cardiac arrest as a result of intraabdominal extravasation of fluid during arthroscopic removal of a loose body from the hip joint of a patient with an acetabular fracture. *J Orthop Trauma.* 1998;12(4):294-299.
5. Fowler J, Owens BD. Abdominal compartment syndrome after hip arthroscopy. *Arthroscopy.* 2010;26(1):128-130.
6. Ilizaliturri VM Jr. Complications of arthroscopic femoroacetabular impingement treatment: a review. *Clin Orthop Relat Res.* 2009;467(3):760-768.
7. Sampson TG. Complications of hip arthroscopy. *Clin Sports Med.* 2001;20(4):831-835.
8. Flierl MA, Stahel PF, Hak DJ, Morgan SJ, Smith WR. Traction table-related complications in orthopaedic surgery. *J Am Acad Orthop Surg.* 2010;18(11):668-675.
9. Byrd JW. Hip arthroscopy by the supine approach. *Instr Course Lect.* 2006;55:325-336.
10. Byrd JW. Hip arthroscopy. *J Am Acad Orthop Surg.* 2006;14(7):433-444.
11. Ochs BC, Herzka A, Yaylali I. Intraoperative neurophysiological monitoring of somatosensory evoked potentials during hip arthroscopy surgery. *Neurodiagn J.* 2012;52(4):312-319.
12. Martin HD, Palmer IJ, Champlin K, Kaiser B, Kelly B, Leunig M. Physiological changes as a result of hip arthroscopy performed with traction. *Arthroscopy.* 2012;28(10):1365-1372.
13. Telleria JJM, Safran MR, Harris AH, Gardi JN, Glick JM. Risk of sciatic nerve traction injury during hip arthroscopy—is it the amount or duration? An intraoperative nerve monitoring study. *J Bone Joint Surg Am.* 2012;94(22):2025-2032.
14. Seldinger SI. Catheter replacement of the needle in percutaneous arteriography: a new technique. *Acta Radiol.* 1953;39(5):368-376.
15. Dienst M, Seil R, Kohn DM. Safe arthroscopic access to the central compartment of the hip. *Arthroscopy.* 2005;21(12):1510-1514.
16. Clarke MT, Arora A, Villar RN. Hip arthroscopy: complications in 1054 cases. *Clin Orthop Relat Res.* 2003;(406):84-88.
17. Griffin DR, Villar RN. Complications of arthroscopy of the hip. *J Bone Joint Surg Br.* 1999;81(4):604-606.
18. McCarthy JC. Hip arthroscopy: applications and technique. *J Am Acad Orthop Surg.* 1995;3(3):115-122.

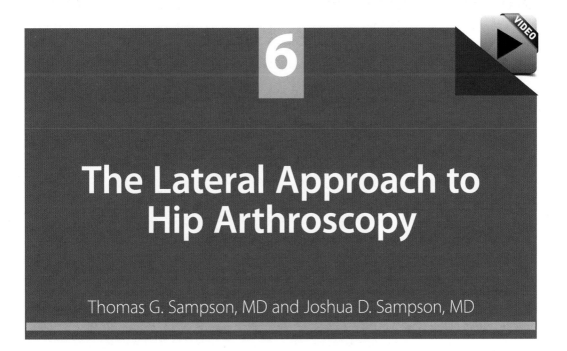

6

The Lateral Approach to Hip Arthroscopy

Thomas G. Sampson, MD and Joshua D. Sampson, MD

INTRODUCTION

In 1931, Burman[1] was the first to arthroscope the hip in a cadaveric study. He was unable to enter the central compartment even with distraction. J. M. Glick, MD, performed 11 cases between 1977 and 1982 and had difficulty accessing the central compartment on 2 occasions in the supine position (personal communication, July 1982). Because experience with the lateral decubitus position in total hip replacements was popular and familiar at the time, the idea of approaching hip arthroscopy with a similar method was developed.[2] Glick and Sampson dissected a cadaver hip to determine the most direct access to the intra-articular space and described the anterior peritrochanteric and posterior peritrochanteric portals (personal communication, July 1982; Figure 6-1). Later, these were referred to as the anterolateral and posterolateral portals. Prior to 1982, there were no accepted techniques or hip-specific instruments for hip arthroscopy. Johnson[3] was one of the first to publish on hip arthroscopy in the first edition of his textbook in 1986, but he did not describe a specific technique. The procedure was first done in the current authors' practice using the supine approach on a fracture table for distraction to enter the intra-articular space, which is now called the central compartment. Simultaneously in Paris, Dorfmann et al[4] were developing methods to get into the peripheral space without traction using the supine position, and in Sweden, Erikkson et al[5] were working on hip distraction to facilitate entering the hip joint. The current authors developed a rope-and-pulley system with weights that they used in shoulder arthroscopy as their first hip distractor (Figure 6-2).

In the authors' early experience, problems getting into the hip joint and complications, including scuffing of the articular cartilage, labral damage, poor maneuverability, and the inability to achieve the anticipated result before extensive fluid extravasation, made the procedure difficult and unpredictable.[6] Specific instruments were not developed, and distraction parameters were not established. As a result, the procedure was neither predictable nor reproducible in entering the central compartment.

Byrd JWT, Bedi A, Stubbs AJ, eds. *The Hip:*
AANA Advanced Arthroscopic Surgical Techniques (pp 71-86).
© 2016 AANA.

Figure 6-1. Original cadaver dissection at Mount Zion Hospital (San Francisco, CA) done by James M. Glick, MD, and Thomas G. Sampson, MD, to develop the portals for hip arthroscopy.

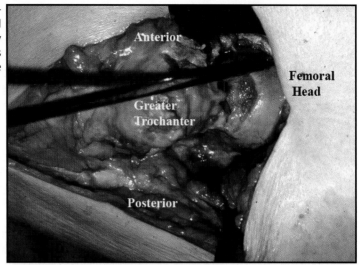

Figure 6-2. Original rope-and-pulley system used for hip distraction adopted from the same system used for shoulder arthroscopy.

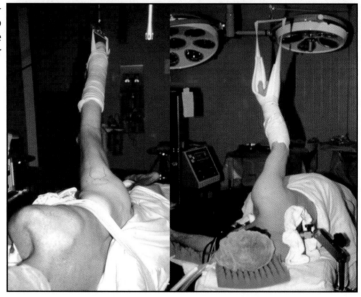

Despite the early hurdles, advantages were observed in the lateral decubitus position. The obese portion of the thigh declines away to expose a prominent greater trochanter. The neurovascular structures are safely away from the portals, and the surgeon is familiar with their locations. The portals offer direct entry into the femoroacetabular joint and do not require imagining the angles of entry as described by Byrd[7] for the supine approach. The few surgeons interested in hip arthroscopy at that time adopted the lateral technique and continue to use it. Although the supine approach has become more popular (as determined by asking participants in courses taught in the past few years), the authors believe that there are advantages to using the lateral approach instead of the supine method. The lateral decubitus position is the most common approach for total hip replacement, the anatomy is familiar, and orientation to the clock face method of orientation, now a zone system, was devised with the lateral position.[8] The trochanter is prominent, and the anterior, peritrochanteric, and posterior structures and deep gluteal spaces are easily accessible. The assistant stands across the table and out of the surgeon's way and may easily control the instruments and scope when necessary without interfering with the surgeon. With the nearly vertical orientation of the scope and instruments, it is rare for them to fall out of the portals, and, in some cases, they may not need to be held while maneuvering the scope. The portals are far away from the femoral and sciatic nerves, and the abdomen is easily palpable to observe for early distension if a retroperitoneal extravasation occurs. The disadvantages are that the patient needs to be turned on the operating table, specialized distractors are needed, and anterior visualization of the peripheral compartment is not enhanced by the posterior displacement of the femoral head by the weight of the buttock as seen in the supine approach.

With industry interest to develop arthroscopic instruments and distractors, the supine approach was once again used and described by Byrd.[7] Editorials, journal articles, and book chapters have been written arguing the advantages of each method. It is now agreed that the approach should be based on the surgeon's training and comfort.[8,9] All hip arthroscopy procedures are done equally well using either technique, and complications are not reported as technique specific.[10,11] A distractor has been designed to be used on any operating table for both techniques (Smith & Nephew), and all instruments designed for hip arthroscopy can be used for either technique; however, the authors have found that shorter, traditional-length instruments work well in the lateral position because the distance from the skin to the depths of the central compartment seem to be shorter due to the soft tissue dropping away from the portals.

The major advancements in getting into the central compartment have come from a better understanding of distraction and the use of cannulated trocars and fluoroscopy. Later, the development of longer arthroscopes, slotted (half-pipe) cannulas, and curved and flexible instruments allowed for advanced techniques (Figure 6-3).

The indications (some of which are controversial), pertinent physical findings, and pertinent imaging are addressed in the other chapters. Byrd said, "The key to successful hip arthroscopy lies in selecting appropriate patients" (personal communication, May 2006). The senior author (TGS) has stated that the patient's expectations should match the surgeon's. Hip arthroscopy in the early 1980s was felt to be a procedure looking for indications. The list of indications has increased with the advancements of the technique.

Currently, the most common reason for arthroscopic surgery of the hip is to treat damage related to femoral acetabular impingement. Prior to 2001, this condition was only treated using a surgical dislocation of the hip with a trochanteric osteotomy as developed by Myers et al.[12] Femoroacetabular impingment was recognized as groin pain from an unintended consequence of overcorrection by a pelvic acetabular osteotomy for developmental dysplasia, from which anterior impingement had occurred.[12] The current authors described an arthroscopic technique to reshape the femoral head-neck junction in 2001 and published it in 2005.[13]

EQUIPMENT

All hip arthroscopy may be accomplished in an outpatient setting, either in a come-and-go unit of a hospital or a surgical center. The operating room should be large enough to accommodate the usual equipment in addition to a fluoroscopic C-arm to facilitate precise portal placement and access to various areas of the hip joint. A standard operating table or a fluoroscopic radiolucent table is most often used. The lateral approach requires a specialized hip distractor specifically designed for hip arthroscopy because fracture tables are not well designed for this approach and may put the sciatic nerve at risk due to pressure from a transverse perineal post. The 2 most popular are designed to be used on a standard table and allow for mobility of the hip in rotation and flexion/extension during hip arthroscopy (Figure 6-4). The force, time, and distance of traction during hip distraction have been compared with the use of a tourniquet, with parameters to not exceed 50 to 75 lb and a time of less than 2 hours to reduce the risks of neuropraxia. An older study by Glick in 1998 that examined hip arthroscopy with the lateral approach using evoked potentials to measure real-time intraoperative sciatic and femoral nerve injuries was reanalyzed with more contemporary statistical methods (personal communication, December 1998). This study found

Figure 6-3. (A) Basic instruments and slotted cannulas, (B) additional instruments, and (C) back table reserve instruments.

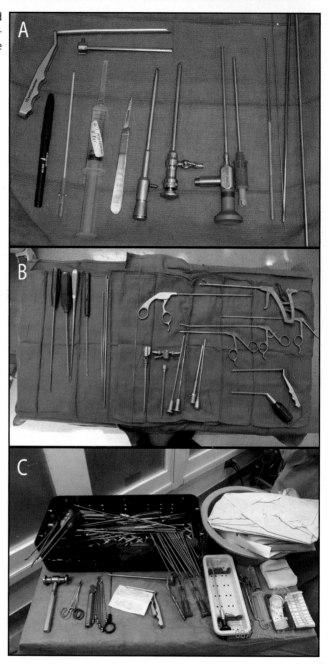

that the amount of force and not time was the predictor of nerve injury.[14] Starting at no distraction, every 1 lb of force increases the risk by 0.45%. For that reason, the current authors advocate their technique of no distraction until the capsulotomy has been completed, which requires less force to separate the head from the acetabulum when traction is applied. Intuitively, they keep the amount of time in distraction to a minimum, although it is not supported by this study.

A standard arthroscopic tower may be used to house all of the electronic equipment and should be placed in a convenient place near the patient's head. The fluoroscopic C-arm is positioned under the table so that it may be rolled in and out of the field when necessary and is out of the surgical

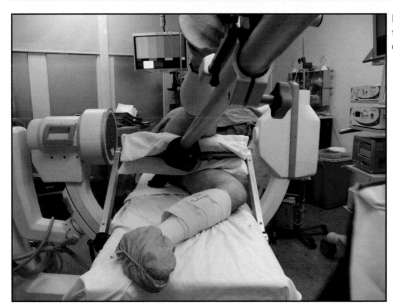

Figure 6-4. Lateral distractor with fluoroscopic C-arm.

field when not needed. A Mayo stand over the patient's shoulder is useful to organize all of the instruments and keep a working inventory of what is needed for each procedure (Figure 6-5).

The essential difference between hip arthroscopy and arthroscopy of other joints is that the hip is located deep within the body cavity surrounded by dense tissue and muscle. Portal placement is done with fluoroscopic observation for accurate portal placement through cannulated trocars. First, a long 17-gauge spinal needle is placed, which is then threaded with a nitinol wire prior to the skin incision and introduction of the cannulated arthroscopic sheath. Standard-length, 4-mm, 30- and 70-degree arthroscopes may be used for most individuals; however, the authors prefer to use slightly longer arthroscopes that may be used on any individual, whether small or large. Interchanging between the 2 angles of vision will allow central and peripheral viewing, which may be constrained by the bony architecture and dense soft tissues. Triangulation appears to be a bit easier with the 30-degree arthroscope, and with capsulotomy, the authors find it rare to use the 70-degree arthroscope except for looking into the extremes of the fovea and the peripheral recesses.

An arthroscopic pump has advantages in providing a high-flow system and will control the exact pressure of fluid irrigation and space distention that may be adjusted to the patient's blood pressure, thereby keeping it at the lowest possible pressure and reducing the risk of extravasation. It is essential that the surgeon be familiar with the pump because they differ from manufacturer to manufacture (Figure 6-6).

Extra-length cannulas—cylindrical and slotted of various types and shapes—are essential for completing the complex procedures currently done in hip arthroscopy. Slotted or half-pipe cannulas allow for curved instruments to be introduced into the hip joint. Bridging cannulas may make it easier to move the scope and operative instruments from portal to portal.

A radiofrequency (RF) probe is vital for coagulating bleeders, cutting through tissue, and congealing frayed material. Shaving equipment is mandatory for debridement, removing tissue, and removing bone with a burr. Standard mechanical instruments are necessary for intra-articular and peripheral compartment work (Figure 6-7). Power instruments are necessary for drilling holes when anchors are used, and sutured devices, such as suture penetrators and sewing devices, facilitate labral, capsular, and muscular repairs.

Figure 6-5. (A) Diagram of the room setup. (B) View of a right hip from above the room setup. (C) Mayo stand above the shoulder that organizes the instruments.

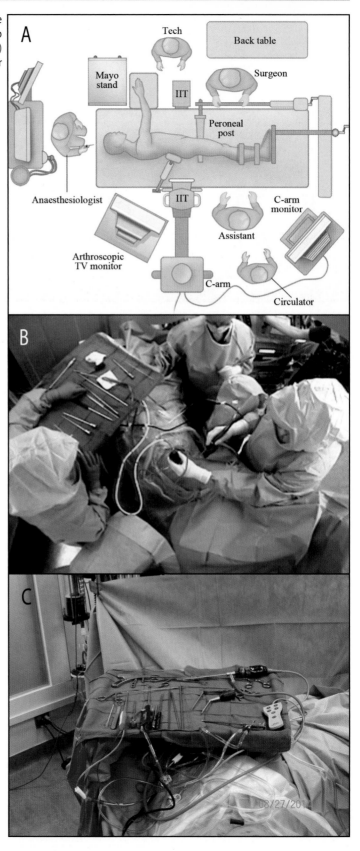

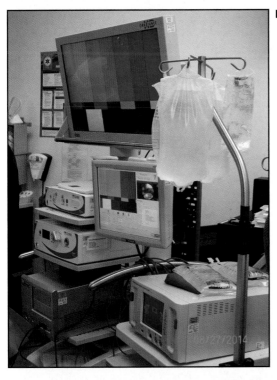

Figure 6-6. Arthroscopic tower with pump.

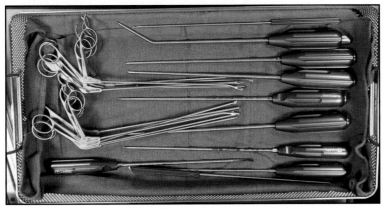

Figure 6-7. Long hip instruments.

POSITIONING

Once adequate anesthesia has been established, the patient is rolled to a lateral decubitus position. Axillary rolls, as well as extra padding for downside bony prominences, are used for safety, and hip positioners stabilize the pelvis. It is essential that the anesthesiologist be secure with the patient's airway because it is more difficult to correct problems in this position once the patient has been prepped and draped (Figure 6-8). The operated leg is then set up in the hip distractor, taking care to adequately pad the foot and provide a large perineal post (Figure 6-9).

Considering most procedures currently require bone resection, the current authors do 6 fluoroscopic views to look for conflict between the head-neck traction of the femur and the acetabular rim. Other subtleties may be picked up with this maneuver, such as previously undetected loose bodies, notch osteophytes, and head-neck bumps (Figure 6-10).

Figure 6-8. Patient positioned and prepped before draping for a right hip (looking from anterior; the head is toward the right).

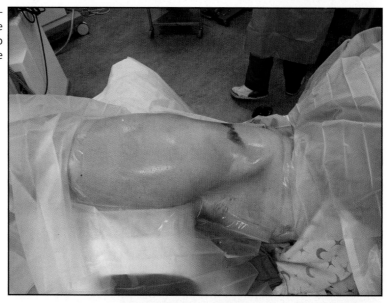

Figure 6-9. Distractor setup with large perineal padded post.

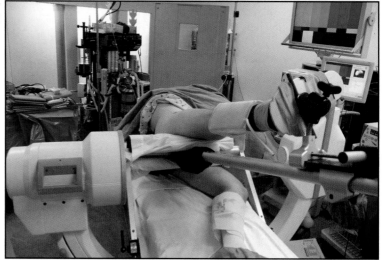

STEP-BY-STEP DESCRIPTION OF THE PROCEDURE

Most hip arthroscopy is initiated by entering the central compartment first, using distraction of the hip and placement of the spinal needle into the central compartment, followed by the nitinol wire, the skin incision, and then the cannulated arthroscopic sheath followed by the arthroscope. The technique is well described in other chapters in this book. The authors feel that a more useful technique, which ensures getting into all hips despite the great variance of the anatomy and tightness between individuals, involves an arthroscopic capsulotomy first, or the out-to-in technique.[15] The advantage is that no distraction is used until the head-neck junction of the femur, the labrum, and the supra-acetabular sulcus are exposed. Distraction is then done under direct vision, allowing for the minimum amount of forces to get enough separation of the head from the acetabulum to drive the arthroscope into the central compartment, and cartilage scuffing and labral damage is minimized during the initial approach (Figure 6-11).

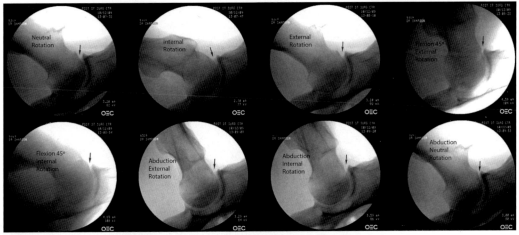

Figure 6-10. Preoperative fluoroscopic views.

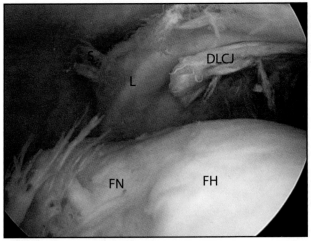

Figure 6-11. Arthroscopic view of a distracted right hip from the peripheral compartment through a capsulotomy. DLCJ = degenerative labrocartilage junction; FH = femoral head; FN = femoral neck; L = labrum; S = synovitis.

Approach to the Central and Peripheral Compartments

Under fluoroscopic control and no distraction, a spinal needle is placed through the anterolateral portal, aiming toward the superior lateral articulation of the head of the femur and acetabulum. After proper positioning, the nitinol wire is placed in the needle, the skin is incised with an 11 blade, and the cannulated arthroscopic trocar and sheath are placed on the external capsule of the hip joint. The second portal is placed mid-anterior, with the spinal needle aimed toward the same position. The nitinol wire is placed through the spinal needle, and the skin is incised more superficially to prevent damage to the lateral femoral cutaneous nerve (Figure 6-12).

A cannulated trocar is then introduced, followed by a switcher stick, then a slotted cannula, and then the operative instruments through the slotted cannula, which is then removed. Insertion of instruments is facilitated with a slotted cannula for the remaining portions of the procedure (Figure 6-13).

The pump is activated, and the space above the capsule is distended to provide a view of the anterior fat pad and the reflected head of the rectus femoris. Just beneath the reflected head and capsule is the labrum. The C-arm is then moved away because fluoroscopy is no longer necessary until the end of the procedure.

Figure 6-12. Creation of the portals into a cadaver right hip. (A) Right hip portals. A = anterior; AI = mid-anterior (ie, anteroinferior); AL = anterolateral; ASIS = anterior superior iliac spine; FAI = far anteroinferior; PL = posterolateral. (B) Creation of an anterolateral portal with a spinal needle and nitinol wire. (C) Creation of a mid-anterior (MA) portal with a spinal needle.

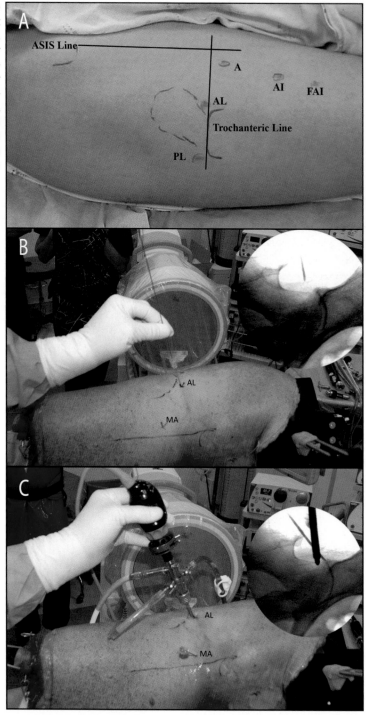

Using an arthroscopic shaver, a portion of the fat pad is excised while protecting the reflected head of the rectus femoris (Figure 6-14). Next, a 50-degree RF suction probe is used to incise the capsule along its anterolateral portion adjacent and through the iliofemoral ligament from the base of the neck to the acetabular rim, further dissecting it laterally and anteriorly, taking care to preserve the labrum. Preoperatively, a decision should be made as to whether the capsule will

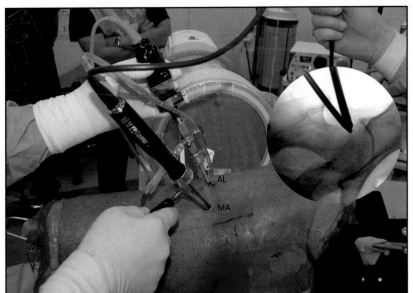

Figure 6-13. Using the slotted cannula and introduction of the shaver. AL = anterolateral portal; MA = mid-anterior portal.

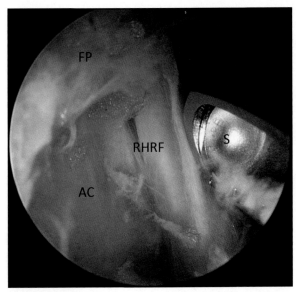

Figure 6-14. Removal of the anterior fat pad (FP) external to the hip capsule (AC), with exposure of the reflected head of the rectus femoris (RHRF) using the shaver (S).

be repaired or excised. A portion of the capsule may be excised and still allow for later repair if the volume of bone is reduced during the femoroplasty and acetabular rim ostectomy procedure (Figure 6-15).

Once the capsulotomy has been completed, the hip is distracted. When adequately opened, the arthroscope is advanced in the central compartment, taking care not to damage the head cartilage, the labrum, or the acetabular cartilage. Occasionally in stiffer hips, flexing the hip to 30 degrees will open up the space adjacent to the labrum and head and make it easier to incise the capsule.

The central compartment is then inspected, beginning with the notch, turning posterior to view the labrum and sulcus, working laterally to view the labrocartilage junction, and finally anteriorly, where most pathology occurs. Attention is then directed to the femoral head, and as much of the fovea as possible is visualized, which may require a 70-degree scope to see. The ligamentum teres is inspected and observed for tensioning during an external rotation maneuver (Figure 6-16).

Figure 6-15. Right hip exposure through a capsulotomy showing the femoral head (FH), labrum (L), acetabular rim (AR), and cut capsule (CC).

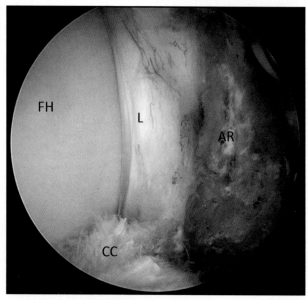

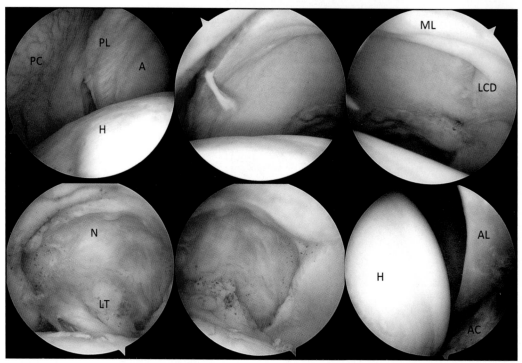

Figure 6-16. Arthroscopic view of a right hip sweeping from posterior (upper left) to anterior (upper right) and then notch (lower left) to very anterior (lower right) showing the posterior capsule (PC), posterior labrum (PL), acetabulum (A), femoral head (H), mid-labrum (ML), labrocartilage junction (LCD), notch (N), ligamentum teres (LT), anterior labrum (AL), and anterior capsule (AC).

A probe is introduced, and the pathology becomes well defined. If there is a labrocartilage junctional delamination or tear, it is repaired with rim trimming and elevation of the defect, followed by microfracture beneath the defect and labral refixation or repair (Figure 6-17).

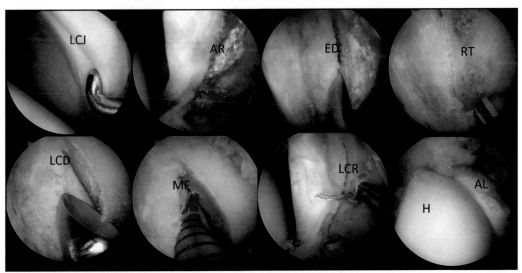

Figure 6-17. Probe on a damaged labrocartilage junction (LCJ) and repair showing the LCJ, acetabular rim (AR), elevation of the defect (ED), rim trimmed (RT), labrocartilage defect (LCD), microfracture (MF), labrocartilage repair (LCR), femoral head (H), and anterior labrum (AL).

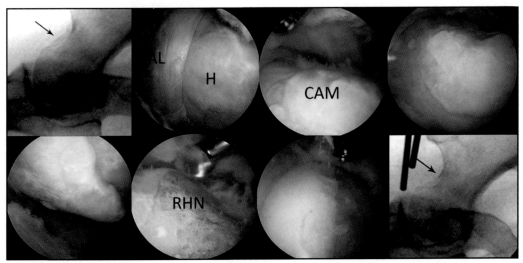

Figure 6-18. Arthroscopic view of a left large head-neck metaplastic bump. Preoperative fluoroscopic view (upper left arrow), anterior labrum (AL), head-neck bump (H), metaplastic head-neck bump (CAM), resected head-neck junction (RHN). Postoperative fluoroscopic view (bottom right arrow).

The head-neck junction of the femur is then explored, the demarcation zones of cartilage indentation or wearing are noted, and excessive bone, such as seen with a cam bump, are defined. The soft tissue is removed with a RF probe, and a femoroplasty is performed using a round burr (Figure 6-18). Loose bodies are easily removed through the capsulotomy, and leaving the capsule open may allow residual loose bodies to exit (Figure 6-19). Synovectomy may be accomplished in all compartments, considering access is through a large incision in the capsule.

The posterolateral portal is less often used because most pathology exists anteriorly, except for access to posterior labral tears and when trimming the acetabular rim with global pincer posteriorly. It is also useful when entering the subgluteal space along with an accessory posterior portal when exploring the pyriformis and sciatic nerve.

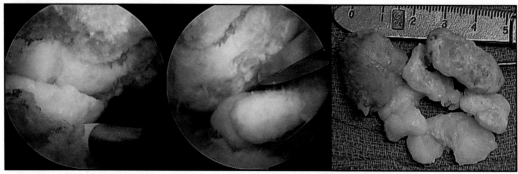

Figure 6-19. Arthroscopic view of removal of loose bodies from a left hip.

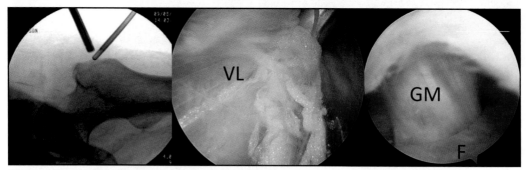

Figure 6-20. Fluoroscopic view of the scope and instruments entering the peritrochanteric space showing the vastus lateralis (VL), gluteus maximus (GM), and femur (F).

The peritrochanteric space is entered under fluoroscopic control by placing the arthroscope near the tip of the greater trochanter beneath the fascia lata and the operative instruments through the mid-anterior portal on the vastus ridge (Figure 6-20). A posterior portal may be added during gluteus medius repair for optimal viewing while placing anchors in the greater trochanter and sutures to the muscle.

Capsular repair may be accomplished in several ways, such as using a suture penetrator, suture relay technique, or suture devices, such as the Scorpion (Arthrex, Inc) or Concept (Conmed Linvatec) suture passers.

Postoperatively, the same 6 fluoroscopic views are taken to determine if the amount of bone removed is as desired. Further resection may be accomplished if needed (Figure 6-21).

POSTOPERATIVE PROTOCOL

Skin closure is done with nylon suture, and a standard bulky dressing is applied for 24 hours to absorb any leakage of irrigation fluid and blood. The dressing is removed the next day, the patient is allowed to shower, and bandages are applied. The patient is given crutches and asked to partially bear weight until he or she is comfortable fully bearing weight.

Rehabilitation starts with a stationary bicycle, followed by an elliptical trainer, with range of motion exercises and a specific rehabilitation protocol. Depending on the procedure, the authors typically have patients doing self-rehabilitation for the first 3 weeks and then assess their needs for range of motion, stability, and strength to determine if formal therapy is required.

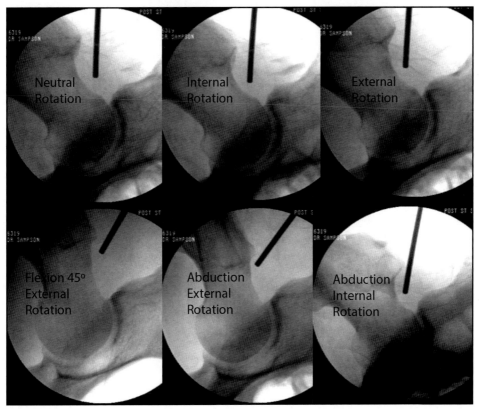

Figure 6-21. Postoperative fluoroscopic views in 6 positions to evaluate femoroplasty and rim trimming of the acetabulum.

POTENTIAL COMPLICATIONS

Complications may be from direct trauma, such as damage to the articular cartilage, labrum, and neurovascular structures; indirect trauma, as with neuropraxias from distraction; retroperitoneal and thigh extravasation from problems with fluid management; and late complications of infection, fracture, and heterotopic bone formation.[16] None of these are surgical-position specific and are discussed in other chapters of this book.

TOP TECHNICAL PEARLS FOR THE PROCEDURE

1. Optimize the surgical environment by training the staff and anesthesiologist to your needs.

2. Position the patient on the table closer to the side on which the surgeon is working for better ergonomics and less surgeon fatigue, and pad the bony prominences on the down side, the perineal nerve, and the foot. Carefully place the axillary roll or axillary protector to protect the brachial plexus, and test the distractor before scrubbing to prevent inadvertent foot slippage.

(continued)

3. Choose special instruments needed prior to the procedure (eg, spinal curettes and heavy graspers for large loose bodies and osteophytectomy; labral refixation anchors).

4. If distraction does not separate the head from the acetabulum despite any amount of distraction in any position, getting into the central compartment may be facilitated by capsulotomy and rim trimming of the acetabulum because capsulotomy facilitates instrument mobility and global exposure.

5. Use distraction judiciously and only when it is necessary to work in the central compartment. Most peripheral compartment work may be performed without distraction.

REFERENCES

1. Burman MS. Arthroscopy or the direct visualization of joints: an experimental cadaver study. 1931. *Clin Orthop Relat Res.* 2001;(390):5-9.
2. Harris WH. Advances in surgical technique for total hip replacement: without and with osteotomy of the greater trochanter. *Clin Orthop Relat Res.* 1980;(146):188-204.
3. Johnson L. *Arthroscopic Surgery: Principles and Practice.* St. Louis, MO: C.V. Mosby; 1986.
4. Dorfmann H, Boyer T, De Bie B. Arthroscopy of the hip [in French]. *Rev Rhum Mal Osteoartic.* 1988;55(1):33-36.
5. Eriksson E, Arvidsson I, Arvidsson H. Diagnostic and operative arthroscopy of the hip. *Orthopedics.* 1986;9(2):169-176.
6. Glick JM, Sampson TG, Gordon RB, Behr JT, Schmidt E. Hip arthroscopy by the lateral approach. *Arthroscopy.* 1987;3(1):4-12.
7. Byrd JW. Hip arthroscopy utilizing the supine position. *Arthroscopy.* 1994;10(3):275-280.
8. Byrd JW. Hip arthroscopy: the supine position. *Clin Sports Med.* 2001;20(4):703-731.
9. Ilizaliturri VM Jr, Byrd JW, Sampson TG, et al. A geographic zone method to describe intra-articular pathology in hip arthroscopy: cadaveric study and preliminary report. *Arthroscopy.* 2008;24(5):534-539.
10. Funke EL, Munzinger U. Complications in hip arthroscopy. *Arthroscopy.* 1996;12(2):156-159.
11. Kim SJ, Choi NH, Kim HJ. Operative hip arthroscopy. *Clin Orthop Relat Res.* 1998;(353):156-165.
12. Myers SR, Eijer H, Ganz R. Anterior femoroacetabular impingement after periacetabular osteotomy. *Clin Orthop Relat Res.* 1999;(363):93-99.
13. Sampson T. Arthroscopic treatment of femoroacetabular impingement. *Tech Orthop.* 2005;20:56-62.
14. Telleria JJ, Safran MR, Harris AH, Gardi JN, Glick JM. Risk of sciatic nerve traction injury during hip arthroscopy—is it the amount or duration? An intraoperative nerve monitoring study. *J Bone Joint Surg Am.* 2012;94(22):2025-2032.
15. Sampson TG. Paper SS-33. Extensive capsulotomy for ideal exposure and treatment in hip arthroscopy. Paper presented at: Annual Meeting of the Arthroscopy Association of North America; May 20-23, 2010; Hollywood, FL.
16. Sampson TG. Complications of hip arthroscopy. *Tech Orthop.* 2005;20(1):63-66.

Please see videos on the accompanying website at

www.ArthroscopicTechniques.com

7

The Use of Intraoperative Fluoroscopy and Dynamic Examination in Hip Arthroscopy

Achieving a Complete Femoroacetabular Impingement Correction

Christopher M. Larson, MD and Rebecca M. Stone, MS, ATC

INTRODUCTION

A thorough correction of the variable hip pathomorphology associated with femoroacetabular impingement (FAI) may be critical to achieve optimal outcomes and minimize failures. Prior studies have reported that residual FAI is the most frequent finding at the time of revision hip preservation surgery.[1-5] In addition, revision FAI correction has been reported to have inferior outcomes compared with primary FAI correction.[4] The use of intraoperative fluoroscopy has been advocated by some surgeons to evaluate the adequacy of FAI correction when performed arthroscopically.[6-10] The current authors have previously published a systematic approach for using intraoperative fluoroscopy to better assess FAI correction.[6] More recently, specific fluoroscopic views of the proximal femur were combined with 3-dimensional computed tomography (3D CT) to evaluate the specific locations that each view represents.[7] The current authors have found that this fluoroscopic evaluation, combined with a thorough arthroscopic dynamic assessment, allows for precise osseous correction as seen on postoperative plain x-rays. This chapter provides a systematic fluoroscopic technique that can be used for accurate osseous FAI corrections.

Byrd JWT, Bedi A, Stubbs AJ, eds. *The Hip: AANA Advanced Arthroscopic Surgical Techniques* (pp 87-102). © 2016 AANA.

Fluoroscopic Technique
for Osseous Correction

To determine the location and degree of osseous resection, it is important to define the hip anatomy and associated pathomorphology. Plain x-rays should be evaluated for acetabular-sided or pincer-type FAI.[10,11] On a well-aligned anteroposterior (AP) x-ray of both hips, the presence of a normal lateral center-edge angle (LCE) and a crossover sign, global overcoverage with an LCE typically greater than 40 degrees, associated rim fractures, and evidence for anterior inferior iliac spine (AIIS) deformities with extension to or beyond the acetabular rim are suggestive of acetabular-sided FAI.[10,11] Plain x-rays should also be evaluated for femoral-sided or cam-type FAI.[9,11] An aspherical head-neck junction as measured with the alpha angle on AP and lateral x-rays, decreased femoral head-neck offset/offset ratio, a low neck-shaft angle/coxa vara on plain x-rays, and femoral retroversion/torsion (magnetic resonance imaging/CT) are suggestive of femoral-sided or cam-type FAI.[9,11] Three-dimensional imaging allows for a more complete evaluation of the extent of the cam morphology and regional/global acetabular coverage.[7,9,12,13]

Limits and Accessibility of Hip Arthroscopy

The majority of the acetabular rim from posteroinferior to anteroinferior and the AIIS are accessible arthroscopically (Figure 7-1). Posterior rim resection and posterior labral management is more challenging and requires more experience in some cases. The anterior femoral head-neck junction is predictably accessed arthroscopically from the medial to the lateral synovial fold. Further distal extension to the level of the greater trochanter and resections beyond the medial and lateral synovial folds (AP deformities) are more challenging but can be accessed with greater experience. More posteriorly based femoral head-neck deformities are not predictably accessed arthroscopically and are better managed with open approaches when symptomatic.

Step-By-Step Description of the Procedure

The current authors perform hip arthroscopy in the supine position with a standard fracture table and custom perineal post. The nonsurgical extremity is abducted approximately 45 degrees, and the fluoroscopic x-ray generator (C-arm) is brought in between the legs at an approximately 45-degree angle. A systematic fluoroscopic assessment of the proximal femur is then performed. A recent study by the current authors evaluated 6 specific fluoroscopic views correlated to radial reformatted CT images with the assistance of a 3D software program.[7] In a series of 50 hips undergoing hip arthroscopy by the current authors, the obtained fluoroscopic views correlated to specific positions on the clock face (according to the right hip; Figure 7-2).[7] AP images of the hip are first obtained with the knee and hip in full extension and the leg in 30 degrees of internal rotation (lateral femoral clock-face position is 11:45), neutral rotation (lateral femoral clock-face position is 12:45), and 30 degrees of external rotation (lateral femoral clock-face position is 1:00; Figure 7-3). These positions are performed by rotating the foot of the operative leg, ensuring that the knee remains in full extension, especially when maximally externally rotated. The images in hip extension provide an evaluation of the lateral and medial head-neck junction with the corresponding lateral clock-face positions. Next, the hip and knee are positioned in approximately 60 degrees of flexion, and images are obtained with the hip in neutral (0 degrees) rotation (anterior femoral clock-face position is 1:30), 40 degrees of external rotation (anterior femoral clock-face position is 2:15), and 60 degrees of external rotation (anterior femoral clock-face position is 2:30;

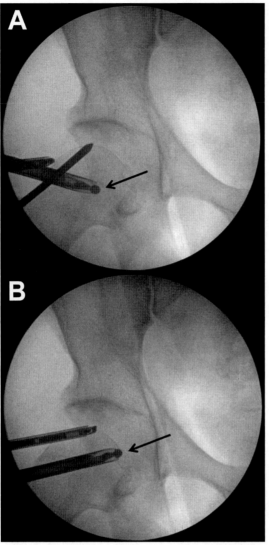

Figure 7-1. (A) AP fluoroscopic image of the right hip showing the posteroinferior extent of the rim resection (arrow) accessed during a global rim resection for the profunda. (B) AP fluoroscopic image of the right hip showing the anteroinferior extent of the rim resection (arrow) accessed during rim resection.

Figure 7-4). The images in flexion provide an evaluation of the anterior and posterior femoral head-neck junction with the corresponding anterior clock-face positions. The fluoroscopic/CT study reported that this technique identified the maximal alpha angle in all 50 cases and provides a reproducible method for evaluating the extent of the cam deformity and cam resection.

Next, the acetabulum is evaluated with intraoperative fluoroscopy. The operative leg is placed in neutral abduction, 0 to 10 degrees of hip flexion, and maximum internal rotation. The anterior superior iliac spines (ASIS) are palpated, and the bed is tilted until the patient is parallel to the floor/ceiling. This orients the pelvis in a neutral medial/lateral position. An AP view of the operative hip is obtained, and the operating table is further positioned with Trendelenburg or reverse Trendelenburg to achieve neutral anterior/posterior pelvic tilt. The goal is to obtain a fluoroscopic image that recreates a well-centered preoperative AP pelvis x-ray.

The authors recommend specific radiographic osseous landmarks to verify appropriate pelvic position. The relationship between the anterior and posterior acetabular rims, as well as the relationship between the ilioischial line and the acetabular teardrop on a well-centered preoperative AP x-ray, are recreated on the AP fluoroscopic image (Figure 7-5). A view of the pubic

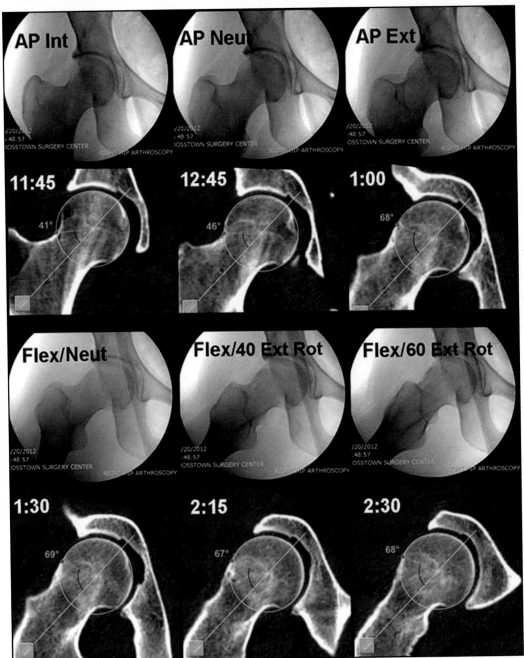

Figure 7-2. A patient's fluoroscopic x-rays with corresponding clock-face positions as determined via alpha angle measurement. AP=anteroposterior; CT=computed tomography; Ext=external; Flex=flexion; Int=internal; Neut=neutral; Rot=rotation. (Reprinted with permission from Ross JR, Bedi A, Stone RM, et al. Intraoperative fluoroscopic imaging to treat cam deformities: correlation with 3-dimensional computed tomography. *Am J Sports Med.* 2014;42[6]:1370-1376.)

symphysis and coccyx are obtained to confirm medial/lateral and anterior/posterior alignment. This technique allows the surgeon to more accurately evaluate acetabular-sided resections that will be reflective of postoperative x-rays. If acetabular resections are performed using poorly aligned fluoroscopic imaging, there may be a risk of over- and underresection. The C-arm is kept in this

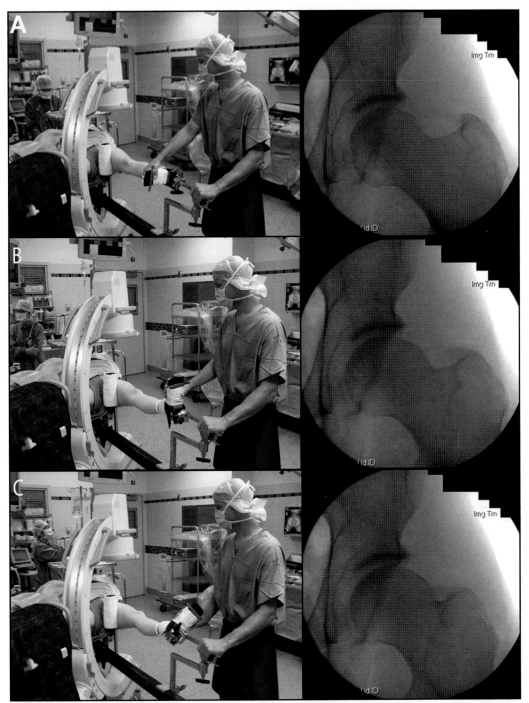

Figure 7-3. Intraoperative positioning with corresponding anteroposterior images (medial and lateral femur) of the left hip are first obtained with the knee and hip in full extension and the leg in (A) 30 degrees of internal rotation (lateral femoral clock-face position is 11:45.) (Reprinted with permission from Larson CM, Wulf CA. Intraoperative fluoroscopy for evaluation of bony resection during arthroscopic management of femoroacetabular impingement in the supine position. *Arthroscopy.* 2009;25[10]:1183-1192.) (B) neutral rotation (lateral femoral clock-face position is 12:45), and (C) 30 degrees of external rotation (lateral femoral clock-face position is 1:00).

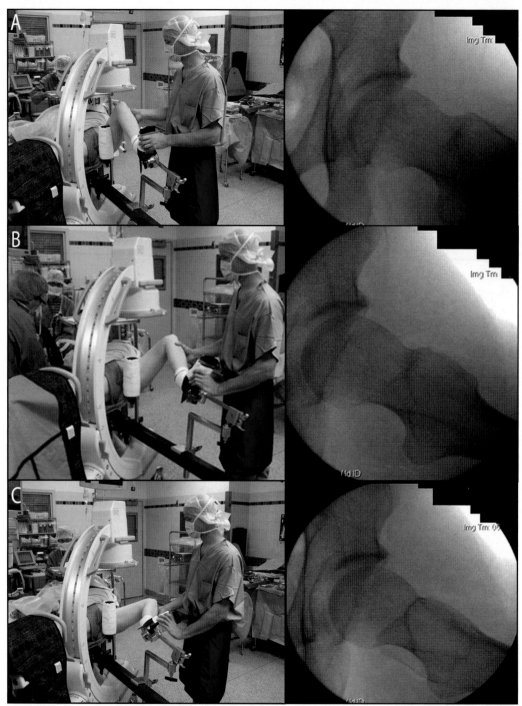

Figure 7-4. Intraoperative positioning with corresponding lateral images (anterior and posterior femur) of the left hip are obtained with the hip and knee in approximately 60 degrees of flexion. Images with the hip in (A) neutral (0 degrees) rotation (anterior femoral clock-face position is 1:30), (B) 40 degrees of external rotation (anterior femoral clock-face position is 2:15), and (C) 60 degrees of external rotation (anterior femoral clock-face position is 2:30. (Reprinted with permission from Larson CM, Wulf CA. Intraoperative fluoroscopy for evaluation of bony resection during arthroscopic management of femoroacetabular impingement in the supine position. *Arthroscopy.* 2009;25[10]:1183-1192.)

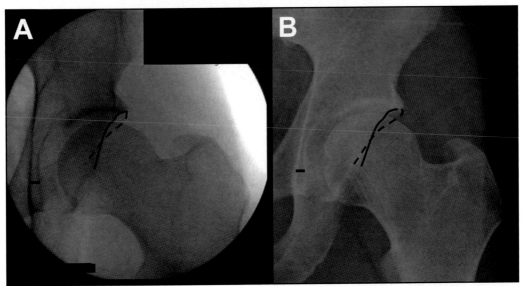

Figure 7-5. The radiographic profile of the operative hip (left hip) is evaluated by comparing the (A) intra-operative fluoroscopic AP view with (B) a properly aligned preoperative AP pelvis view. Specific attention is paid to reproducing the level and degree of acetabular crossover (with the posterior wall represented by a solid line and the anterior wall represented by a dashed line) and the relationship between the tear-drop and ilioischial line (horizontal line) on fluoroscopic and preoperative AP pelvis images. (Reprinted with permission from Larson CM, Wulf CA. Intraoperative fluoroscopy for evaluation of bony resection during arthroscopic management of femoroacetabular impingement in the supine position. *Arthroscopy.* 2009;25[10]:1183-1192.)

position throughout the surgery, and the surgical extremity is moved into various positions to evaluate osseous resections rather than changing the position of the C-arm.

RIM RESECTION FLUOROSCOPY TECHNIQUE

The current authors typically perform central compartment work prior to peripheral compartment procedures. The labral seal is gently released with traction or a spinal needle, and an anterolateral and mid-anterior portal is used for all cases, with the use of a posterolateral portal if more extensive posterior rim resections are required. After portal placement, a capsulotomy from just medial/inferior to the mid-anterior portal to the anterolateral/posterolateral portal is made. Rim resection is then performed if indicated based on preoperative imaging and intraoperative findings. Fluoroscopy can be used to locate the portion of the rim currently being treated with a motorized burr (see Figure 7-1). Rim fractures and areas of labral calcific change/ossification, as well as the AIIS, can also be precisely located. If there is apparent extension of the anterior acetabular rim beyond/lateral to the burr when placed on the edge of the anterior rim, one should consider the possibility of AIIS/subspine deformity contributing to radiographic anterior overcoverage or crossover sign. The AIIS often has a sclerotic cortex and can overlap the anterior rim resulting in a sclerotic crescent appearance on fluoroscopic images (Figure 7-6). In the setting of subspine impingement, the distal portion of the AIIS can be felt with the burr and localized using fluoroscopy (see Figure 7-6). Typically, the AIIS is resected back to the level of the acetabular sourcil as seen on the intraoperative AP fluoroscopic image, resulting in the removal of the sclerotic crescent (see Figure 7-6). Ultimately, the amount of subspine decompression is based on preoperative imaging and intraoperative findings. The surgeon should be aware that the operative hemipelvis will

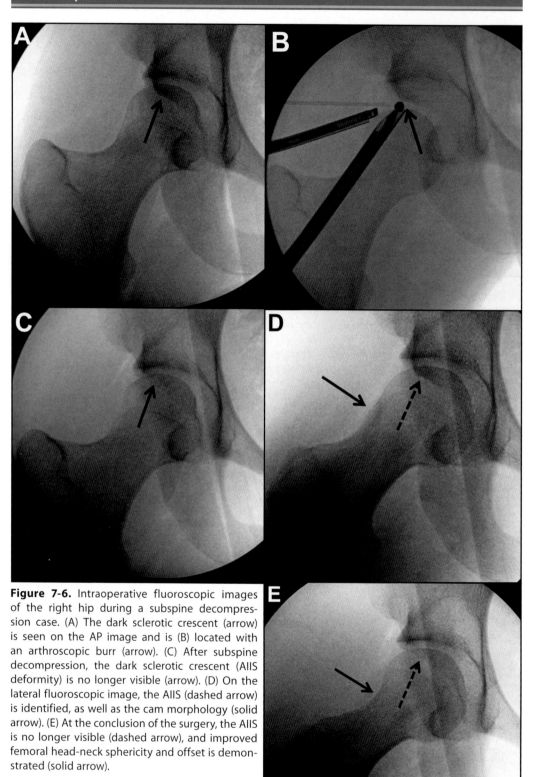

Figure 7-6. Intraoperative fluoroscopic images of the right hip during a subspine decompression case. (A) The dark sclerotic crescent (arrow) is seen on the AP image and is (B) located with an arthroscopic burr (arrow). (C) After subspine decompression, the dark sclerotic crescent (AIIS deformity) is no longer visible (arrow). (D) On the lateral fluoroscopic image, the AIIS (dashed arrow) is identified, as well as the cam morphology (solid arrow). (E) At the conclusion of the surgery, the AIIS is no longer visible (dashed arrow), and improved femoral head-neck sphericity and offset is demonstrated (solid arrow).

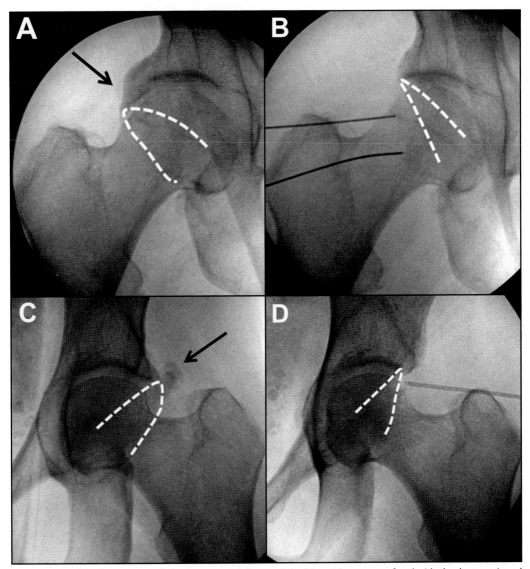

Figure 7-7. (A) Intraoperative fluoroscopy revealing a right hip with coxa profunda (dashed arrows) and (B) after global rim resection (dashed arrows). (C) Intraoperative fluoroscopy revealing a left hip with protrusio acetabula (dashed arrows) and a large labral calcific deposit (arrow) and (D) after global rim resection (dashed arrows).

sometimes tilt farther laterally/anteriorly with traction, which can create the appearance of greater retroversion/subspine extension and should be taken into account when evaluating resections. The anterosuperior rim and AIIS are resected with the burr in the mid-anterior portal, and the lateral rim is resected with the burr in the anterolateral portal. If more posterior rim resection is required, as seen in cases of global overcoverage (profunda/protrusio; Figure 7-7), resection can be performed via the posterolateral portal. Posterior rim resections can be facilitated by increasing the length of the capsulotomy and temporarily increasing the degree of traction. For more extensive rim resections laterally and posteriorly, it can be difficult to evaluate femoral head coverage by the acetabulum with the hip distracted. In these cases, it can be helpful to release traction and verify appropriate anterior, lateral, and posterior coverage in an effort to avoid overresection or residual deformity prior to labral refixation/repair.

Figure 7-8. Intraoperative fluoroscopic images of a left hip with the hip in flexion and neutral rotation defining the medial extent of the femoral resection osteoplasty with a burr moving from the (A) posteromedial to the (B) anterolateral head-neck junction. The medial extent of the femoral resection typically runs from the posteromedial femoral head-neck junction along a line (dashed line) roughly perpendicular to the femoral neck axis. (Reprinted with permission from Larson CM, Wulf CA. Intraoperative fluoroscopy for evaluation of bony resection during arthroscopic management of femoroacetabular impingement in the supine position. *Arthroscopy.* 2009;25[10]:1183-1192.)

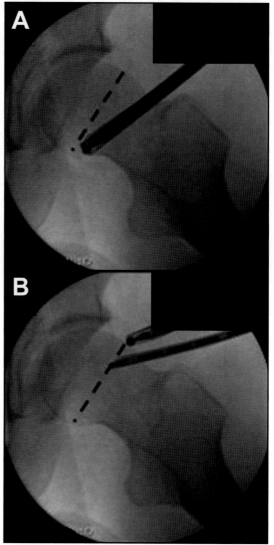

FEMORAL RESECTION FLUOROSCOPY TECHNIQUE

Once the central compartment work is complete, traction is released, the femoral head-neck junction is inspected, and dynamic assessment is performed as discussed in the next section. The depth and extent of femoral resection is planned based on preoperative imaging and is ultimately confirmed with intraoperative dynamic assessment. The current authors typically begin the resection medially in the region of the medial synovial fold. The arthroscope is in the mid-anterior portal and the burr is introduced via the anterolateral portal with the hip in 20 to 30 degrees of flexion. Fluoroscopy can help define the proximal extent of the resection, beginning at the more normal posterior head-neck junction and extending laterally along a line that runs roughly perpendicular to the femoral neck axis (Figure 7-8). This reference is used along with direct inspection of the head-neck junction and dynamic assessment. The goal of the correction is to achieve a relatively spherical femoral head-neck junction that maintains the labral seal and results in impingement-free range of motion (ROM). The anterior resection is performed in flexion, and the hip is then extended to access the lateral femoral deformity. Occasionally, it is necessary to place the hip in traction to work around the lateral retinacular vessels for posterolateral extension. Fluoroscopy can identify the medial, anterior, lateral, posterior, proximal, and distal positions of the burr and extent of resection. It is important to recognize that when working on a given area, the hip requires repositioning to evaluate the adequacy of resection. For example, when working in flexion on the anterior head-neck junction, the hip should be further flexed, externally rotated, or both to assess the resection. Similarly, if residual deformity is seen at the anterior or lateral head-neck junction on fluoroscopy, the hip should be extended, internally rotated, or both to access this particular region. At the completion of the femoral resection, the 6 previously described fluoroscopic views (3 in extension and 3 in flexion) are obtained to evaluate sphericity and offset (Figure 7-9).

ARTHROSCOPIC DYNAMIC ASSESSMENT

Arthroscopic dynamic assessment ultimately confirms the adequacy of bony resections and impingement-free ROM. This assessment should be performed before and after osseous resection and consists of direct arthroscopic visualization of the labrum/acetabular rim and femoral head-neck junction, assessment for improved hip ROM, and the quality or feel of the ROM and the endpoint. Dynamic assessments in varying hip positions should be performed to confirm global impingement-free ROM.

The current authors use a systematic evaluation in 3 primary positions that assess different areas of contact between the proximal femur and acetabular rim. The first dynamic assessment is performed by abducting the fully extended hip. This position evaluates contact between the lateral femur and lateral acetabular rim. The second dynamic assessment is performed by abducting the flexed (20 to 30 degrees) hip. This position evaluates contact between the lateral femur and posterolateral rim. Greater degrees of flexion/abduction result in contact farther posterior along the acetabular rim. The third dynamic assessment is performed with greater than 90 degrees of hip flexion and adduction/internal rotation. This position evaluates contact between the anterior femur and anterior acetabular rim. Appropriate and complete osseous correction is confirmed when the fluoroscopic images reveal improved femoral sphericity and offset and normal anterior/lateral/posterior acetabular depth and when dynamic assessment reveals normalized and smooth ROM, a soft endpoint feel, and no evidence of impingement. The current authors have found that the described fluoroscopic evaluation, when combined with a thorough arthroscopic dynamic assessment, allows for precise osseous correction as seen on postoperative plain x-rays (Figures 7-10 and 7-11).

POTENTIAL COMPLICATIONS

Complications associated with osseous corrections on the acetabular side include iatrogenic instability secondary to overresection.[14-17] Complications on the femoral side include femoral neck fractures, loss of the labral seal secondary to overresection, or both.[18] It is critical to have an appropriate preoperative diagnosis when contemplating osseous resections. In addition, one must be aware of the appropriate use and limitations of fluoroscopy for hip arthroscopy. There are learning curves with regard to accessing more challenging regions and with fluoroscopic evaluation. When resections performed are not visible on fluoroscopic imaging, this can be secondary to inappropriate pelvic alignment or improper repositioning of the hip to evaluate the resections. In these situations, further resections based on fluoroscopy are ill advised.

Figure 7-9. Intraoperative fluoroscopic evaluation in extension evaluating the lateral femoral head-neck deformity (A,C) pre- and (B,D) postresection. Intraoperative fluoroscopic evaluation of the anterior femoral head-neck deformity (E,G) pre- and (F,H) postresection. Intraoperative fluoroscopic evaluation of the anterior femoral head-neck deformity (E,G) pre- and (F,H) postresection.

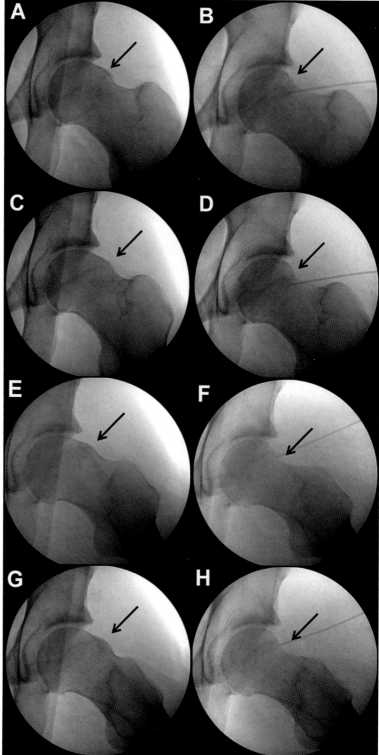

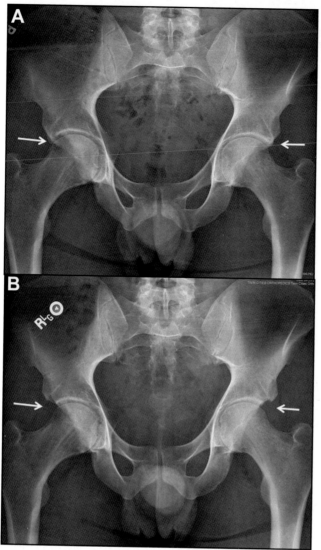

Figure 7-10. (A) Preoperative AP pelvis x-ray revealing bilateral profunda/retroversion pincer-type FAI (arrows). (B) Postoperative AP pelvis x-ray after bilateral rim resection and subspine decompression bilaterally revealing normalized acetabular coverage (arrows).

CONCLUSION

Achieving accurate arthroscopic FAI correction requires a thorough understanding of hip pathomorphology and can be challenging. The surgeon must put multiple arthroscopic views together in an effort to achieve a 3D understanding of the hip. Intraoperative fluoroscopy can be a helpful adjunct to evaluate acetabular- and femoral-sided deformities and resections. Similar to concepts in fracture reduction, one's resection is only as good as the image with the poorest correction. Fluoroscopic evaluation with the hip in multiple positions can give a global/3D evaluation in an effort to optimize the correction. Ultimately, a combination of appropriate preoperative plain x-rays, 3D imaging, intraoperative assessment of the pathology present, a systematic fluoroscopic evaluation, and dynamic assessment are critical to achieve impingement-free ROM and accurate bony correction.

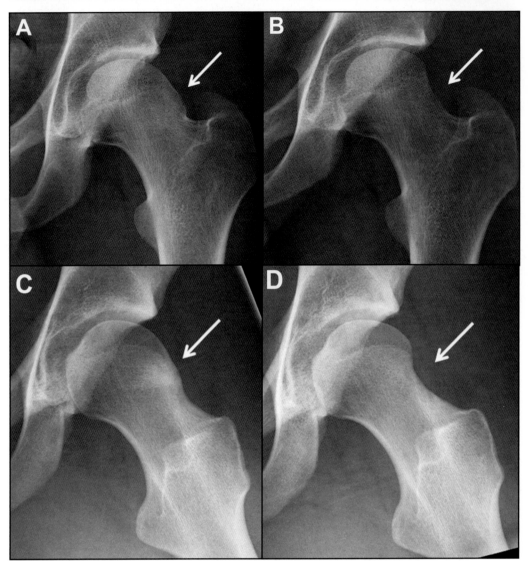

Figure 7-11. (A) Plain AP pelvic x-ray revealing a posterolateral cam deformity (arrow) and (B) improved sphericity and offset (arrow) postarthroscopic femoral resection. (C) Lateral plain x-ray reveals anterior cam-type deformity (arrow) and (D) improved sphericity and offset (arrow) post arthroscopic femoral resection.

TOP TECHNICAL PEARLS FOR THE PROCEDURES

Intraoperative Fluoroscopy

1. Recreate a well-centered AP pelvis image intraoperatively to more accurately assess acetabular resections.

2. Release traction intermittently for larger rim resections to better evaluate femoral head coverage.

3. When resecting the anterior cam deformity, the hip should then be flexed, externally rotated, or both to fluoroscopically confirm the resection.

4. If fluoroscopy fails to confirm the resections being performed, the pelvis, femur, or both should be repositioned to avoid iatrogenic overresections.

5. Femoral head-neck sphericity and offset should be evaluated and confirmed on all extension and flexion images.

Intraoperative Dynamic Assessment

1. Abduction of the extended hip assesses the lateral femur and lateral rim.

2. Abduction of the flexed hip assesses the lateral femur and posterolateral rim.

3. The FADIR test at 90 degrees assesses the anterior femur and the anterior rim.

4. Using a small perineal post or temporarily removing the perineal post improves the ability to dynamically assess the hip.

5. Use tactile sensation to evaluate for smooth ROM, improved ROM, and the quality and feel of the ROM endpoint.

REFERENCES

1. Heyworth BE, Shindle MK, Voos JE, Rudzki JR, Kelly BT. Radiologic and intraoperative findings in revision hip arthroscopy. *Arthroscopy*. 2007;23(12):1295-1302.

2. Philippon MJ, Schenker ML, Briggs KK, Kuppersmith DA, Maxwell RB, Stubbs AJ. Revision hip arthroscopy. *Am J Sports Med*. 2007;35(11):1918-1921.

3. Domb BG, Stake CE, Lindner D, El-Bitar Y, Jackson TJ. Revision hip preservation surgery with hip arthroscopy: clinical outcomes. *Arthroscopy*. 2014;30(5):581-587.

4. Larson CM, Giveans MR, Samuelson KM, Stone RM, Bedi A. Arthroscopic hip revision surgery for residual femoroacetabular impingement (FAI): surgical outcomes compared with a matched cohort after primary arthroscopic FAI correction. *Am J Sports Med*. 2014;42(8):1785-1790.

5. Clohisy JC, Nepple JJ, Larson CM, Zaltz I, Millis M; Academic Network of Conservation Hip Outcome Research (ANCHOR) Members. Persistent structural disease is the most common cause of repeat hip preservation surgery. *Clin Orthop Relat Res*. 2013;471(12):3788-3794.

6. Larson CM, Wulf CA. Intraoperative fluoroscopy for evaluation of bony resection during arthroscopic management of femoroacetabular impingement in the supine position. *Arthroscopy*. 2009;25(10):1183-1192.

7. Ross JR, Bedi A, Stone RM, et al. Intraoperative fluoroscopic imaging to treat cam deformities: correlation with 3-dimensional computed tomography. *Am J Sports Med*. 2014;42(6):1370-1376.

8. Matsuda DK. Fluoroscopic templating technique for precision arthroscopic rim trimming. *Arthroscopy*. 2009;25(10):1175-1182.

9. Larson CM, Stone RM. Femoroacetabular impingement arthroscopic management of the proximal femur. In: Clohisy J, Beaule P, DellaValle C, Callaghan JJ, Rosenberg AG, Rubash HE, eds. *The Adult Hip: Hip Preservation Surgery*. Vol 3. Philadelphia, PA: Wolters Kluwer Health; 2015:553-565.

10. Larson CM. Arthroscopic management of pincer-type impingement. *Sports Med Arthrosc*. 2010;18(2):100-107.

11. Clohisy JC, Carlisle JC, Beaulé PE, et al. A systematic approach to the plain radiographic evaluation of the young adult hip. *J Bone Joint Surg Am*. 2008;90 suppl 4:47-66.

12. Milone MT, Bedi A, Poultsides L, et al. Novel CT-based three-dimensional software improves the characterization of cam morphology. *Clin Orthop Relat Res*. 2013;471(8):2484-2491.

13. Larson CM, Moreau-Gaudry A, Kelly BT, et al. Are normal hips being labeled as pathologic? A CT-based method for defining normal acetabular coverage. *Clin Orthop Relat Res*. 2015;473(4):1247-1254.

14. Matsuda DK. Acute iatrogenic dislocation following hip impingement arthroscopic surgery. *Arthroscopy*. 2009;25(4):400-404.

15. Ranawat AS, McClincy M, Sekiya JK. Anterior dislocation of the hip after arthroscopy in a patient with capsular laxity of the hip. *J Bone Joint Surg Am*. 2009;91(1):192-197.

16. Benali Y, Katthagen BD. Hip subluxation as a complication of arthroscopic debridement. *Arthroscopy*. 2009;25(4):405-407.

17. Mei-Dan O, McConkey MO, Brick M. Catastrophic failure of hip arthroscopy due to iatrogenic instability: can partial division of the ligamentum teres and iliofemoral ligament cause subluxation? *Arthroscopy*. 2012;28(3):440-445.

18. Ayeni OR, Bedi A, Lorich DG, Kelly BT. Femoral neck fracture after arthroscopic management of femoroacetabular impingement: a case report. *J Bone Joint Surg Am*. 2011;93(9):e47.

8

Portal Placement in Hip Arthroscopy

Anatomic Considerations and Access to the Central, Peripheral, and Peritrochanteric Spaces

Geoffrey D. Abrams, MD; Joshua D. Harris, MD; and Marc R. Safran, MD

INTRODUCTION

In performing hip arthroscopy, portal placement is arguably the most important component of the procedure. Given the constrained nature of the hip joint, even small errors in the location of the portals can limit access to intra- and extra-articular structures. Anatomic landmarks are used, and fluoroscopy is commonly used to ensure accurate portal placement. This allows the surgeon to access all areas of the hip joint and surrounding structures while avoiding iatrogenic injury to the cartilage and neurovascular structures. Numerous portals have been described for hip arthroscopy in the central and peripheral compartments.

Anatomy

Although a variety of portals have been described, the one thing that remains constant is the location of anatomic landmarks and neurovascular structures around the hip. A thorough knowledge of the location of these structures is important to guide positioning of the portals and help avoid complications.

The 2 most important surface landmarks that serve as reference points for portal placement are the anterior superior iliac spine (ASIS) and the greater trochanter. In general, points medial and distal to the ASIS serve as potential locations where the femoral neurovascular bundle, lateral femoral cutaneous nerve (LFCN), and ascending branch of the lateral femoral circumflex artery (LCFA) can be injured. The commonly used initial anterolateral portal is adjacent to the anterosuperior corner of the greater trochanter. Posterior to the greater trochanter lies the sciatic nerve, whereas superior to the tip of the trochanter is the superior gluteal nerve.

Byrd JWT, Bedi A, Stubbs AJ, eds. *The Hip:*
AANA Advanced Arthroscopic Surgical Techniques (pp 103-112).
© 2016 AANA.

Figure 8-1. Intraoperative photo demonstrating patient setup following prepping and draping for a right hip arthroscopy in the supine position. The right leg is in traction with the left leg abducted approximately 45 degrees. The C-arm is positioned on the contralateral side of the table to aid in the establishment of portal placement and acetabular and cam lesion resection.

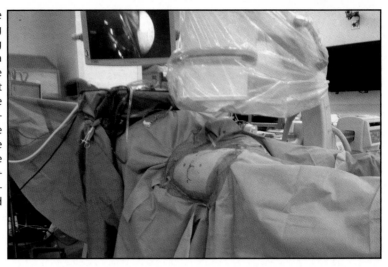

One difference between portal placement in the hip vs other joints is the large soft tissue envelope surrounding the hip. When placing the trocar into the hip joint, one must first penetrate the large muscular envelope around the joint. Following this, the thick hip capsule itself is encountered, which may provide considerable resistance against the trocar.[1] The capsule contains discreet thickenings that comprise the capsuloligamentous stabilizers of the joint—the iliofemoral (also known as the Y ligament of Bigelow), ischiofemoral, and pubofemoral ligaments.[2,3]

The hip joint is divided into the central and peripheral compartments, with the acetabular labrum marking the division between the 2 spaces. The central compartment contains the cartilage-covered articular surfaces of the femoral head and acetabulum, whereas the peripheral compartment contains the area surrounding the femoral neck, including the femoral head-neck junction. Thus, the central compartment is where the ligamentum teres and labral and articular cartilage injuries are identified and treated, whereas the peripheral compartment is where resection of a cam lesion may be performed. It is also one location for iliopsoas lengthening and where loose bodies and synovial pathology are often found.[4] The labrum is an important structure and serves to increase articular surface area[5] and oppose the flow of synovial fluid into and out of the central compartment.[6,7] These functions allow for enhanced stability of the hip by maintaining negative intra-articular pressure,[8] maintaining joint fluid within the central compartment for nutrition to the chondrocytes,[7] providing more equal distribution of forces across the articular cartilage,[9] and allowing for a smooth gliding surface.[10]

POSITIONING AND PORTALS

Hip arthroscopy can be performed in the supine and lateral positions.[11] The authors prefer placing the patient in the supine position on a fracture table or traction attachment apparatus so as to allow traction on the operative leg (Figure 8-1). General anesthesia with muscle relaxation is recommended, as well as a well-padded peroneal post to minimize the occurrence of pudendal nerve or peroneal skin injury.[12] Gentle traction is placed on the operative leg to allow for approximately 1 cm of distance between the femoral head and acetabulum. This will allow space for the cannulae within the central compartment without damage to articular surfaces. The hip should be in neutral flexion-extension and slight abduction to neutral abduction-adduction. Some prefer approximately 15 to 20 degrees of internal rotation of the hip to offset the normal anteversion of the femoral neck, whereas others may place the hip in 10 to 20 degrees of flexion. After proper positioning, the ASIS, greater trochanter,

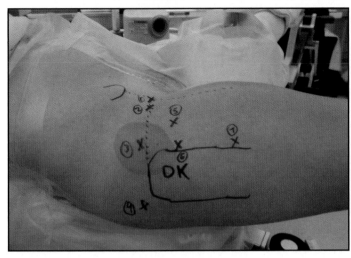

Figure 8-2. Intraoperative photograph showing provisional skin markings for portal placement in a right hip (head to the left, foot to the right). The ASIS and the greater trochanter are marked with a dashed line extending distally and posteriorly from the ASIS. The portals are (1) anterior, (2) anterior peritrochanteric, (3) anterolateral and proximal peritrochanteric, (4) posterolateral, (5) mid-anterior, (6) distal anterolateral, and (7) distal peritrochanteric.

and future portal sites should be marked (Figure 8-2). Although it may seem obvious, the trochanter should not be outlined until after traction is applied because it moves distally with traction.

Although some vent the hip after prepping and draping, others prefer to perform this procedure prior to skin preparation to eliminate the vacuum phenomenon created with the leg in traction. This is done for the following 2 reasons: to assure the hip can be adequately distracted and to reduce the amount of force necessary to distract the hip.[13] This technique involves putting the leg in traction, using sterile technique and fluoroscopy, and placing a larger-bore (17- or 18-gauge) 6-inch spinal needle at the location of the anterolateral portal. The needle is introduced with the long end of the bevel away from the femoral head to reduce the risk of gouging the articular cartilage. The path of the needle is such that the tip of the needle should end at the upper portion of the cotyloid fossa and the junction of the medialmost aspect of the sourcil, with the shaft of the needle adjacent to the femoral head (Figure 8-3A). This will serve as a guide for proper positioning and trajectory of the anterolateral portal. When the tip of the needle is in the correct location within the central compartment, the stylus is removed to eliminate the negative intra-articular pressure created by the joint distraction. While confirming the air arthrogram with the fluoroscope (Figure 8-3B), one will also notice the relaxation of the quadriceps muscle as air initially enters the joint, indicative of relaxation of the capsule and its proprioceptive mechanoreceptors.

Hip arthroscopy portals used for working within the central compartment, peripheral compartment, and peritrochanteric space will be described. Most surgeons prefer 2 or 3 portals for standard hip arthroscopy involving the central and peripheral compartments. Additional accessory portals may be added as needed.

The greatest risk in portal placement includes injury to the neurovascular structures and iatrogenic injury to the cartilage and labrum. The structures at greatest risk are discussed individually with each portal description. The most recent literature indicates major and minor complication rates of 0.6% and 7.5% following hip arthroscopy, respectively, with complication rates specifically related to portal placement of 0.5% to 0.6%.[12,14]

Anterolateral Portal

The anterolateral portal is usually the first portal established because it lies most centrally in the safe zone for hip arthroscopy. Positioning of the other portals within the central compartment is facilitated by viewing through this portal. The closest structure is the superior gluteal nerve at an average of 4.4 cm proximally.[15] The entry point on the skin is adjacent to the anterosuperior border of the greater trochanter. Under fluoroscopic guidance (see Figure 8-3), the spinal needle

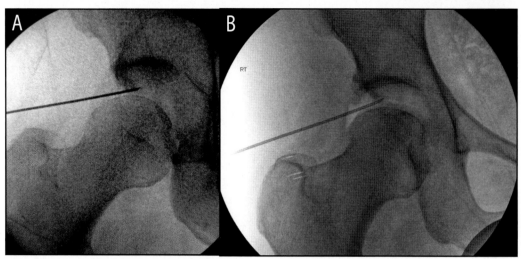

Figure 8-3. (A) Fluoroscopic image of a spinal needle used for localization of the initial anterolateral portal following joint distraction. Note the trajectory of the needle adjacent to the femoral head (vs the acetabulum) so as to avoid penetration of the labrum. (B) Fluoroscopic image of a spinal needle following removal of the stylus demonstrating the air arthrogram created and indicating intra-articular placement of the needle.

is directed through the gluteus medius muscle belly at approximately 15 degrees cranially and 20 to 30 degrees posteriorly to position the tip of the needle close to the femoral head but without injuring the cartilage. These are general guidelines because the soft tissue envelope, femoral version, femoral neck length, and neck-shaft angle vary between patients. Another technique to identify the starting position and cranial-caudal angle is to overlay the needle on the skin. Using fluoroscopy, the needle is positioned to determine the skin entry point and angle of inclination by overlying the tip of the needle at the junction of the cotyloid fossa and sourcil, having the shaft of the needle next to the femoral head. Following the needle laterally along the skin will identify where the entry point should be in the proximal-distal axis.

Fluoroscopy (the needle should be adjacent to the femoral head; see Figure 8-3A) and tactile sensation are used to avoid piercing the labrum with the spinal needle because subsequent placement of the trocar in this position will damage the labrum.[13] Although minimal resistance is provided by the gluteus medius muscle belly, the hip capsule is a thick structure and provides greater resistance to needle penetration. Once the tip of the needle has penetrated the capsule, resistance should again be minimal as it enters the space of the central compartment. Again, the long end of the bevel of the needle should be away from the femoral head. Continued resistance will be experienced if the needle pierces the labrum or comes in contact with the femoral head or acetabulum.

The stylus of the spinal needle is then removed, and a nitinol guidewire is placed through the needle. Leaving the guidewire in place, the needle is removed, and a cannula with a cannulated obturator is placed over the guidewire. Some prefer to dilate the soft tissue around the portal with progressively larger obturators for easier placement of the final cannula. After a second portal is established (typically the modified anterior or posterolateral portal) within the central compartment, a 70-degree arthroscope is inserted through this second portal to confirm appropriate placement of the anterolateral portal between the femoral head and acetabulum with avoidance of the labrum. If the anterolateral portal needs to be adjusted because of injury to the labrum, this can be done with a spinal needle under direct visualization through the second portal.

Using a 70-degree arthroscope through the anterolateral portal, most of the structures within the central compartment can be visualized. Nearly the entire acetabular labrum can be seen; however, this portal provides the best visualization to the anterior and superior portions of this structure (Figure 8-4). The articular cartilage surfaces of the femoral head and posteromedial

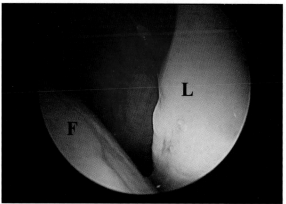

Figure 8-4. Arthroscopic image with a 70-degree arthroscope of the initial view through the anterolateral portal showing the anterior triangle with the anterosuperior labrum on the right (L), femoral head on the left (F), and capsuloligamentous structure centrally.

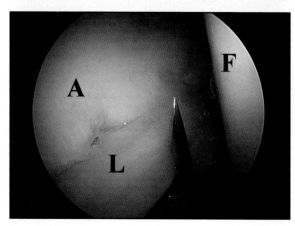

Figure 8-5. Arthroscopic image with a 70-degree arthroscope from the anterolateral portal demonstrating spinal needle localization of the posterolateral portal. The acetabular cartilage (A) and labrum (L) and the femoral head articular cartilage (F) can be seen.

acetabulum are also well visualized (Figure 8-5). Other structures that can be seen best through this portal are the cotyloid fossa (Figure 8-6) and ligamentum teres, capsular-labral recess, and anterior triangle (Figure 8-7). The anterior triangle is made up of the intra-articular portion of the iliofemoral ligament and capsule, the anterosuperior portion of the femoral head, and the acetabular labrum. Visualization of this space is particularly important because it allows for direct viewing of the spinal needle for creation of the anterior and/or mid-anterior portals.

The anterolateral portal can also be used to work within and/or visualize the peripheral compartment of the hip. To access this compartment, traction is released, and the camera is placed through the anterolateral portal at the femoral head-neck junction (Figure 8-8). Fluoroscopy can be useful to confirm the correct location. The femoral neck and anterior and superior aspects of the nonarticulating portion of the femoral head can be visualized for eventual cam resection with an instrument through an additional accessory portal.

The most significant risk in the placement of an anterolateral portal is not the superior gluteal nerve, which lies an average of more than 4 cm proximal, but rather iatrogenic chondrolabral injury because it is the only portal placed without direct visualization. The utilization of fluoroscopy and tactile sensation is important in the placement of this portal to avoid damage to the intra-articular structures.

Anterior Portal

This portal originates at the intersection of, or just lateral to, a line drawn distally from the ASIS and a transverse line from the tip of the greater trochanter (see Figure 8-2). It is approximately

Figure 8-6. Arthroscopic image from the anterolateral portal demonstrating the cotyloid fossa on the right with a flexible electrothermal ablation instrument and the femoral head on the left.

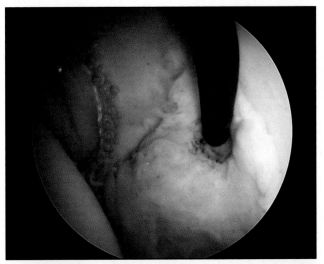

Figure 8-7. Arthroscopic image with a 70-degree arthroscope from the anterolateral portal showing needle localization of the mid-anterior portal through the anterior triangle. The anterosuperior labrum (L) is on the left, the femoral head is on the right (F), and the needle is piercing the capsuloligamentous structure.

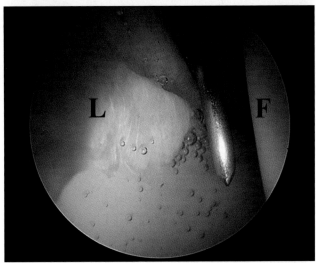

Figure 8-8. Image from the anterolateral portal with traction released. The acetabular labrum (with labral repair sutures) can be seen on the left with the suction-seal effect recreated. The femoral head-neck junction, which will be the site of potential cam lesion resection, is on the right.

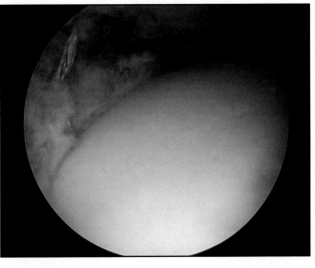

6.3 cm distal to the ASIS. When inserting the spinal needle in this location, the portal is aimed approximately 40 degrees cephalad and 25 to 30 degrees toward the midline. The muscle bellies of the sartorius and the rectus femoris are traversed before entering the hip through the anterior capsule. With the 70-degree arthroscope in the anterolateral portal and with a clear view of the anterior triangle, this portal is localized under direct visualization with a spinal needle.

When it is the second portal created, one should first view through the anterior portal to confirm that the anterolateral portal is in the correct location and has not pierced the labrum. It can also be used as a working and/or viewing portal for evaluation and treatment of associated pathology. The anterior portion of the femoral head, the ligamentum teres, the acetabular fossa, and the superior labrum can be visualized from this location. The authors typically create a mid-anterior portal rather than a traditional anterior portal, but the senior author (G.D.A.) uses the anterior portal position for labral takedown and retraction as an accessory portal when indicated.

The LFCN is at greatest risk with this portal because it is located only 3 mm from the portal.[15] The femoral nerve and the ascending branch of the LFCA are approximately 4 cm away. Terminal branches of the LFCA, however, may be as close as 2 mm.[15] Because of the proximity of the LFCN, a superficial skin incision should be made, followed by blunt dissection to protect the nerve. As long as the portal is not medial to the line drawn distally from the ASIS, the femoral artery and vein should not be at risk. Localization of this portal with a spinal needle under arthroscopic visualization, typically through the anterolateral portal, minimizes the risk of cartilage or labral injury.

Mid-Anterior Portal

Given the proximity of the anterior portal to the LFCN and the recent interest in labral repair, the mid-anterior portal is becoming increasingly used instead of the traditional anterior portal. The authors regularly use this portal, along with the anterolateral portal, when performing hip arthroscopy. This portal is placed using an outside-in technique similar to the placement of the anterior portal. It is located 5 to 7 cm distal to the anterolateral portal at a 45-degree angle (see Figure 8-2). This allows for the same visualization of structures as would be obtained through the anterior portal but with less risk to the LFCN[16] and an improved angle for placement of superior and anterior anchors for labral repair (Figure 8-9). It also allows for easier and safer access in cases of more pronounced pincer impingement with significant anterior acetabular overcoverage.

Posterolateral Portal

The posterolateral portal is placed 1 cm posterior to the superoposterior tip of the greater trochanter and under arthroscopic visualization through one of the anterior portals (see Figure 8-5). The portal traverses just posterior to the gluteus medius and minimus and proximal to the piriformis tendon.[17] As the hip is more internally rotated, the trajectory of this portal becomes more parallel with the floor. However, internal rotation brings the sciatic nerve closer to the joint capsule, increasing the risk of injury to the nerve. External rotation should also be avoided because that brings the greater trochanter more posterior. This reduces the zone of safety with regard to the sciatic nerve. It should also be approximately parallel to the anterolateral portal.

This portal provides visualization to the weight-bearing dome of the acetabulum, the posteromedial and anterolateral labrum, and the femoral head. The posterior labral recess, floor of the acetabular fossa, and inferior gutter can also be seen and are common areas for loose bodies to be found. In addition, this portal allows for work anteriorly and laterally without having to move the arthroscopic camera between the anterolateral and mid-anterior portals (if working with only 2 portals).

There is minimal risk to the neurovascular structures when the portal is in the appropriate position. The sciatic nerve is, on average, 2.9 cm away,[15] whereas the deep branch of the medial femoral circumflex artery is just more than 1 cm away, assuming normal trochanteric anatomy.[18] The risk to

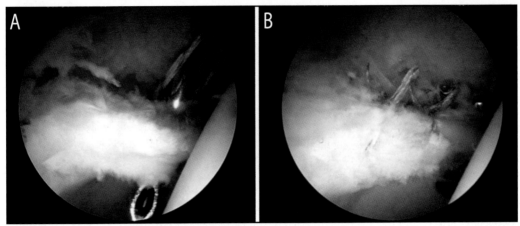

Figure 8-9. Arthroscopic images from the anterolateral portal with a 70-degree arthroscope demonstrating labral repair. (A) A suture shuttling device is placed through the mid-anterior portal following anchor placement through this same portal. (B) Knots are tied through the mid-anterior portal to achieve a secure repair.

the sciatic nerve is increased with hip internal or external rotation. Given that the portal is placed under direct arthroscopic visualization, the risk of iatrogenic injury to articular structures is low.

Accessory Portals

Proximal and Distal Anterolateral Portals

The authors prefer to use proximal and/or distal anterolateral portals when working in the peripheral compartment for a cam lesion resection, iliopsoas release, or lesser trochanter resection for ischiofemoral impingement. For a cam resection, visualization with a 30-degree arthroscope is performed though the standard anterolateral portal. An accessory proximal or distal anterolateral portal is created in line with and approximately 3 to 4 cm proximal or distal to the anterolateral portal (see Figure 8-2). In some cases, a shaver is first introduced through the proximal anterolateral portal to remove soft tissue overlying the capsule prior to capsulotomy. Alternatively, the distal anterolateral portal may be used to incise the capsule for later repair. Once the cam lesion has been identified at the femoral head-neck junction, a burr is used for resection through these working portals.

The distal anterolateral accessory portal may also be used for percutaneous suture anchor placement during anterior and anterolateral labral repair. For more distal pathology, including iliopsoas release and lesser trochanteric resection for isciofemoral impingement, a distal anterolateral portal is made 3 to 5 cm distal to the anterolateral portal and 1 to 2 cm anterior. This allows easier access to the lesser trochanter or release of the iliopsoas at the level of the lesser trochanter.

Peritrochanteric Space Portals

Anterior Peritrochanteric Portal

The anterior peritrochanteric portal (different from the standard anterior portal previously described) offers visualization of the peritrochanteric space. This portal is placed 1 cm lateral and slightly distal to the ASIS and is inserted between the tensor fascia lata and sartorius (see Figure 8-2). With the leg in neutral flexion-extension and adduction-adduction and slight internal rotation, a small skin incision is made, and the cannula is bluntly directed posteriorly into the peritrochanteric space.[19] The cannula is swept back and forth between the iliotibial band (ITB) and the greater trochanter to open up this area. If done properly, one should clearly be able to see the greater trochanter and ITB with the 70-degree arthroscope. Tears of the gluteus medius and minimus tendons can also be seen through this portal.

Distal Peritrochanteric Portal

This portal allows for access distally and proximally for procedures such as ITB release, trochanteric bursectomy, and gluteus medius and minimus repairs (see Figure 8-2). In addition, a third portal can be placed proximal to the tip of the greater trochanter in line with the distal posterior portal to further facilitate access to the peritrochanteric space and serve as an additional working portal for these procedures.

CONCLUSION

Given the articular congruity of the hip joint, accurate portal placement is critical to avoid iatrogenic neurovascular injury and to visualize and address hip pathology. The anterolateral portal is distant from neurovascular structures, but because it is the only portal not placed under direct visualization, it has the highest risk of iatrogenic chondral and labral injury. The anterior portal provides the greatest risk for nerve injury during portal placement, with the LFCN an average of 3 mm away. Although the traditional anterolateral and posterolateral portals are still commonly used and relatively safe, the mid-anterior portal is gaining in popularity over the anterior portal because it offers less risk of LFCN injury and offers an improved angle for suture anchor placement in labral repairs. Accessory portals include the proximal and distal anterolateral portals, and they may be used for cam lesion resection, suture anchor placement for labral repair, iliopsoas release, and lesser trochanteric resection in ischiofemoral impingement. Peritrochanteric space portals prove useful when arthroscopically addressing gluteus medius and minimus tears, external snapping hip, and trochanteric bursitis.

TOP TECHNICAL PEARLS FOR THE PROCEDURE

1. Mark out skin landmarks after traction has been applied.
2. Venting the hip prior to prepping and draping may allow for improved distraction of the hip.
3. Initial anterolateral portal placement is critical because it is the only one that is made without direct visualization.
4. Iatrogenic cartilage and/or labral injury is most common with placement of the anterolateral portal.
5. If using an anterior portal, care must be taken to incise only skin so as to protect the lateral femoral cutaneous nerve.

REFERENCES

1. Roy DR. Arthroscopy of the hip in children and adolescents. *J Child Orthop.* 2009;3(2):89-100.

2. Wagner FV, Negrão JR, Campos J, et al. Capsular ligaments of the hip: anatomic, histologic, and positional study in cadaveric specimens with MR arthrography. *Radiology.* 2012;263(1):189-198.

3. Telleria JJ, Lindsey DP, Giori NJ, Safran MR. An anatomic arthroscopic description of the hip capsular ligaments for the hip arthroscopist. *Arthroscopy.* 2011;27(5):628-636.

4. Dienst M, Seil R, Kohn DM. Safe arthroscopic access to the central compartment of the hip. *Arthroscopy.* 2005;21(12):1510-1514.

5. Seldes RM, Tan V, Hunt J, Katz M, Winiarsky R, Fitzgerald RH Jr. Anatomy, histologic features, and vascularity of the adult acetabular labrum. *Clin Orthop Relat Res.* 2001;(382):232-240.

6. Ferguson SJ, Bryant JT, Ganz R, Ito K. The acetabular labrum seal: a poroelastic finite element model. *Clin Biomech (Bristol, Avon).* 2000;15(6):463-468.

7. Ferguson SJ, Bryant JT, Ganz R, Ito K. An in vitro investigation of the acetabular labral seal in hip joint mechanics. *J Biomech.* 2003;36(2):171-178.

8. Crawford MJ, Dy CJ, Alexander JW, et al. The 2007 Frank Stinchfield Award. The biomechanics of the hip labrum and the stability of the hip. *Clin Orthop Relat Res.* 2007;465:16-22.

9. Safran MR. The acetabular labrum: anatomic and functional characteristics and rationale for surgical intervention. *J Am Acad Orthop Surg.* 2010;18(6):338-345.

10. Song Y, Ito H, Kourtis L, Safran MR, Carter DR, Giori NJ. Articular cartilage friction increases in hip joints after the removal of acetabular labrum. *J Biomech.* 2012;45(3):524-530.

11. Pollard TC, Khan T, Price AJ, Gill HS, Glyn-Jones S, Rees JL. Simulated hip arthroscopy skills: learning curves with the lateral and supine patient positions: a randomized trial. *J Bone Joint Surg Am.* 2012;94(10):e68.

12. Harris JD, McCormick FM, Abrams GD, et al. Complications and reoperations during and after hip arthroscopy: a systematic review of 92 studies and more than 6,000 patients. *Arthroscopy.* 2013;29(3):589-595.

13. Byrd JW. Avoiding the labrum in hip arthroscopy. *Arthroscopy.* 2000;16(7):770-773.

14. Clarke MT, Arora A, Villar RN. Hip arthroscopy: complications in 1054 cases. *Clin Orthop Relat Res.* 2003;(406):84-88.

15. Byrd JW, Pappas JN, Pedley MJ. Hip arthroscopy: an anatomic study of portal placement and relationship to the extra-articular structures. *Arthroscopy.* 1995;11(4):418-423.

16. Robertson WJ, Kelly BT. The safe zone for hip arthroscopy: a cadaveric assessment of central, peripheral, and lateral compartment portal placement. *Arthroscopy.* 2008;24(9):1019-1026.

17. Byrd JW. Hip arthroscopy. *J Am Acad Orthop Surg.* 2006;14(7):433-444.

18. Sussmann PS, Zumstein M, Hahn F, Dora C. The risk of vascular injury to the femoral head when using the posterolateral arthroscopy portal: cadaveric investigation. *Arthroscopy.* 2007;23(10):1112-1115.

19. Voos JE, Rudzki JR, Shindle MK, Martin H, Kelly BT. Arthroscopic anatomy and surgical techniques for peritrochanteric space disorders in the hip. *Arthroscopy.* 2007;23(11):1246.e1-1246.e5.

9

Alternative Approaches to Access to the Hip Joint

Starting in the Peripheral Compartment

Matthias Kusma, MD and Michael Dienst, MD

INTRODUCTION

Portal placement in the hip joint is a demanding and crucial step during hip arthroscopy.[1-3] This is related to the following various anatomic features: a thick soft tissue mantle; a strong articular capsule; the constrained ball and socket architecture of the joint; a relatively small intra-articular volume; and the additional sealing of the deep, central part of the joint by the acetabular labrum. In particular, the anatomy of the acetabular labrum must be considered before accessing the hip joint. It separates the hip joint into the central compartment (CC) and the peripheral compartment (PC).[4]

Even with the knowledge of current techniques for avoiding the labrum and cartilage in hip arthroscopy,[3] occasionally some degree of damage is unavoidable.[2] The highest risk of iatrogenic damage is during the first access to the CC under traction. Here, only fluoroscopy and the surgeon's feeling when penetrating the soft tissues and articular capsule help not to penetrate the labrum and scratch the hyaline cartilage of the femoral head. In addition, there are situations in which direct access to the CC under traction at the beginning of arthroscopy is not possible due to insufficient distraction of the hip joint. This may be caused by a stiff and thickened capsule or a bony overhang of the acetabular rim as is frequently found in femoroacetabular pincer impingement with advanced ossifications of the acetabular labrum.

With this experience, the authors have developed the PC-first technique. The portals are placed in the PC first, without traction and without the risk of injury to the acetabular labrum and femoral head cartilage. For arthroscopy of the CC, further portal placement is controlled arthroscopically. This chapter describes the current PC-first technique, including a discussion of advantages and disadvantages.

Byrd JWT, Bedi A, Stubbs AJ, eds. *The Hip:*
AANA Advanced Arthroscopic Surgical Techniques (pp 113-122).
© 2016 AANA.

INDICATIONS

The PC-first technique is the authors' routine approach to the hip and is applicable for every patient. In the authors' experience, this technique should be used particularly for the following:

▶ When starting with hip arthroscopy to get over the learning curve with fewer complications during the first arthroscopic access to the joint

▶ In patients with limited hip distraction in order to perform a capsular release and improve subsequent distraction for CC arthroscopy

▶ In patients in whom CC access is hindered by an osseous bony overhang because it is frequently found in coxa profunda and pincer femoroacetabular impingement (FAI) with labral ossifications

EQUIPMENT

For the PC-first technique, special equipment is not necessary. The same positioning devices and instruments that are routinely used for the classic CC-first arthroscopy are used for the PC-first technique.

POSITIONING

Hip arthroscopy with and without traction can be performed with the patient in the lateral or supine position. In the authors' experience, the decision of whether to use the lateral or supine position is more a matter of individual training and habit of use. However, because of the almost exclusive use of the proximal and distal anterolateral and anterior portals during hip arthroscopy without traction, the authors prefer the supine position, using a standard traction table used for fracture management.

STEP-BY-STEP DESCRIPTION OF THE PROCEDURE

PC Access

In contrast to arthroscopy of the CC, mostly no distraction is used for portal placement to the PC and subsequent therapeutic PC arthroscopy. For the first proximal anterolateral portal placement, the hip is in neutral rotation, the knee is straight, and the hip flexed to 10 to 20 degrees without abduction (Figure 9-1). Only minimal traction is applied to hold the knee straight and the hip in position. Avoiding more flexion for the first portal placement keeps the capsule somewhat tensed to ease penetration with the needle. As soon as the arthroscope confirms a correct intra-articular position, the hip can be flexed and rotated to relax the strong iliofemoral ligament and increase the intracapsular joint volume.[5]

In some cases, 2 portals are sufficient for complete diagnostic round and therapeutic procedures in the PC. The standard viewing portal is placed proximal anterolaterally and the standard instrumentation portal is placed anteriorly. To address lateral and posterolateral areas of the femoral head and neck, such as in the pistol-grip deformity of cam FAI, an additional classic anterolateral or lateral portal needs to be placed for instrumentation.

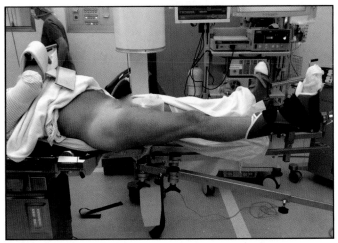

Figure 9-1. The patient in the supine position.

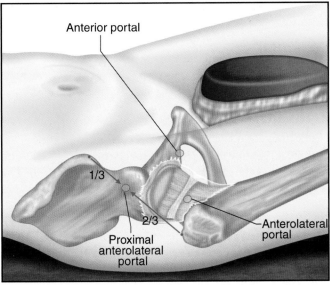

Figure 9-2. Standard portals to the PC.

Portal Placement

Proximal Anterolateral Portal

The classical anterolateral portal can be used as the first access and main viewing portal for arthroscopy of the PC. However, the authors prefer a more proximal position of the anterolateral portal to the PC. This allows for better maneuverability of the arthroscope and easier viewing of the lateral and posterolateral areas of the femoral neck.[6]

The skin incision is on the line connecting the anterior superior iliac spine (ASIS) and greater trochanter on the transition of the proximal to the middle third (Figure 9-2). A soft spot is palpable, representing the transition from the gluteus medius to the tensor fasciae lata muscles. Aiming approximately 30 degrees caudal and 20 degrees posterior, the portal penetrates the posterior parts of the tensor fasciae lata muscle.[6] The anterolateral area is safe regarding the femoral and sciatic nerves. However, the proximal anterolateral portal is closer to the branches of the superior gluteal nerve than the classical anterolateral portal. This portal is placed with fluoroscopic control. A 2-mm needle perforates the capsule on the femoral head-neck junction anterolaterally,

Figure 9-3. Placement of the proximal antero-lateral portal to the PC. The needle (arrow) is perpendicular to the femoral neck axis, perforating the capsule at the anterolateral head-neck transition. The nitinol wire passed through the needle bounces against the medial capsule.

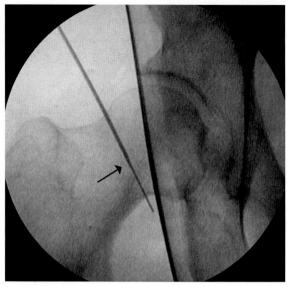

perpendicular to the neck axis. It is important to perforate the capsule at about 1 o'clock to have a better overview of the anterolateral head-neck junction and anterolateral rim, where most pathologies can be found. If the perforation is more anterior, viewing of this part of the PC may be limited. In addition, the perforation should not be distal at the neck area to avoid entering the PC distal to the zona orbicularis. If the portal is placed at this position, motion of the arthroscope and inspection of the anterolateral head is limited by the tight zona orbicularis.

After distension with 20 mL of saline, a nitinol wire is placed through the needle. The wire is inserted until the soft but distinct resistance of the medial capsule is palpable (Figure 9-3). The trocar of the arthroscope is then placed over the wire.

Anterior Portal

With the arthroscope in the proximal anterolateral portal, the anterior portal is placed under arthroscopic control. The skin incision of the anterior portal is the same used for the anterior portal to the CC, lying 4 to 6 cm distal and 2 to 3 cm lateral from the ASIS,[7] aiming approximately 0 to 10 degrees cephalad and 10 to 20 degrees medially (Figure 9-4). It penetrates parts of the tensor fasciae lata and rectus femoris muscles.[6] Ideally, the capsule is perforated anteriorly to the femoral neck and just proximal to the orbicular zone. This allows reaching medial and lateral areas with relatively good maneuverability. Byrd et al[7] reported that this portal is always close to at least one branch of the lateral femoral cutaneous nerve. The minimum distance to the lateral edge of the femoral nerve is 2.7 cm.[7]

The incision of the portal may vary depending on the main pathology. In synovial disease, it may be beneficial to choose the skin entry site on the vertical line from the ASIS to have easier access to the medial head and neck area for synovectomy and chondroma removal. In cam FAI, a skin incision 2 to 3 cm lateral to the vertical line allows better access to the lateral part of the femoral head-neck junction for easier resection of the cam deformity.

Classical Anterolateral Portal

The classical anterolateral portal facilitates addressing the lateral and posterolateral aspects of the head-neck junction in pistol grip deformity cases of cam FAI (Figure 9-5). In addition, the classical anterolateral portal is used as the first access portal to the CC.

This portal incision is located at the anterosuperior margin of the greater trochanter approximately 1 cm proximal and 1 cm anterior to the tip of the greater trochanter (Figure 9-6).[8] Aiming

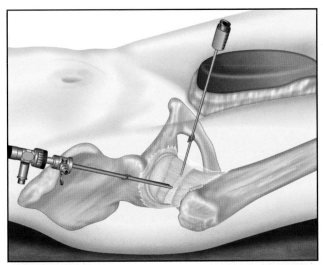

Figure 9-4. Placement of the anterior portal to the PC: the needle is aiming approximately 0 to 10 degrees cephalad and 10 to 20 degrees medially.

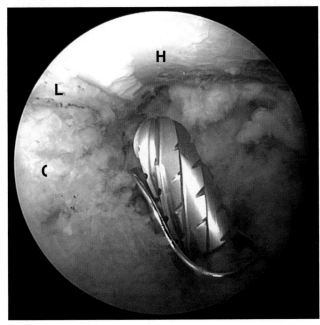

Figure 9-5. With the burr in the distal anterolateral portal, lateral aspects of the cam deformity can be addressed. Viewing portal: proximal anterolateral portal. C = capsule; H = femoral head; L = labrum.

approximately 15 degrees cephalad and 15 degrees posteriorly, the anterolateral portal penetrates the gluteus medius muscle before entering the lateral aspect of the capsule. The anterolateral portal is in the safe zone of the hip, with a comfortable distance to the femoral and sciatic nerve.[7,9] The only structure of significance relative to the anterolateral portal is the superior gluteal nerve, with a minimal distance of 3.2 mm.[7]

The direction of the portal and site of the capsular penetration depends on its purpose. If the posterolateral cam needs to be addressed, the capsular penetration needs to be at the height of the lateral bump. If the CC needs to be accessed under arthroscopic control, the capsular penetration needs to be close to the free edge of the acetabular labrum to shoot away from the prominent femoral head cartilage.

Figure 9-6. Standard portals to the CC.

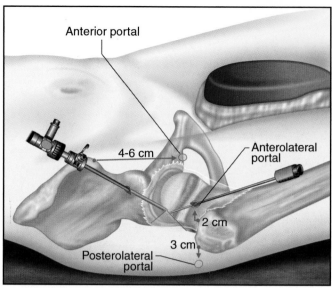

Central Compartment Access Under Peripheral Compartment Control

Portal placement to the CC under arthroscopic control from the PC can be done in different ways. When the authors started with this technique, the anterior portal was placed to the CC as the first viewing portal in the CC. The disadvantage of this technique is the difficulty viewing the needle or cannulated trocar after passing the gap between the acetabular labrum and femoral head. Over the past few years, the following technique of anterolateral portal placement has shown advantages with less risk of cartilage damage of both head and socket.

After completion of the diagnostic round or arthroscopic work in the PC, the arthroscope is lying in the proximal anterolateral portal viewing the lateral labrum and lateral head. A switching stick is introduced almost vertically from the anterior portal, pushing the lateral capsule away from the lateral femoral head and neck to increase the joint space in this tight part of the PC. It may be necessary to release a tight anterolateral zona orbicularis to have sufficient access to this area.

The hip is brought into full extension. Under arthroscopic control, the classic anterolateral portal to the CC is established. The capsule needs to be perforated at about 12 o'clock, directly next to the free edge of the labrum. Traction is applied until a sufficient space between the acetabular labrum and femoral head can be identified. The metal cannula is kept at the position of the labrum and not further advanced to avoid scratching the femoral head cartilage. Instead, a nitinol guidewire is introduced and advanced to the acetabular fossa (Figure 9-7). Subsequently, the cannula is removed, and the arthroscopy sheath with the cannulated trocar is advanced over the guidewire into the joint. After switching the arthroscope to the anterolateral portal to the CC, further portal placement is controlled arthroscopically without the need for additional fluoroscopic radiation.

Switching Between the Compartments

The order of arthroscopy with and without traction depends on different parameters (Figure 9-8). The authors always start in the PC. Depending on the volume and visibility within the PC space, a synovectomy and capsular release of various extent is performed to allow a complete diagnostic round in the PC. In standard cases in which the diagnosis is clear from preoperative physical and radiological imaging, therapy in the PC, such as a chondroma removal, cam resection,

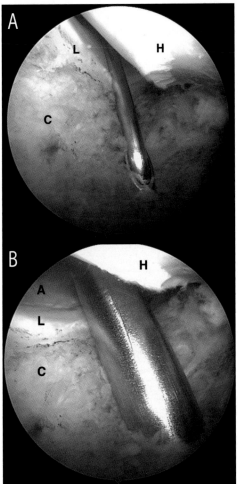

Figure 9-7. Placement of the anterolateral portal to the CC in the right hip under arthroscopic control. Anterolateral aspect of the femoral head after distraction, inspected via the PC. (A) A nitinol guidewire is placed between the labrum and the head under direct arthroscopic control. (B) After further distraction, the cannulated arthroscopy sheath is placed in the CC. A = lunate cartilage of the acetabulum; C = capsule; H = femoral head; L = labrum.

or removal of prominent ossifications or calcification from the peripheral side of the labrum, is completed. For accessing the lateral or posterolateral head-neck junction, traction is applied, staying with the arthroscope and instruments in the PC.

Under arthroscopic control from the PC, traction can be sequentially increased until the distraction of the femoral head from the labrum is sufficient. With the arthroscope in the proximal anterolateral portal, the classic anterolateral portal is established to the CC, avoiding the labrum and femoral head cartilage. The arthroscopy sheath in the proximal anterolateral portal can be kept on the neck to allow a continuous fluid outflow. After switching the arthroscope to the anterolateral portal to the CC, further portal placement to the CC can be checked arthroscopically. After completion of the work in the CC, the arthroscope and instruments should be moved back to the PC, the traction released, and an adequate work on the labrum or complete chondroma removal confirmed before the joint is evacuated.

Occasionally, the preoperative diagnosis is unclear. If diagnostic PC arthroscopy shows no obvious pathology, the diagnostic round should be completed, including the CC, before further treatment in the PC is initiated. In these cases, portals to the CC should be placed and a diagnostic arthroscopy of the CC performed. Depending on the type of rim damage or other potential pathology, the correct treatment should be indicated and completed in the CC before going back to the PC.

However, there are cases in which the distraction of the hip is limited and portal placement to the CC is too risky or impossible for the labrum or cartilage. Such situations are frequent in pincer

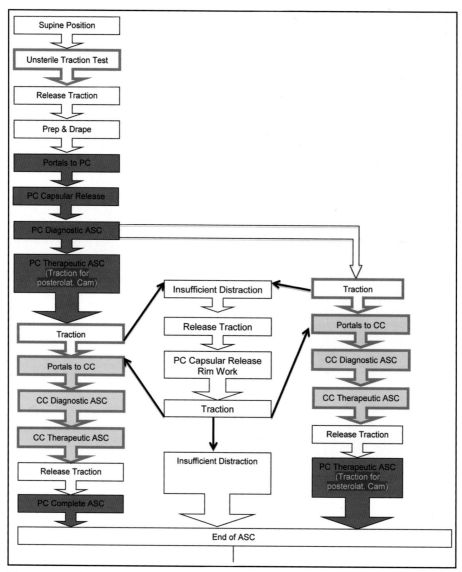

Figure 9-8. Flow chart. ASC = arthroscopy; CC = central compartment; PC = peripheral compartment.

FAI, in which the rim is significantly overhanging or the labrum is subtotally or totally ossified. Here, portal placement to the CC must not be forced. In most cases, traction should be released and a more extensive release of the articular capsule performed. In addition, rim work can be initiated from the PC, without and with traction. Peeling off the labrum from the bony rim can be done without traction, allowing a precise assessment of the residual labral width and decision as to whether debridement or refixation of the labrum is beneficial. Also, rim trimming can be started without traction but needs to be advanced under traction. This can be done with only a limited distraction of the head from the rim. Frequently, with progressive work on the capsule and rim, distraction will improve, allowing switching of the arthroscope and instruments into the CC.

A few cases remain where distraction is still not sufficient. Here, arthroscopy of the PC should only be considered to avoid iatrogenic damage of the acetabular labrum and the femoral head cartilage during portal placement to the CC.

POSTOPERATIVE PROTOCOL

The postoperative rehabilitation protocol is based on the pathology encountered and the procedure performed. It is not influenced by the way the hip is initially accessed.

POTENTIAL COMPLICATIONS

If the hip is fully or nearly extended and the first portal is placed toward the head, there is a risk of damaging the anterior head cartilage. This can be easily avoided by slight flexion of the hip of 10 to 20 degrees and aiming the cannula toward the head-neck junction.

In rare cases in which there is a connection between the joint and the iliopectineal bursa, the nitinol wire and cannulated instruments can be easily advanced into the bursa without the typical resistance from the anteromedial capsule. Thus, if no resistance is felt, the position of the wire and subsequent instrumentation should be checked fluoroscopically.

There is a risk of early fluid extravasation during arthroscopy of the PC if the pump pressure is too high and fluid leakage from the joint is blocked. The authors recommend starting with low pressure and monitoring the outflow of fluid. In addition, resection of the anteromedial capsule should be avoided to limit fluid extravasation via the iliopectineal bursa into the medial thigh and along the psoas into the retroperitoneum. In consequence, psoas tendon evaluation and eventual tenotomy should be performed at the end of the operation.

CONCLUSION

The PC-first access technique and complete arthroscopically controlled CC portal placement technique offer a beneficial alternative to the classic CC-first access technique. The risk of iatrogenic injury to the labrum and femoral head cartilage is reduced, and the primary work in the PC eases working in the CC.

TOP TECHNICAL PEARLS FOR THE PROCEDURE

1. Check correct positioning by distraction test before draping: after patient positioning, apply traction and check for sufficient distraction with fluoroscopy.

2. First portal: proximal anterolateral portal to the PC placed without traction under fluoroscopic control with a needle pointing toward the head-neck junction anterolaterally, perpendicular to the neck axis.

3. Establish the anterior portal and a distal anterolateral portal.

4. When doing a capsular release first, the traction force needed for accessing the CC will be decreased.

5. Place 2 portals (anterior and anterolateral) to the CC under direct arthroscopic control after applying traction.

REFERENCES

1. Byrd J. Hip arthroscopy: portal technique and arthroscopic anatomy [in German]. *Orthopade.* 2006;35(1):44-50.
2. Dienst M, Seil R, Kohn D. Safe arthroscopic access to the central compartment of the hip. *Arthroscopy.* 2005;21(12):1510-1514.
3. Byrd JW. Avoiding the labrum in hip arthroscopy. *Arthroscopy.* 2000;16(7):770-773.
4. Dorfmann H, Boyer T. Arthroscopy of the hip: 12 years of experience. *Arthroscopy.* 1999;15(1):67-72.
5. Dienst M, Gödde S, Seil R, Hammer D, Kohn D. Hip arthroscopy without traction: in vivo anatomy of the peripheral hip joint cavity. *Arthroscopy.* 2001;17(9):924-931.
6. Dienst M. Portale. In: Dienst M, ed. *Hüftarthroskopie.* München, Germany: Elsevier GmbH; 2009:97-118.
7. Byrd JW, Pappas JN, Pedley MJ. Hip arthroscopy: an anatomic study of portal placement and relationship to the extra-articular structures. *Arthroscopy.* 1995;11(4):418-423.
8. Byrd JW. Hip arthroscopy utilizing the supine position. *Arthroscopy.* 1994;10(3):275-280.
9. Robertson WJ, Kelly BT. The safe zone for hip arthroscopy: a cadaveric assessment of central, peripheral, and lateral compartment portal placement. *Arthroscopy.* 2008;24(9):1019-1026.

Please see videos on the accompanying website at

www.ArthroscopicTechniques.com

SECTION III

Central and Peripheral Compartments

Approaches to Capsulotomy and Capsular Management in Hip Arthroscopy

Jeffrey J. Nepple, MD; Asheesh Bedi, MD;
and Christopher M. Larson, MD

INTRODUCTION

Adequate arthroscopic access and visualization are vital to the thorough and precise treatment of femoroacetabular impingement (FAI). Inadequate correction of bony deformity is thought to be the most common cause of failure of arthroscopic treatment.[1-7] Similarly, the complications of overresection are now more commonly recognized. The type and extent of arthroscopic hip capsulotomy affects the arthroscopic visualization and maneuverability of instruments. However, equally important are the effects of capsulotomy and subsequent capsular repair on the postoperative stability and kinematics of the hip joint.

Hip stability has become a topic of interest with the increased ability to address intra-articular pathology via hip arthroscopy.[1,3,8,9] Hip stability relies on a complex interplay between bony congruency, the labral suction seal, dynamic muscular forces, and capsular/ligamentous restraints. The hip joint is generally considered an inherently stable joint due to its degree of bony congruency in comparison with other joints, such as the shoulder. Larson et al[10] recently established normative values of acetabular coverage of the femoral head on computed tomography of asymptomatic subjects.[8] Mean global coverage of the femoral head was $39.9\% \pm 2.4\%$, with mean anterior coverage of $31.0\% \pm 3.5\%$, superior coverage of $60.0\% \pm 3.2\%$, and posterior coverage of $49.4\% \pm 3.7\%$.

The acetabular labrum further increases the functional coverage of the femoral head. The function of the acetabular labrum in hip stability and biomechanics was previously questioned.[11] However, a growing body of literature supports the important function of the acetabular labrum in the hip fluid seal.[12-18] Sealing of the central compartment from the peripheral compartment with compressive loading appears to be important to minimize load transmission, improve load distribution, and maintain normal hip kinematics and stability.

Dynamic muscular forces also supplement the stability of the hip joint. The muscular envelope around the hip joint creates significant compressive forces across the hip joint, even at rest. The

Byrd JWT, Bedi A, Stubbs AJ, eds. *The Hip: AANA Advanced Arthroscopic Surgical Techniques* (pp 125-137).

anterior hip is significantly less constrained than the lateral and posterior hip but is supported by dynamic musculature of the iliopsoas and iliocapsularis. In the setting of hip dysplasia (acetabular dysplasia or increased femoral anteversion), the iliopsoas muscle is increasingly used for dynamic anterior hip stability and commonly presents with symptoms secondary to overuse. The iliocapsularis has only recently been recognized as a potentially important structure that may function to dynamically tension the hip capsule and affect hip stability.[19,20]

An accurate understanding of the ligamentous anatomy of the hip is important. The hip capsule originates circumferentially proximal to the bony attachment of the acetabular labrum, creating the normal capsulolabral recess. The hip capsule inserts circumferentially at the distal aspect of the femoral neck, including anteriorly at the intertrochanteric line, superiorly at the base of femoral neck proximal to the retinacular branches of the medial femoral circumflex artery, and posteriorly to the intertrochanteric crest. The ligamentous organization of the hip capsule is best considered as the following 4 components: iliofemoral ligament (IFL), pubofemoral ligament, ischiofemoral ligament, and zona orbicularis (ZO).[1,3,5]

The IFL (also called the Y ligament of Bigelow) is located anteriorly and is the strongest and thickest portion of hip capsule. The IFL is the most clinically relevant portion of the hip capsule, and the ligament is routinely violated during arthroscopy with an interportal capsulotomy.[5] It originates below the anterior inferior iliac spine and has medial and lateral arms that create the shape of an inverted Y. The medial arm is oriented vertically and inserts along the intertrochanteric line. The lateral arm is oriented obliquely and inserts more proximally along the intertrochanteric line.

The ischiofemoral ligament is the primary component of the posterior hip capsule; it originates from the ischial portion of the acetabular rim and inserts onto the intertrochanteric crest. The ischiofemoral ligament is significantly weaker than either arm of the IFL. The ischiofemoral ligament provides stability to hip internal rotation and adduction.

The pubofemoral ligament is the primary component of the medial hip capsule and blends into the medial arm of the IFL. The pubofemoral ligament originates from the pubic portion of the acetabular rim and obturator crest. It inserts into the inferior portion of the intertrochanteric line, distal posteromedial femoral neck, and intertrochanteric crest proximal to lesser trochanter. The pubofemoral ligament provides stability to external rotation (ER) in hip extension, in addition to the IFL.

The ZO is a condensation of the internal portion of the hip capsule that encircles the femoral neck, creating a narrowing in the capsular envelope. It provides significant restraint to hip distraction by acting as a constricted ring around the femoral neck.[8] The proximal-distal location of the ZO relative to arthroscopic anatomy has not been as clearly defined as other hip capsular ligaments. The anterior extension of the ZO is less distinct because it blends into the thicker fibers of the anterior IFL. Ito et al[8] described the ZO as a portion of the proximal and middle aspects of the capsule, with no extension to the distal aspect of the capsule. Imaging studies generally suggest that the ZO lies at the narrowest portion of the femoral neck (middle aspect of the capsule).[2,4,6,7,21]

The incompetence of any of the previously noted structures can decrease the degree of hip stability and put increasing demands on secondary hip stabilizers. Nepple et al[18] demonstrated a similar interplay between the stabilizing effect of the labrum and capsular ligaments of the hip in a biomechanical cadaveric study.[1,3,9] Stability to distractive forces was contributed by the labrum and the capsular ligaments (with the labrum being the primary stabilizer to the first few millimeters of distraction). However, in the setting of capsular incompetence, the labrum is required to exert increasing demands to resist distraction.

The interportal and T capsulotomies are the most commonly used types during hip arthroscopy. The interportal capsulotomy is performed by connecting the sites of capsular penetration of the anterolateral/posterolateral and mid-anterior portals and keeping the cut of the capsulotomy parallel to the acetabular rim. The interportal capsulotomy can be extended farther anteriorly or posteriorly depending on the need of the arthroscopic procedure. Telleria et al[5] described the arthroscopic anatomy of the hip capsular ligaments and reported the IFL to be located from 12:45 to 3 o'clock (anterior, in a right hip).[10] Thus, increasing the anterior extension of the interportal capsulotomy from the mid-anterior portal violates additional portions of the medial arm of the IFL. However, posterior extension from the anterolateral portal can be performed without additional violation of major ligaments until the ischiofemoral ligament is encountered at 10:30 o'clock (posterior, in a right hip). When considering capsular closure, the interportal cut should be made 5 to 10 mm distal to the labrum to maximize the size of the proximal capsular leaflet.

The T capsulotomy incorporates a vertical component of the capsulotomy performed parallel to the femoral neck. This approach is generally performed when entering the peripheral compartment over the region of maximal cam deformity. The vertical limb is best performed in the intramuscular plane between the gluteus minimus and iliocapsularis and can be carefully defined prior to division of the ligament. This not only minimizes iatrogenic muscular injury but maintains appropriately sized medial and lateral flaps for later anatomic closure. For extensile exposure, the vertical limb is carried distally through to the trochanteric insertion. This technique allows for full visualization of the superior and inferior retinacular vessels and may be selectively used in cases with extensive loss of distal head-neck offset and posterolateral extension of the deformity. Alternatively, a limited vertical limb can be used that does not violate the ZO. Proponents of the larger T capsulotomy prefer the large peripheral compartment exposure that it allows, which may make osteoplasty more efficient, and generally use some form of capsular closure. Partial capsular closure is defined as closure of the vertical limb of the T capsulotomy without closure of the interportal portion. Complete capsular closure is defined as closure of both limbs.

Capsulotomy without closure has been used for many years, with negative results reported in a small subset of patients. Traditionally, capsulectomy to some degree has also been performed to aid in visualization. Several case reports of hip dislocation after hip arthroscopy with unclosed capsulotomy have been reported.[11,22-25] Most cases had one or more contributing factors, including occult acetabular dysplasia, excessive acetabular rim trimming, or underlying connective tissue disorder. Although overt dislocation is an obvious complication after capsulotomy, microinstability of the hip is an evolving concept. In the authors' experience, postoperative microinstability of the hip presents with vague complaints of residual hip pain, muscular fatigue, and overload due to suspected subtle underlying instability.

Capsular Plication

Technical differentiation between arthroscopic capsular closure and capsular plication is poorly defined. Capsular closure generally implies a capsulotomy, debridement of capsular tissue, and subsequent side-to-side capsule-based repair, which likely results in a small amount of capsular tightening (Figure 10-1). However, capsular plication generally refers to the surgical advancement of the distal capsular limb to decrease the redundancy of the capsular envelope. In addition, some authors advocate oblique advancement of the distal capsule to maximize the reduction in capsular volume.[9,12-18] This inferior shift is performed by relative lateral advancement of the distal capsular arm compared with its native position. In addition, thermal capsulorrhaphy has been reported but is less commonly used due to concerns of chondrolysis, as experienced with its use in shoulder arthroscopy.[26]

The indications for capsular plication lack evidence-based outcomes, with the diagnosis of microinstability being subjective and surgeon dependent. In addition, in the setting of coexisting FAI, it is difficult to differentiate the relative effects of the treatment of FAI and capsular plication. Despite a lack of literature on the issue, capsular plication is likely indicated in a small subset of patients, such as those with underlying connective tissue disorders or severe ligamentous laxity.

The senior author has used arthroscopic capsular plication routinely in the setting of Ehlers-Danlos syndrome.[19,20,27] Fifteen patients (20 hips) were treated for atraumatic hip instability, generally in the setting of coexistent FAI. Preoperative modified Harris Hip Score averaged

Figure 10-1. Arthroscopic visualization of the posterolateral extent of a capsulotomy through the mid-anterior portal demonstrating the (A) extent of capsulotomy and (B) complete capsular closure. D=distal capsular arm; L=labrum, P=proximal capsular arm.

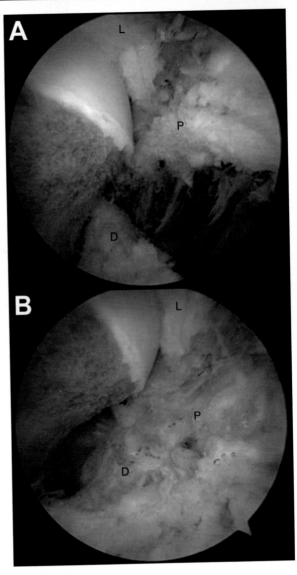

46 points, reflecting the significant disability in this population. Following arthroscopic treatment, which included capsular plication, excellent results were seen, with an average modified Harris Hip Score of 89 points. One patient needed a revision surgery for recurrent instability. Further research is needed to better define the indications for capsular plication in this population.

INDICATIONS

Preoperative physical examination and x-rays help to assist in capsular management decision making. Capsulotomies are important to maximize exposure and allow for more challenging resection of the posterolateral femur (seen on anteroposterior x-rays) and those cases with significant loss of head-neck offset that extends distally (Figure 10-2) and some cases of global acetabular overcoverage (Figure 10-3). Extensile capsulotomies have been used during hip arthroscopy for some time, but debate remains regarding the role for capsular closure and plication. There are

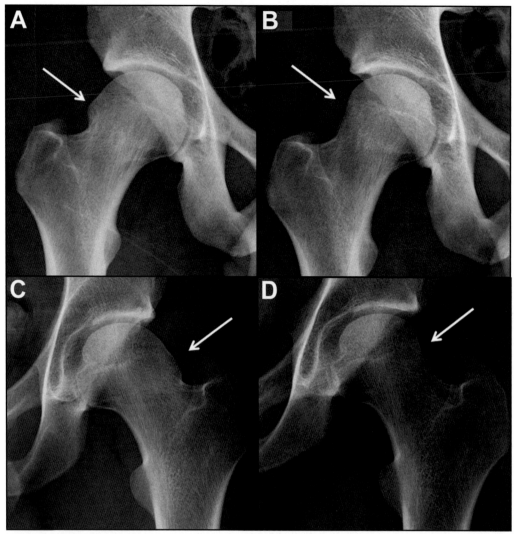

Figure 10-2. Pre- (A, C) and postoperative (B, D) coned anteroposterior pelvis x-rays of 2 cases with large posterosuperior extensions of cam deformity (arrow) treated adequately with arthroscopy using an interportal capsulotomy.

several preoperative findings that, if present, may compel the surgeon to consider a complete capsular closure (or plication) (Table 10-1). If the hip is considered to be borderline dysplastic or if soft tissue laxity/capsular hypermobility/incompetence is present, a capsular repair (or plication) may be considered. Intraoperative findings that may lead the surgeon to consider capsular repair or plication include easy entry through the capsule with minimal resistance, visualization of a patulous and/or thin capsule upon entry into the central compartment, and excessive mobility of the distal limb of the capsule after capsulotomy, which is present if the capsule can be pulled to or beyond the acetabular rim at the conclusion of the procedure.

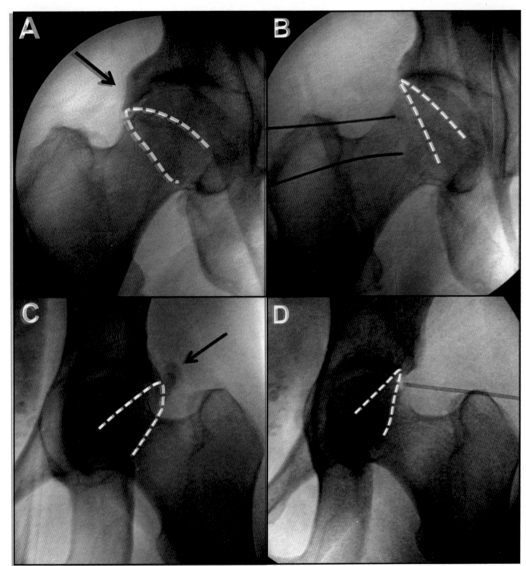

Figure 10-3. Pre- (A, C) and postoperative (B, D) anteroposterior fluoroscopic images demonstrating correction of global acetabular overcoverage using arthroscopy with an interportal capsulotomy.

STEP-BY-STEP DESCRIPTION OF THE TECHNIQUE

Interportal Capsulotomy (Current Authors' Technique)

The senior author performs hip arthroscopy in the supine position with a standard fracture table and custom perineal post. A capsulotomy is performed in all cases from the mid-anterior to the anterolateral/posterolateral portal and is repaired (or plicated), if indicated, at the conclusion of surgery more than 95% of the time. Initially, the anterolateral portal is established under fluoroscopic guidance with care to avoid labral penetration or femoral head chondral injury. A spinal needle is inserted in the location of the posterolateral portal under fluoroscopic guidance and is used for outflow. The mid-anterior portal is then established, and an arthroscopic Beaver blade

---

Table 10-1. Preoperative Findings for Which a Capsular Repair or Plication May Be Considered

▶ Borderline dysplastic findings: lateral center-edge angle 20 to 25 degrees, anterior center-edge angle 15 to 20 degrees, Tönnis angle 10 to 15 degrees, coxa valga (neck-shaft angle > 140 degrees), increased femoral anteversion > 25 degrees, increased acetabular anteversion

▶ Prior traumatic hip dislocation/subluxation (often with underlying FAI)

▶ Hypermobility: generalized hypermobility, connective tissue disorders (eg, Ehlers-Danlos syndrome), globally increased hip ROM (hip flexion > 110 degrees, rotational arc > 100 degrees in hip flexion)

▶ Increased passive ER and lack of a firm endpoint with supine log rolling

▶ Apprehension with hip extension/ER in the absence of significant osseous dysplastic findings

▶ Extreme ROM and laxity-induced instability: dancers, gymnasts, and yoga and martial arts students

▶ Prior hip arthroscopy with unrepaired capsulotomy/capsular incompetence

---

(Smith & Nephew) is introduced via the mid-anterior portal. An anterior capsulotomy is initially performed approximately 5 to 10 mm distal to the acetabular rim from just medial/inferior to the mid-anterior portal and is extended to the anterolateral portal. Maintaining the capsulotomy slightly distal to the indirect head of the rectus tendon is important to allow for later closure. The arthroscope is then placed into the mid-anterior portal, and the capsulotomy is extended from the anterolateral portal to the posterolateral portal approximately 1 cm distal to the acetabular rim (Figure 10-4A). Making the capsulotomy further distal to the acetabular rim allows the surgeon to access the more distal regions of the head-neck junction and femoral neck, which can be a primary site of impingement, particularly for extreme range of motion (ROM) impingement–induced instability and capsular laxity/hypermobility patterns.

At this point, the arthroscope is switched back to the anterolateral portal, and the arthroscopic knife is again introduced via the mid-anterior portal to complete the capsulotomy from just anterior or medial to the mid-anterior portal to the posterolateral portal. The interportal cut described here cuts the majority of the IFL (with a variable amount maintained anteriorly), with the primary restraint to anterior hip translation and ER. At this point, central compartment work is performed with care to elevate the capsule adjacent to the acetabular rim and avoiding aggressive capsular debridement. The goal is to elevate the capsule to expose the acetabular rim and anterior inferior iliac spine, when indicated, without excising excessive capsule peripherally in an effort to leave adequate medial and lateral capsular limbs for later repair. After the central compartment pathology is addressed, traction is released, and any cam-type deformity is addressed. Again, care is taken to avoid excessive capsular resection that might limit the ability to repair the capsule. At the conclusion of the peripheral compartment procedure, a decision is made regarding capsular repair or plication. The current authors routinely repair the capsule more than 95% of the time with 3 to 6 absorbable sutures.

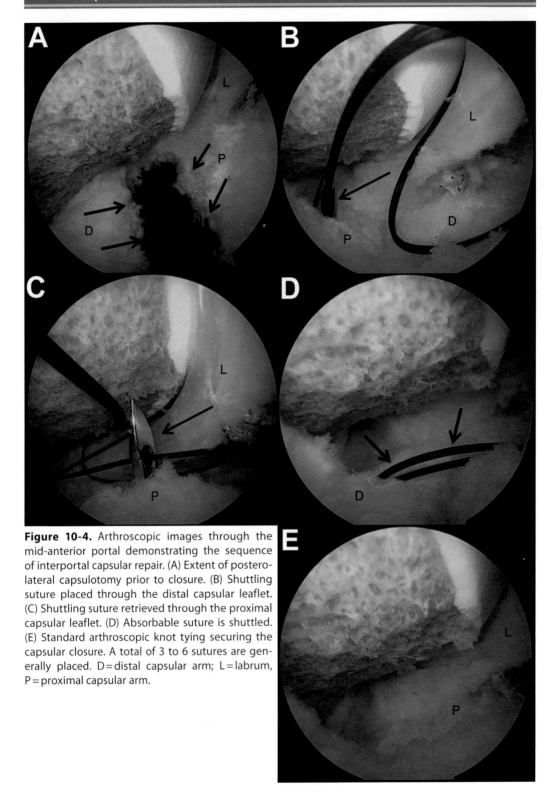

Figure 10-4. Arthroscopic images through the mid-anterior portal demonstrating the sequence of interportal capsular repair. (A) Extent of posterolateral capsulotomy prior to closure. (B) Shuttling suture placed through the distal capsular leaflet. (C) Shuttling suture retrieved through the proximal capsular leaflet. (D) Absorbable suture is shuttled. (E) Standard arthroscopic knot tying securing the capsular closure. A total of 3 to 6 sutures are generally placed. D=distal capsular arm; L=labrum, P=proximal capsular arm.

CAPSULAR CLOSURE/PLICATION

The capsule is repaired or plicated with the hip in a position of 10 to 20 degrees of flexion and some degree of ER (20 to 30 degrees). The capsular limbs reapproximate with internal rotation of the hip and separate further with ER of the hip. This hip position might be important when closing the capsule to avoid overtensioning or "capturing" the hip with resultant loss of ER ROM or capsular disruption during postoperative rehabilitation. The senior author typically begins with the arthroscope in the mid-anterior portal and a large cannula for suture management in the anterolateral portal (see Figure 10-4A). A curved or angled suture-passing device is used to initially shuttle a monofilament (or final) suture from the distal capsular limb toward the proximal/rim side capsular limb (Figure 10-4B). This device can be used to gauge the tension or laxity in the capsule to determine whether to use a repair or plication technique. A penetrating grasper is then used to retrieve the suture through the proximal limb, and a #2 absorbable suture is then shuttled across the capsule with the monofilament looped suture (Figures 10-4C and D). The suture is then tied with standard arthroscopic knot-tying techniques, with the knot placed on the superficial capsular surface (Figure 10-4E). No effort is made to further expose or clear muscle/fat from the superficial capsule; instead, a minimal dissection is preferred, and the cannula is placed adjacent to the capsule to avoid capturing soft tissues more superficially. If significant laxity is present, the distal capsular limb can be further debrided, large bites can be taken with the suture, and/or a shift-type procedure can be performed. The type of suture is at the surgeon's discretion. The senior author prefers #2 absorbable sutures in the absence of instability findings, alternating between absorbable and nonabsorbable braided sutures for capsular plications, and all nonabsorbable braided sutures for patients with connective tissue disorders (ie, Ehlers-Danlos syndrome). Two or 3 sutures are initially placed approximately 1 cm apart, taking care to check capsular tension after each suture is placed to avoid over- or undertensioning the capsule. At this point, the arthroscope and cannula could be exchanged to complete the anterior capsular closure. However, the senior author does not typically exchange portals but instead repositions the cannula more anteriorly and then places more sutures (total of 4 to 6 sutures) to complete the capsular repair or plication. A curved penetrating grasper can be helpful for the final 1 or 2 anteromedial sutures using this technique. The last sutures are placed while visualizing the superficial side of the capsule. Once complete, the hip is put through ROM, including flexion ER and extension ER to assess the stability of the repair and hip ROM.

T Capsulotomy

The arthroscopic setup for using a T capsulotomy is initially identical to that described above. A standard interportal capsulotomy is initially created as previously described. A distal accessory anterolateral portal (DALA) is then placed under direct arthroscopic visualization with the arthroscope in the mid-anterior portal. This portal is typically in line and approximately 4 to 5 cm distal to the proximal anterolateral portal along the anterior margin of the greater trochanter. Upon transitioning to the peripheral compartment, the amount of additional exposure is estimated based on visualization and the size of the cam deformity. The superficial surface of the capsule is cleared through the DALA portal to identify the intermuscular plane between the iliocapsularis and gluteus minimus. The T capsulotomy is then extended from the interportal cut in line with this plane (roughly between the medial and lateral arms of the IFL) and centered over the maximal cam deformity. This exposure can initially be performed with electrocautery to maintain hemostasis and is then completed sharply (Figure 10-5). The amount of T-extension of the capsulotomy affects the degree to which the ZO is violated. The ZO can be difficult to identify in the anterior hip because it blends with the thick anterior capsule of the IFL. The ZO is generally located at the narrowest portion of the femoral neck but is typically greater than 1 cm proximal to the insertion of the capsule on the femur. A limited T-extension may represent an intermediate

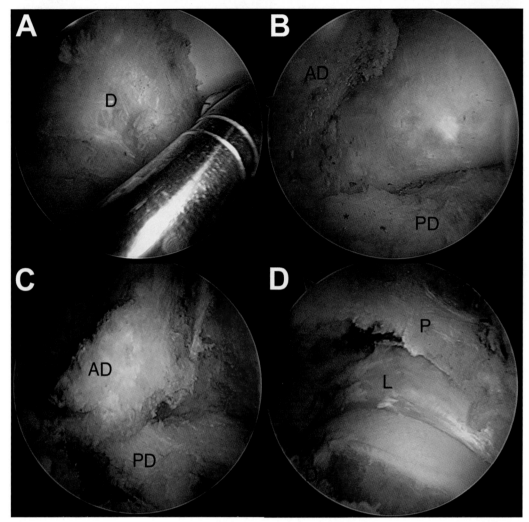

Figure 10-5. Arthroscopic images through the mid-anterior portal demonstrating the sequence of T capsulotomy and repair. (A) Extension of T capsulotomy performed through the DALA portal. (B) Typical visualization for osteoplasty as capsular flaps naturally retract. (C) Side-to-side repair performed through the DALA portal. (D) Arthroscopic visualization after knot tying. A total of 3 to 4 sutures are generally used for the T-extension closure. Closure of the interportal cut is then performed. AD = anterior portion of distal capsular arm; D = distal capsular arm; L = labrum; P = proximal capsular arm; PD = posterior portion of distal capsular arm; * = region of zona orbicularis.

between a simple interportal capsulotomy and a full T capsulotomy. Once the T-extension of the capsulotomy is created in the correct intermuscular plane, the medial and lateral limbs of the capsule tend to retract to allow excellent exposure. Exposure can be improved by placing a switching stick (Smith & Nephew) via the proximal anterolateral portal to retract the lateral capsule. Care is taken to preserve capsular tissue during the peripheral compartment exposure to facilitate subsequent repair.

Capsular closure starts with closure of the T-extension. This is generally performed through the DALA portal (with the arthroscope remaining in the mid-anterior portal) in a similar fashion to that described for the interportal capsulotomy. A curved hook (ACCU-PASS; Smith & Nephew) allows for capture of the medial capsular limb, and a tissue penetrator (ARTHRO-PIERCE; Smith & Nephew) can be passed via the proximal anterolateral portal through to the lateral limb to retrieve the stitch and place horizontal mattress sutures. Three to 4 sutures are generally used to close a full T-extension, progressing from distally to proximally. Some surgeons only close the T-extension of this type of capsulotomy, but the current authors generally prefer to perform a complete capsular closure by subsequently closing the interportal capsulotomy. This portion of the procedure is performed as described previously, generally with absorbable sutures.

POSTOPERATIVE PROTOCOL

In the absence of significant laxity or hypermobility, physical therapy and unrestricted ROM begins on postoperative day 0 or 1 with no brace or other precautions. If a significant capsular plication is performed for capsular laxity, hypermobility, or incompetence, a hip brace or orthosis is used for 3 to 4 weeks to limit hip extension beyond neutral. Hip ER and extension precautions are used for 3 to 4 weeks postoperatively, and pain is used as the primary guide for ROM. Passive hip extension and the extremes of ER are discouraged for 4 weeks postoperatively in physical therapy. Crutches and protected weight bearing are used for 2 to 4 weeks and are based on osseous resections and bone quality rather than labral or capsular procedures. The senior author does not use continuous passive motion devices unless the procedure is performed in a revision surgery setting with the treatment of associated adhesions.

POTENTIAL COMPLICATIONS

No complications directly related to capsular closure have been reported in the literature. However, capsular repair is technically challenging for surgeons not experienced with this technique, and complications may occur. First, capsular repair initially results in longer operative times, with the potential for greater fluid extravasation into the soft tissues. With operative experience, this portion of the procedure can generally be completed more quickly, lessening the extravasation risk. Second, additional iatrogenic trauma to the hip capsule may increase the incidence of heterotopic ossification (HO). Overall rates of HO after hip arthroscopy have been reported to be 1% to 2%, with a decreased risk associated with use of anti-inflammatory prophylaxis. As such, HO prophylaxis should be considered in the setting of capsular repair. Third, overtightening of the capsule could theoretically restrict ROM or lead to global stiffness. In addition, the indirect head of the rectus femoris could be tethered by the capsular repair, which could lead to persistent pain. Some surgeons use absorbable suture (and avoid nonabsorbable suture) during capsular closure for this reason. Finally, complete visualization during capsular closure can be difficult, and iatrogenic trauma to the femoral head cartilage or acetabular labrum may result.

CONCLUSION

Adequate visualization is important to achieve accurate and precise resection of proximal femoral cam deformities and more complex global acetabular overcoverage. Interportal and T capsulotomies are commonly used to optimize visualization. Extensive capsulotomies may increase the risk of iatrogenic hip subluxation, dislocation, and subtle instability. Consideration should be given to repair of capsulotomies, especially in patients at increased risk of instability. Capsular plication may play a role in patients with underlying hyperlaxity or connective tissue disorders, but accepted indications are evolving. Further research will continue to define the role of capsular management in an effort to optimize outcomes after arthroscopic interventions.

Top Technical Pearls for the Procedure

1. Intraoperative findings consistent with instability/laxity include minimal capsular resistance while making portals, visualization of capsular redundancy with traction on, and increased mobility of the lateral limb of the capsulotomy.

2. Care must be taken to minimize capsular debridement during exposure and throughout the case to preserve enough capsule for repair/plication.

3. Capsular overtightening should be avoided by repairing with the hip near extension (10 to 30 degrees of flexion) and in ER (20 to 30 degrees) to prevent postoperative motion loss or disruption of capsular repair.

4. Making the capsulotomy farther from the acetabular rim provides more capsule for later repair and facilitates femoral resection more distally without the need for an additional T-cut.

5. Passing the looped suture initially through the distal limb and shuttling the suture adjacent to the rim allows for more predictable suture retrieval than passing in the opposite manner, which requires more challenging shuttling of the suture between the femoral neck and capsule.

References

1. Martin HD, Savage A, Braly BA, Palmer IJ, Beall DP, Kelly B. The function of the hip capsular ligaments: a quantitative report. *Arthroscopy*. 2008;24(2):188-195.
2. Larson CM, Giveans MR, Samuelson KM, Stone RM, Bedi A. Arthroscopic hip revision surgery for residual femoroacetabular impingement (FAI): surgical outcomes compared with a matched cohort after primary arthroscopic FAI correction. *Am J Sports Med*. 2014;42(8):1785-1790.
3. Bedi A, Galano G, Walsh C, Kelly BT. Capsular management during hip arthroscopy: from femoroacetabular impingement to instability. *Arthroscopy*. 2011;27(12):1720-1731.
4. Heyworth BE, Shindle MK, Voos JE, Rudzki JR, Kelly BT. Radiologic and intraoperative findings in revision hip arthroscopy. *Arthroscopy*. 2007;23(12):1295-1302.
5. Telleria JJ, Lindsey DP, Giori NJ, Safran MR. An anatomic arthroscopic description of the hip capsular ligaments for the hip arthroscopist. *Arthroscopy*. 2011;27(5):628-636.
6. Philippon MJ, Schenker ML, Briggs KK, Kuppersmith DA, Maxwell RB, Stubbs AJ. Revision hip arthroscopy. *Am J Sports Med*. 2007;35(11):1918-1921.
7. Clohisy JC, Nepple JJ, Larson CM, Zaltz I, Millis M; Academic Network of Conservation Hip Outcome Research (ANCHOR) Members. Persistent structural disease is the most common cause of repeat hip preservation surgery. *Clin Orthop Relat Res*. 2013;471(12):3788-3794.
8. Ito H, Song Y, Lindsey DP, Safran MR, Giori NJ. The proximal hip joint capsule and the zona orbicularis contribute to hip joint stability in distraction. *J Orthop Res*. 2009;27(8):989-995.
9. Domb BG, Philippon MJ, Giordano BD. Arthroscopic capsulotomy, capsular repair, and capsular plication of the hip: relation to atraumatic instability. *Arthroscopy*. 2013;29(1):162-173.
10. Larson CM, Moreau-Gaudry A, Kelly BT, et al. Are normal hips being labeled as pathologic? A CT-based method for defining normal acetabular coverage. *Clin Orthop Relat Res*. 2015;473(4):1247-1254.
11. Konrath GA, Hamel AJ, Olson SA, Bay B, Sharkey NA. The role of the acetabular labrum and the transverse acetabular ligament in load transmission in the hip. *J Bone Joint Surg Am*. 1998;80(12):1781-1788.
12. Ferguson SJ, Bryant JT, Ganz R, Ito K. The influence of the acetabular labrum on hip joint cartilage consolidation: a poroelastic finite element model. *J Biomech*. 2000;33(8):953-960.
13. Ferguson SJ, Bryant JT, Ganz R, Ito K. An in vitro investigation of the acetabular labral seal in hip joint mechanics. *J Biomech*. 2003;36(2):171-178.

14. Smith MV, Panchal HB, Ruberte Thiele RA, Sekiya JK. Effect of acetabular labrum tears on hip stability and labral strain in a joint compression model. *Am J Sports Med.* 2011;39 suppl:103S-110S.

15. Greaves LL, Gilbart MK, Yung AC, Kozlowski P, Wilson DR. Effect of acetabular labral tears, repair and resection on hip cartilage strain: a 7T MR study. *J Biomech.* 2010;43(5):858-863.

16. Cadet ER, Chan AK, Vorys GC, Gardner T, Yin B. Investigation of the preservation of the fluid seal effect in the repaired, partially resected, and reconstructed acetabular labrum in a cadaveric hip model. *Am J Sports Med.* 2012;40(10):2218-2223.

17. Philippon MJ, Nepple JJ, Campbell KJ, et al. The hip fluid seal—part I: the effect of an acetabular labral tear, repair, resection, and reconstruction on hip fluid pressurization. *Knee Surg Sports Traumatol Arthrosc.* 2014;22(4):722-729.

18. Nepple JJ, Philippon MJ, Campbell KJ, et al. The hip fluid seal—part II: the effect of an acetabular labral tear, repair, resection, and reconstruction on hip stability to distraction. *Knee Surg Sports Traumatol Arthrosc.* 2014;22(4):730-736.

19. Ward WT, Fleisch ID, Ganz R. Anatomy of the iliocapsularis muscle: relevance to surgery of the hip. *Clin Orthop Relat Res.* 2000;(374):278-285.

20. Babst D, Steppacher SD, Ganz R, Siebenrock KA, Tannast M. The iliocapsularis muscle: an important stabilizer in the dysplastic hip. *Clin Orthop Relat Res.* 2010;469(6):1728-1734.

21. Wagner FV, Negrão JR, Campos J, et al. Capsular ligaments of the hip: anatomic, histologic, and positional study in cadaveric specimens with MR arthrography. *Radiology.* 2012;263(1):189-198.

22. Benali Y, Katthagen BD. Hip subluxation as a complication of arthroscopic debridement. *Arthroscopy.* 2009;25(4):405-407.

23. Austin DC, Horneff JG III, Kelly JD IV. Anterior hip dislocation 5 months after hip arthroscopy. *Arthroscopy.* 2014;30(10):1380-1382.

24. Matsuda DK. Acute iatrogenic dislocation following hip impingement arthroscopic surgery. *Arthroscopy.* 2009;25(4):400-404.

25. Mei-Dan O, McConkey MO, Brick M. Catastrophic failure of hip arthroscopy due to iatrogenic instability: can partial division of the ligamentum teres and iliofemoral ligament cause subluxation? *Arthroscopy.* 2012;28(3):440-445.

26. Philippon MJ. The role of arthroscopic thermal capsulorrhaphy in the hip. *Clin Sports Med.* 2001;20(4):817-829.

27. Larson CM, Stone RM, Grossi EF, Giveans MR, Cornelsen GD. Ehlers-Danlos syndrome: arthroscopic management for extreme soft-tissue hip instability [published online ahead of print July 18, 2015]. *Arthroscopy.*

Please see videos on the accompanying website at

www.ArthroscopicTechniques.com

Arthroscopic Labral Debridement, Repair, and Stitch Configurations

Andrew B. Wolff, MD and Matthew Mantell, MD

INTRODUCTION

This chapter reviews the current indications for operative management of labrum tears and the pertinent history and physical findings associated with this pathology. The different stitch configurations and technical aspects are covered, along with the author's preferred technique and surgical pearls.

INDICATIONS

The indication is a simple tear of the base of the labrum that is unstable to probing in a patient with symptoms consistent with hip pain, absence of osteoarthritis, or significant dysplasia and for whom conservative management has failed.

Controversial Indications

▶ Complex chronic labral tears (may be better served with debridement and/or segmental reconstruction)

▶ Labral tears with intrasubstance cystic or synovitic changes (may be better served debridement and/or segmental reconstruction)

▶ Labral tears in the setting of osteoarthritis (may be better served with nonoperative therapy or arthroplasty)

▶ Labral tears in the setting of dysplasia (may need concomitant proximal femoral and/or acetabular osteotomy)

Byrd JWT, Bedi A, Stubbs AJ, eds. *The Hip:*
AANA Advanced Arthroscopic Surgical Techniques (pp 139-146).
© 2016 AANA.

Pertinent Physical Findings

▶ Reproduction of groin pain with passive flexion to 90 degrees, adduction, and internal rotation (FADIR [anterior impingement test]).[1,2]

▶ Flexion, abduction, external rotation (FABER) demonstrating an increased distance from the lateral aspect of the knee to the examining table on the affected side compared with the unaffected side. This maneuver may also elicit pain.[1,2]

Pertinent Imaging

▶ Plain x-rays to assess bony pathology include the following[3]:

  ▷ Anteroposterior pelvis

  ▷ 90- and 45-degree modified Dunn lateral

  ▷ False profile

▶ Magnetic resonance imaging with or without arthrography[4]

Positioning and Equipment

Although multiple surgeons have reported reliably good outcomes with lateral positioning, the preponderance of hip preservation surgeons perform hip arthroscopy in the supine position. Several table options are available to facilitate the procedure, from standard fracture tables to commercially available tables designed for anterior-approach total hip arthroplasty to commercially available table attachments that are affixed to standard operating tables. The table used is largely a function of preference and availability at the surgeon's facility. The required features must include a well-padded perineal post; secure and padded holders for the feet; and the ability to flex, extend, abduct, and adduct the limb; internally and externally rotate the hip; and apply traction (Figure 11-1).

Following the administration of anesthesia—which typically includes complete muscle relaxation of the muscles of the lower extremity—the patient is placed supine on the operating table. The ipsilateral arm is placed across the chest and the contralateral arm is placed on an armboard to the side. The table is tilted 10 degrees away from the operative side and may be placed in some Trendelenburg so as to decrease the amount of pressure on the pudendal nerve. The hip is flexed approximately 10 degrees in approximately 15 degrees of internal rotation with the knee straight. Traction is applied with the hip in slight abduction. The hip is then brought into slight adduction against the padded post to create a lateral vector to displace the femoral head inferiorly and laterally. Distraction of the femoral head with 30 to 50 lb of traction applied creates 8 to 10 mm of joint space.[1] This is visualized via large C-arm fluoroscopy prior to sterile prepping and draping. Traction may then be released during prepping and draping. Draping is most easily accomplished with a commercially available shower curtain drape, as is used in hip fracture fixation, fortified by surgeon preference (see Figure 11-1).

Equipment

A wide array of commercially available surgical equipment is necessary to successfully perform arthroscopic surgery of the hip to address labral pathology. A 70-degree arthroscope is necessary,

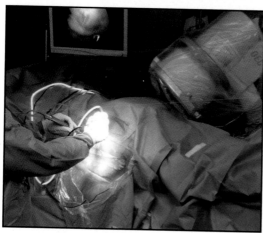

Figure 11-1. Draping is accomplished with a shower curtain drape fortified as necessary over the patient, who is supine on a commercially available table. The required features must include a well-padded perineal post; secure and padded holders for the feet; and the ability to flex, extend, abduct and adduct the limb, as well as internally and externally rotate the hip and apply traction. The C-arm can be positioned between the legs or across the body.

as are elongated cannulas for access into the joint. Spinal needles, nitinol guidewires, and extra-long suture-passing devices similar to those used in the shoulder are also needed. These are used along with penetrating passers, looped graspers, locking serrated graspers, and other suture-passing, -shuttling, and -grasping instruments per surgeon preference. A cannula of sufficient length and diameter (typically at least 7 mm in diameter and 6 cm in length) for suture management, an elongated arthroscopic probe, an arthroscopic knot pusher, motorized shavers, burrs, and electrocautery devices are key instruments in completing any labral repair.

STEP-BY-STEP DESCRIPTION OF THE PROCEDURE

After the patient is positioned, prepped, and draped as described in the previous section, traction is applied. The distracted hip is visualized fluoroscopically (approximately 8 to 10 mm of joint space is typically adequate). A spinal needle is used to set the anterolateral portal. This is typically placed approximately 1 cm anterior and superior to the tip of the greater trochanter but should be adjusted so as to have a useful portal that does not penetrate the labrum or injure the femoral head. This is visualized fluoroscopically to ensure optimal position.

A Seldinger technique is used to create an anterolateral portal using a nitinol wire passed through the spinal needle, which is then removed. An arthroscopic cannula is then placed over this guidewire. The camera is inserted into the joint. At this point, arthroscopic fluid is avoided if possible because there is no outflow portal. A spinal needle is used to localize the mid-anterior portal, which is placed at approximately the mid-point in the medial-lateral plane between the tip of the greater trochanter and the anterior superior iliac spine and approximately 7 cm distal to the anterolateral portal. The placement of this portal is variable and dependent on anatomy. Fluoroscopy is of limited utility. In general, if you are having trouble, consider that this portal is placed much more in line with your anterolateral portal than you might think. There are commercially available devices to help with placement of this portal if necessary; however, practice and familiarity with the procedure are your best tools.

Typically, the next step is to perform an interportal capsulotomy connecting the anterolateral and mid-anterior portals. This is done with a banana knife or Beaver blade. This step is occasionally unnecessary in patients for whom peripheral compartment work is not indicated and/or patients for whom instability is an issue. When performing the capsulotomy, be sure to leave a sufficient capsule on the acetabular side so that it may be repaired at the end of the procedure.

At this point, the entire central compartment is visible and should be inspected, and the labrum should be probed to assess for tears and instability. If a labral tear is encountered, it should be

Figure 11-2. The distal antero-lateral portal in a left hip arthroscopy. This can be a useful portal to ensure safe positioning as close to the articular surface as possible without violating the articular cartilage. This portal can also be useful for manipulation of the labrum with a grasper during repair to establish appropriate tension and placement of the labrum on the rim. It can also be useful when placing multiple suture anchors at one time for efficiency of placement and suture management.

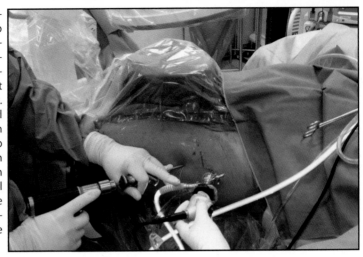

assessed for extent and whether it is amenable to repair. Tears with instability at the base should be repaired. Peripheral fraying of the labrum should be debrided. In patients with complex degenerative tears with significant intrasubstance tearing and synovitis, consideration should be given to resection and reconstruction. This is also true for patients with diminutive and severely damaged labra. The indications for labral reconstruction are evolving. Few published data support primary labral reconstruction at this time.[5] Debridement of irreparable tears remains a viable option.[6-12] If labral debridement is indicated, it is performed with an arthroscopic motorized shaver, electrocautery device, and/or arthroscopic biter. If a labral repair is performed, the next step is to identify the acetabular rim, to which the labrum is usually still at least partially attached.

The bone of the acetabulum is exposed with a shaver and/or an electrocautery device, with careful attention paid to labral preservation. If there is significant damage at the chondrolabral junction or a significant acetabuloplasty is to be performed based on preoperative imaging demonstrating significant pincer-type femoroacetabular impingement, then burring of the acetabular rim is undertaken to effect an appropriate pincer correction or to eliminate the area of damage at the chondrolabral junction. Do not overresect the acetabular rim because this will destabilize the hip.[13] Burring is then undertaken to correct the bony aspect of the pathology and to create a bleeding bony interface for healing.[14] Damaged labra and damaged or redundant articular cartilage is then resected with an arthroscopic biter, shaver, and/or electrocautery device. If there is no detachment or significant damage on the articular side of the chondrolabral junction and there is no need for a significant acetabuloplasty, the chondrolabral junction may be preserved. In this case, burring is performed only to the extent necessary to get to a surface of bleeding bone for labral repair/refixation.

Place anchors into the acetabular rim. This can be done through either of the existing portals or through a distal anterolateral portal localized with a spinal needle and placed approximately 8 cm distal to the anterolateral portal (Figure 11-2). It is often easier to place all of the anchors at one time and then proceed to the repair because the acetabulum is most exposed at this time. Once anchors have been placed and their sutures passed around the labrum, exposure to the acetabular rim is a bit more challenging. The drill guide should be positioned as close as possible to the acetabular rim to effect anatomic repair. The surgeon should consider drilling these holes for the purposes of tactile feedback while the assistant holds the camera focused on the acetabular articular surface to ensure that there is no violation of same. Similarly, the holes for anchor placement should not violate the extra-articular portion of the bone, particularly anteriorly because the bone is thin in this area, and a protruding anchor can be an irritant to the psoas tendon.

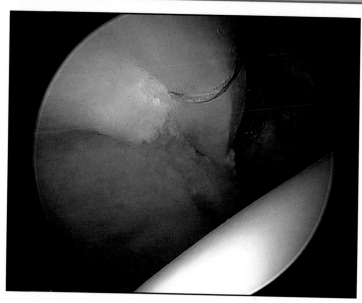

Figure 11-3. Vertical mattress or base refixation suture placement of the posterosuperior labrum of a right hip. The relative meniscoid shape of this labrum lends itself to a vertical mattress configuration. The lead suture has already been placed through the chondral-labral junction and is now being retrieved through the labrum more peripherally. The post suture is not pictured because it is in the cannula.

Place a clear cannula for suture management into the mid-anterior portal for more anterior tears and an anterolateral portal for more lateral and posterior tears. Retrieve the postsuture limb from the anteriormost suture anchor. Pass the other suture limb from the most anterior anchor through the chondrolabral junction. Grasp this suture limb and retrieve it through the cannula. It is at this point that the surgeon must decide whether to use a simple loop suture or a vertical mattress (also known as a base-refixation suture).[15,16] Both are acceptable. Most hip surgeons feel that the anatomy of the patient's labrum ought to dictate the suture configuration (Figure 11-3). For more cylindrical and smaller labra or cases with marginal tissue quality, a simple loop suture is preferable. For more hypertrophic and/or meniscoid labra with robust tissue quality, a vertical mattress is preferable to restore the original anatomic configuration (Figures 11-4 and 11-5). The base configuration has been shown to better preserve the suction-seal.

Sutures are then tied using a standard arthroscopic knot-tying technique. In large, detached tears, it can be beneficial to use an arthroscopic grasper placed through the distal accessory portal to hold appropriate tension on the labrum during suture fixation. Alternatively, the sutures for labral repair can be placed first and then passed through knotless anchors that are then placed into the acetabular rim.

POSTOPERATIVE PROTOCOL

For simple labral repairs, patients are kept protected weight bearing with crutches for 2 to 3 weeks until their gait has normalized. Weight bearing will be more restricted for a longer duration of time based on concomitant procedures (eg, chondral restorative procedure, capsular plication, osteoplasty, and periacetabular osteotomy). Passive motion is begun immediately with a continuous passive motion machine or with a stationary bike without resistance. Time to initiation of physical therapy is variable among practitioners but usually begins within 1 week. Gentle range of motion and isometric exercises are begun in the early phases, with progression to more active strengthening focused on the core and gluteal musculature as weeks progress. Manual therapy can be a valuable adjunct during the recovery phase.

Depending on the goals and rate of progress of the patient, a gradual return to running can begin at 10 to 12 weeks. Although some authors have reported a successful return to competitive

Figure 11-4. The labrum after 2 vertical mattress sutures have been placed.

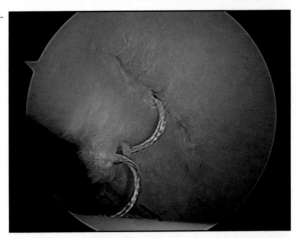

Figure 11-5. Labral repair performed in a right hip with a simple loop suture more superiorly and a vertical mattress suture more anteriorly. This was done because the anterior labrum was more meniscoid, whereas the superior labrum was more cylindrical.

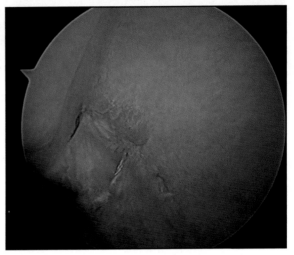

athletics as early as 3 months, most advocate a minimum of 4 to 6 months, particularly for high hip–demand sports, such as football, lacrosse, hockey, basketball, soccer, crew, ballet, or wrestling.

POTENTIAL COMPLICATIONS

Many of the potential complications that are specifically related to the surgical management of the labrum are difficult to assess in any specific patient. Technical errors can occur, such as anchor penetration into the joint, anchor breakage and retention in the joint, and anchor placement that abrades the iliopsoas tendon. Most complications are likely not true complications but more the result of suboptimal technique, decision making, and/or anatomy. For instance, a complete labral resection in a young female with borderline dysplasia does not meet the criteria for a complication but represents an adverse event. Similarly, repair of a chronically damaged and irreparable labrum introduces an unnecessarily high likelihood of failure. Such tears are likely better treated with debridement or reconstruction.

As understanding of hip pathology has progressed, it is likely that more subtle decisions are made that create marginal differences in case series but likely represent real differences in individual patients. These potential complications include everting the labrum away from the rim of the acetabulum and thus not reestablishing the seal with the femoral head (typically caused by anchor placement far from the acetabular surface); repair performed on an irreparable labrum; a loop stitch placed around a large hypertrophic labrum, which distorts its anatomy and compromises the suction-seal; failure to recognize and debride damaged and synovitic tissue within the labrum; and resection of the labrum in a patient who relied on his or her labrum for stability.

TOP TECHNICAL PEARLS FOR THE PROCEDURE

1. Do not struggle with anchor placement. Have a low threshold to use a distal anterolateral portal for anchor placement. This portal can also be useful for placement of the labrum in an anatomic position while securing suture fixation. A more distal portal minimizes the risk of joint penetration while permitting anchor placement close to the rim margin.

2. Place anchors as close to the articular surface as possible for anatomic repair.

3. Stay in the bone. Watch the acetabular articular surface during anchor placement. Do the drilling and anchor placement yourself for tactile feedback while the assistant holds the camera.

4. Place a nitinol guidewire down the drilled anchor hole to ensure that the distal end of the drill hole is still in the bone. This is important in the anterior acetabulum where the bone is thin and a protruding anchor can irritate the iliopsoas tendon.

5. Let the shape of the labrum dictate the stitch configuration. In smaller, more cylindrical labra, use a loop stitch configuration. In larger, more meniscoid labra, use a vertical mattress stitch.

REFERENCES

1. Troelsen A, Mechlenburg I, Gelineck J, Bolvig L, Jacobsen S, Søballe K. What is the role of clinical tests and ultrasound in acetabular labral tear diagnostics? *Acta Orthop.* 2009;80(3):314-318.
2. Martin RL, Enseki KR, Draovitch P, Trapuzzano T, Philippon MJ. Acetabular labral tears of the hip: examination and diagnostic challenges. *J Orthop Sports Phys Ther.* 2006;36(7):503-515.
3. Delaunay S, Dussault RG, Kaplan PA, Alford BA. Radiographic measurements of dysplastic adult hips. *Skeletal Radiol.* 1997;26(2):75-81.
4. Sutter R, Zubler V, Hoffman A, et al. Hip MRI: how useful is intraarticular contrast material for evaluating surgically proven lesions of the labrum and articular cartilage? *Am J Roentgenol.* 2014;202(1):160-169.
5. Philippon MJ, Briggs KK, Hay CJ, Kuppersmith DA, Dewing CB, Huang MJ. Arthroscopic labral reconstruction in the hip using iliotibial band autograft: technique and early outcomes. *Arthroscopy.* 2010;26(6):750-756.
6. Byrd JW, Jones KS. Hip arthroscopy and labral pathology: prospective analysis with 10-year follow-up. *Arthroscopy.* 2009;25(4):365-368.
7. Espinosa N, Rothenfluh DA, Beck M, Ganz R, Leunig M. Treatment of femoro-acetabular impingement: preliminary results of labral refixation. *J Bone Joint Surg Am.* 2006;88(5):925-935.
8. Farjo LA, Glick JM, Sampson TG. Hip arthroscopy for acetabular labral tears. *Arthroscopy.* 1999;15(2):132-137.
9. Krych AJ, Thompson M, Knutson Z, Scoon J, Coleman SH. Arthroscopic labral repair versus selective labral debridement in female patients with femoroacetabular impingement: a prospective randomized study. *Arthroscopy.* 2013;29(1):46-53.

10. Larson CM, Giveans MR. Arthroscopic debridement versus refixation of the acetabular labrum associated with femoracetabular impingement. *Arthroscopy.* 2009;25(4):369-376.

11. Larson CM, Giveans MR, Stone RM. Arthroscopic debridement versus refixation of the acetabular labrum associated with femoroacetabular impingement: mean 3.5-year follow-up. *Am J Sports Med.* 2012;40(5):1015-1021.

12. Ferguson SJ, Bryant JT, Ganz R, Ito K. An in vitro investigation of the acetabular labral seal in hip joint mechanics. *J Biomech.* 2003;36(2):171-178.

13. Philippon MJ, Wolff AB, Briggs KK, Kuppersmith DA, Zehms CT, Hay C. Correlation of pre- and postoperative center-edge angles with the extent of acetabular rim resection. *Arthroscopy.* 2010;25(6):756-761.

14. Wenger DE, Kendell KR, Miner MR, Trousdale RT. Acetabular labral tears rarely occur in the absence of bony abnormalities. *Clin Orthop Relat Res.* 2004;(426):145-150.

15. Fry R, Domb B. Labral base refixation in the hip: rationale and technique for an anatomic approach to labral repair. *Arthroscopy.* 2010;26(9 suppl):S81-S89.

16. Philippon MJ, Briggs KK, Fagrelius T, Patterson D. Labral refixation: current techniques and indications. *HSS J.* 2012;8(3):240-244.

Please see videos on the accompanying website at

www.ArthroscopicTechniques.com

12

Arthroscopic Management of Focal Chondral Injuries in the Hip

Thomas H. Wuerz, MD, MSc and Shane J. Nho, MD, MS

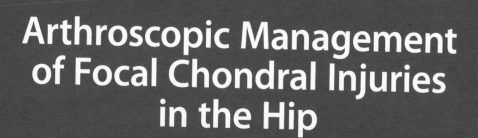

INTRODUCTION

The treatment of focal chondral defects (FCD) remains a challenge in any weight-bearing joint due to its inherent limited capacity to regenerate or heal. The management of cartilage defects has historically been the focus of biologic approaches to joint preservation, including chondral debridement, marrow-stimulating techniques, autologous chondrocyte implantation, osteochondral autograft, and osteochondral allograft. Restoring the biologic and biomechanical properties of articular cartilage remains to be achieved. The depth, joint congruity, and geometry of the hip joint make the treatment of FCD technically challenging. Although long-term outcome studies on knee cartilage replacement and restoration are prevalent in the literature, definitive evidence-based treatment guidelines for FCD of the hip have only recently received more attention with the increased use of open and arthroscopic hip preservation techniques.[1-4]

Oftentimes, FCDs are identified at the time of surgery to address labral injury and osteochondroplasty of the acetabulum and femoral head-neck junction. Depending on the size, location, and International Cartilage Repair Society (ICRS) grade, chondral injuries can be treated, for example, with arthroscopic debridement for partial-thickness lesions or arthroscopic microfracture for full-thickness lesions.

Ilizaliturri et al[5] developed a geographic zone method to describe intra-articular pathology, which was found to be more reproducible than the clock-face method.[6] Two vertical lines are drawn across the acetabulum in line with the anterior and posterior border of the acetabular notch. A horizontal line is drawn along the superior limit of the notch perpendicular to the vertical lines. The acetabulum is therefore divided into 6 zones. Numbers for each zone are assigned consecutively. Zone 1 is the anteroinferior acetabulum. The numbers increase around the notch. Zone 5 is assigned to the posteroinferior acetabulum. Zone 6 is the acetabular notch. The same method is applied to the femoral head.

Byrd JWT, Bedi A, Stubbs AJ, eds. *The Hip: AANA Advanced Arthroscopic Surgical Techniques* (pp 147-162). © 2016 AANA.

Table 12-1. Beck Classification of Cartilage Defects

0	Macroscopically normal cartilage
1	Malacia: roughening of surface, fibrillation
2	Pitting malacia: roughening, partially thinning, and full-thickness defects of deep fissuring to bone
3	Debonding: loss of fixation to subchondral bone, macroscopically sound cartilage (carpet phenomenon)
4	Cleavage: loss of fixation to subchondral bone, frayed edges, thinning of cartilage
5	Defect: full-thickness defect

Apart from the general ICRS grade and Outerbridge classification, Beck et al[7] developed a short and pragmatic system (Table 12-1). Sampson[4] proposed a more detailed system that is distinct for the acetabular and femoral sides, respectively.

There is a diverse etiology of cartilage damage in the hip, including trauma, femoroacetabular impingement (FAI), labral tears, hip dysplasia, slipped capital epiphysis, osteochondritis dissecans, loose bodies, osteonecrosis, and degenerative joint disease.[8-12] Early recognition of FCDs, particularly in younger patients, and management with joint-preserving techniques may slow down or ideally revert subsequent degenerative changes.

Advances in the understanding of the pathomechanism of FAI are helping to elucidate the etiology of cartilage damage in the hip. Cam deformities, in which the femoral head-neck junction has an abnormal protrusion causing impingement on the anterior acetabulum, have been shown to cause chondral damage to the anterior acetabulum near the rim in a fairly predictable and progressive manner.[11] Pincer deformity, in which a retroverted or deep acetabulum makes abnormal contact with the femoral neck, may result in chondral damage to the femur and a posteromedial acetabular contrecoup injury.[13,14] FAI frequently presents as a mixed form, with elements of cam and pincer impingement. As more information has been gathered through arthroscopy on the patterns of chondral injury in hips, new classification systems have recently been published. These attempt to grade acetabular chondral defects in a way that more accurately guides treatment.[15] Konan et al[16] found good intra- and interobserver validity of a classification system by Ilizaliturri et al[5] that divided the acetabulum into 6 anatomical zones with varying degrees of cartilage injury and location in each zone.

Some authors have reported that once cartilage injury has occurred, the cartilage will not show signs of improvement even after correction of the underlying osseous deformity. Second-look arthroscopy after pelvic osteotomies found no improvement in the majority of cases with regard to articular cartilage lesions present at the time of the index operation.[17] The current trend is to correct symptomatic hip pathomorphology in younger patients in an attempt to prevent irreversible chondrolabral injury and progression to advanced osteoarthritic changes. Labral tears occur in the setting of abnormal morphology with FAI and have been associated with the progression of osteoarthritis by increasing joint contact stress by up to 92%.[14] It has also been shown that most cartilage injuries of the hip are associated with a torn acetabular labrum.[8] The morphologic changes associated with FAI have been associated with being a major contributing factor to osteoarthritis in the hip and have also been reported to have a high association with patients younger than 50 years undergoing total hip arthroplasty.[16,18]

A variety of joint-preserving treatments options are available for chondral and osteochondral lesions of the hip. These include chondroplasty,[19,20] microfracture,[9-11,13,14,19] autologous chondrocyte transplantation (ACI) and matrix-induced ACI (MACI),[20-22] osteochondral autograft transplantation

(OATS) and mosaicplasty,[3,23-25] osteochondral allograft transplantation,[26,27] partial-resurfacing prostheses,[28] and suturing techniques,[19] as well as fixation with a fibrin adhesive for delamination lesions.[29,30] However, only chondroplasty, microfracture, and MACI have been applied to hip arthroscopy to a significant extent based on the current literature. Microfracture has most commonly been used for full-thickness cartilage lesions and requires intact subchondral bone on which a stable marrow clot can form.[13,19] Osteochondral autografts and allografts and mosaicplasty have been used for defects that involve a combination of cartilage and subchondral bone destruction[3,23,27]; however, these techniques required an open approach due to the limitations of hip arthroscopy.

ACI requires articular harvest of chondrocytes with subsequent cell culture expansion at an off-site facility. The cultivated and expanded chondrocytes are then implanted into the targeted chondral defect. There are few reports on the use of ACI in the hip, partially related to the fact that the field of hip arthroscopy is fairly young, but most likely also because harvesting arthroscopically in the hip is more challenging compared with the knee.

The initial ACI technique in the knee used a periosteal patch to contain the solution with the cultured chondrocytes injected into the defect. Subsequent to that, synthetic patches were developed and applied.[31-33] MACI is a newer technique based on the use of biodegradable 3-dimensional scaffolds for chondrocyte delivery. The benefits of that delivery system are twofold in that the chondrocyte phenotype more closely resembles the original articular cartilage matrix and chondrocytes and that no patches are needed to contain the cells in the defect.[20,22,32,33]

A multitude of treatment options are available for chondral defects in the hip; however, no clear evidence-based guidelines currently exist with regard to which technique should be applied for specific chondral defects. This chapter highlights arthroscopic microfracture but also includes cartilage repair, chondroplasty, and MACI. Some of the techniques described are experimental, particularly as they pertain to applications in the fairly new field of hip preservation surgery.

INDICATIONS

The indications have largely been derived from the knee literature because there is a lack of long-term outcomes data on the hip.

- Chondroplasty
  - ▷ Minimal signs of osteoarthritis (Tönnis grade ≤ 1)
  - ▷ Focal, well-contained lesion measuring less than 2 cm^2
  - ▷ Partial-thickness cartilage defects (ICRS grade 1 to 3) or loose flaps
- Microfracture
  - ▷ Minimal signs of osteoarthritis (Tönnis grade ≤ 1)
  - ▷ Focal, well-contained lesion measuring less than 4 cm^2
  - ▷ Full-thickness defects with intact subchondral bone
- MACI
  - ▷ Minimal signs of osteoarthritis (Tönnis grade ≤ 1)
  - ▷ Focal, well-contained lesion measuring 4 to 10 cm^2
  - ▷ Full-thickness defects with intact subchondral bone

Controversial Indications

Because there is a lack of long-term clinical outcomes data in the hip, all techniques and their respective indications presented in this chapter might be considered controversial. In the authors' view, however, all of the techniques presented are perhaps not so much controversial but rather cutting edge and less established. The authors will limit their discussion on what is available in the current literature.

Pertinent Physical Findings

Presentation

▶ Most patients with FCD also have evidence of FAI and become symptomatic when the labrum becomes injured.

▶ Patients with cam deformities have repetitive sheer stress across the anterosuperior acetabulum, which causes chondral delamination and chondrolabral separation.

▶ Patients with pincer deformities have intrasubstance injury to the labrum and injury to the posteromedial aspect of the acetabulum.[34]

▶ Patients with FCD are typically indistinguishable from patients with labral tears secondary to FAI.

▶ Typically, anterior groin pain may also radiate into the posterior gluteal region (C sign) or down the medial thigh.

▶ Patients have a baseline level of dull, achy pain that can become sharp with activities such as sitting, squatting, twisting or turning, getting in and out of a car, and recreational activities.

▶ Patients sometimes have a history of mechanical symptoms of catching and locking, which can be attributed to loose bodies or labral pathology.

Physical Examination

▶ As with any evaluation of hip pain, the focus is on differentiating potential intra- from extra-articular etiologies.

▶ Assess symmetry, gait, and active and passive range of motion (ROM) in combination with a neurologic and vascular assessment of the lower extremities.

▶ There are no distinct physical examination maneuvers that assess specifically for FCD.

▶ Although not specific to FCD, maneuvers for assessing intra-articular etiologies elicit positive findings.

▶ Intra-articular sources of hip pain, such as FAI or FCD, will likely have difficulty, pain, and decreased ROM in flexion and internal rotation compared with the opposite side.

▶ Anterior impingement test:
  ▷ The hip is dynamically brought into flexion, adduction, and internal rotation.
  ▷ Positive if the patient has reproducible groin pain with this movement.
  ▷ Typically signifies the presence of intra-articular pathology.

▶ Posterior impingement test:
  ▷ Hip extension and external rotation
  ▷ Can indicate a posteriorly located FCD
  ▷ Any reproducible signs of mechanical symptoms while taking the hip through ROM may indicate intra-articular loose bodies or delamination.

PERTINENT IMAGING

Plain X-Rays

The authors prefer to routinely obtain anteroposterior (AP) pelvis, false-profile, and Dunn lateral views of the hip for initial assessment.

Routine Radiographic Parameters

- Lateral center-edge angle (on AP)
- Tönnis angle (on AP)
- Alpha angle measured on all views

Magnetic Resonance Imaging

- Important for assessment of soft tissue and articular cartilage of the hip.
- T1- and T2-weighted images are useful for assessment of chondral surfaces of the acetabulum and femoral head.
- T2-weighted fat-suppressed images are helpful for identification of underlying subchondral marrow edema.

Magnetic Resonance Arthrogram

- Better for identifying articular cartilage or labral defects.
- Shown to accurately diagnose only 76% of acetabular labral tears and 62.7% of articular cartilage lesions when compared with arthroscopy.[17]
- Can be supplemented with diagnostic anesthetic joint injection during the magnetic resonance arthrogram procedure to help identify whether the origin of pain is intra- or extra-articular.[4]

Delayed Gadolinium-Enhanced Magnetic Resonance Imaging

- Potential to accurately diagnose FCDs in a noninvasive manner, but the gold standard remains direct visualization by arthroscopy.
- In general, advanced imaging is more reliable at detecting the severity of labral damage and less reliable at delineating the full extent of articular surface pathology for the clinician.

EQUIPMENT

Apart from the general hip arthroscopy equipment, specific instruments for the mentioned procedures include the following:

- Ringed and regular arthroscopic curettes
- Microfracture awls
- Microfracture drills
- Drill guides of varying angles (45, 70, and 90 degrees)
- Depth caps (4 to 7 mm) for the guide handle to allow for drilling to a predetermined depth

POSITIONING

The patient is placed in a supine position. Traction is used in combination with a well-padded perineal post. Fluoroscopy is used to confirm adequate portal position at the start of the procedure as well as for confirmation of adequate acetabular and femoral bone resection later on. The hip is distracted in neutral extension using adduction maneuvers.

STEP-BY-STEP DESCRIPTION OF THE PROCEDURE

Arthroscopic Evaluation of Focal Chondral Defects and Debridement

At the authors' institution, hip arthroscopy is performed with the patient in the supine position, utilizing traction, a well-padded perineal post, and fluoroscopy. The hip is distracted in neutral extension and adduction maneuvers. Typically, the following 3 portals are used for this procedure: anterolateral, mid-anterior, and distal accessory anterolateral (approximately 4 cm distal to antero-lateral portal). These portals are created in standard fashion using cannulated instruments (spinal needle, guidewire, and metal trocars). Once the portals are established, a diagnostic arthroscopy is performed with the use of a 70-degree arthroscope. Viewing through the anterolateral portal, the arthroscope is directed toward the ligamentum teres, and the adjacent articular surface is visualized in the anterior half of the acetabulum. The arthroscope can be slowly backed out to allow the peripheral aspect of the articular surface and labrum to be evaluated. Next, place the arthroscope in the mid-anterior portal to visualize the posterior half of the acetabulum, and use the same technique to visualize the entire articular surface. A thorough diagnostic evaluation of the articular cartilage surface is performed to identify and characterize the FCD.

The authors prefer to perform acetabular rim trimming and labral refixation before address-ing FCD. For partial-thickness cartilage defects (ICRS grade 1 to 3) or loose flaps, the goal is to create a stable surface and prevent the likelihood of loose cartilage bodies. The chondral surface is debrided with an arthroscopic shaver, and the authors prefer a curved shaver to assist in access-ing areas of the chondral surface that may be difficult to reach. Using the shaver through the mid-anterior portal may allow access to the anteromedial portion of the acetabulum, whereas the anterolateral portal may allow access to the posterolateral portion. To access femoral head lesions, additional portals may need to be created using a spinal needle to localize the exact location.

Microfracture Using Awls

Before proceeding to microfracture, the extent of the FCD needs to be assessed with a probe and documented accordingly. The decision to perform a microfracture is reserved for full-thick-ness cartilage defects (ICRS grade 4). Unstable segments are resected using an arthroscopic shaver. The base of the defect and the rim are carefully prepared using ringed curettes to create a clearly demarcated lesion with stable shoulders of surrounding intact articular cartilage. Vertical walls help contain the marrow clot and create a load-bearing transition zone. The location of the FCD may vary but is generally located in the anterosuperior quadrant of the hip joint. The chondral defect is measured with an arthroscopic probe to determine the length, width, and depth. Next, arthroscopic curettes are used to remove the calcified cartilage layer. Removal of the calcified layer affords better clot adhesion. Care is taken not to disrupt the underlying subchondral plate. Then, an arthroscopic awl is used in a perpendicular fashion to create several holes penetrating into the subchondral bone. Deep enough penetration into the subchondral bone allows pluripotent marrow cells and concomitant growth factors to fill into the chondral defect area with the goal of

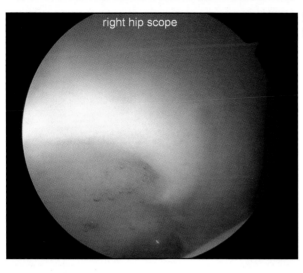
right hip scope

Figure 12-1. Wave sign in a right hip viewed from the anterolateral portal.

creating fibrocartilage healing. Bleeding from the holes should be seen and documented. This can be facilitated by stopping the water pump or decreasing the pump pressure.

Microfracture Using Arthroscopic Drilling

Following preparation of the FCD, a flexible arthroscopic microfracture drill is used to make multiple perforations in the exposed subchondral bone. Drill guides of varying angles (45, 70, and 90 degrees) are used to gain access to the lesion, but the authors prefer to use the 70-degree curved drill guide. Depth caps (4 to 7 mm) are assembled to the guide handle to allow for drilling to a predetermined depth. The authors' preferred depth is 7 mm to ensure adequate depth to penetrate the subchondral plate. The drill guide is placed against the surface of the lesion at a 90-degree angle. The hole is made by drilling through the drill guide continuously on full forward speed to a hard stop at the depth. After the hard stop, the drill is removed while continuing on full forward speed. Drill holes are first made around the periphery of the defect, adjacent to the healthy cartilage. Next, the defect is perforated with additional holes spaced approximately 3 to 4 mm from each other to avoid combining the holes. As irrigation pressure is decreased, fat and blood droplets should be observed exiting the drill holes.[35]

Addressing focal cartilage lesions with microfracture has been a well-established technique in the knee with good outcomes.[31,36,37] Clinical outcomes data on microfracture in the hip at this point are fairly limited, with no long-term data, small sample sizes, and lack of control groups.

Based on the current literature, microfracture appears to be a simple and effective treatment option for management of FCD in the hip in patients with minimal osteoarthritis and a focal, contained lesion smaller than 4 cm^2 in size.[9,36-43] However, further well-controlled and long-term outcomes studies are necessary for evidence-based recommendations on its effectiveness.

Articular Cartilage Repair

Cartilage delamination is observed during arthroscopy in the form of a positive wave sign (Figure 12-1) and can represent a full-thickness[42] or partial-thickness separation from the subchondral bone frequently associated with anterosuperior labral tears and FAI. When there is only a partial-thickness chondral lesion, this can be managed by simple chondroplasty. With full-thickness delaminations, however, the delaminated cartilage can be resected, resulting in exposure of the underlying subchondral bone. Lesions less than 3 cm^2 can be addressed with microfracture.[43] Lesions larger than 3 cm^2 are more difficult to manage. There are reports of attempted repairs

Figure 12-2. Anchor placement in a right hip viewed from the mid-anterior portal.

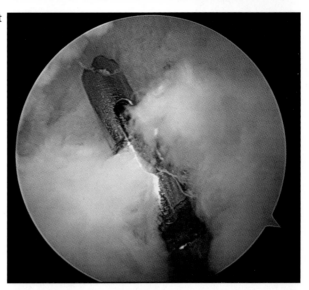

Figure 12-3. Tissue-penetrating device inserted adjacent to the rim in a right hip viewed from the mid-anterior portal.

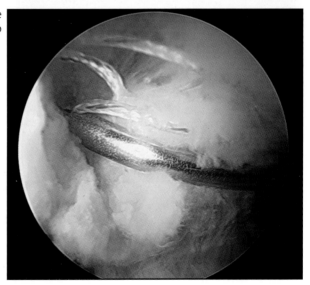

of unstable but healthy-appearing delaminated cartilage using fibrin adhesives or fixation with sutures or fibrin adhesive.[29,30]

The authors' preferred technique to address cartilage delamination is to incorporate the delaminated cartilage flap into the labral repair. After preparation of the chondrolabral junction and of the acetabular rim with a shaver and burr, single-loaded anchors are placed in the usual fashion close to the chondrolabral junction (Figure 12-2). The initial anchor is placed at the lateral extent of the chondrolabral injury while viewing from the mid-anterior portal, and the drill guide is used through the anterolateral portal. The authors prefer to use 1.4-mm suture anchors to allow placement as close to the articular cartilage surface as possible without penetrating the articular surface. Once the anchor is secured within the bone tunnel, a tissue-penetrating device is used to grasp one suture limb and is passed through the delaminated full-thickness cartilage distal to the labrum to incorporate the delaminated cartilage into the labral repair (Figure 12-3). Next, the tissue-penetrating device is passed through the widest portion of the labrum and is used to retrieve the suture. The mattress stitches are tied using reverse half hitches and alternating posts to secure

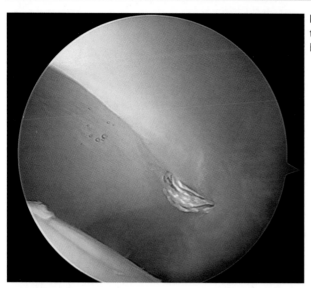

Figure 12-4. Mattress stitch incorporating the area of cartilage delamination in a right hip viewed from the mid-anterior portal.

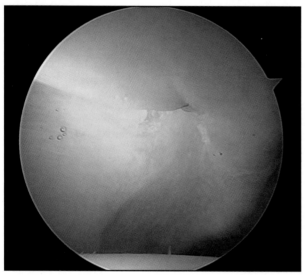

Figure 12-5. Chondrolabral refixation of the posterolateral rim in a right hip viewed from the mid-anterior portal.

the knot (Figures 12-4 and 12-5). The arthroscope is placed in the anterolateral portal, the drill guide is placed through the distal accessory anterolateral portal to place the anterior anchors, and a plastic cannula is placed through the mid-anterior portal. Once the suture anchor is secured, a tissue-penetrating device is placed through the mid-anterior portal and is used to penetrate just adjacent to the acetabular rim to ensure that the delaminated cartilage can be incorporated. The suture is retrieved after piercing the widest portion of the labrum to create a mattress stitch configuration when possible (Figure 12-6). If the labral tissue is hypotrophic or degenerative, a simple stitch configuration can be used. The authors typically do not perform concomitant microfracture; however, there have been anecdotal reports of microdrills being used for microfracture through the delaminated cartilage.

Based on the current literature, repair of delaminated articular cartilage in the hip with suture repair in combination with microfracture and/or fibrin adhesive appears to be feasible only for small lesions of focal delamination of otherwise healthy-appearing cartilage.[29,30,43] The fibrin adhesive used in these studies is not currently approved for use in the United States.

Figure 12-6. Chondrolabral refixation of the anteromedial rim in a right hip viewed from the anterolateral portal.

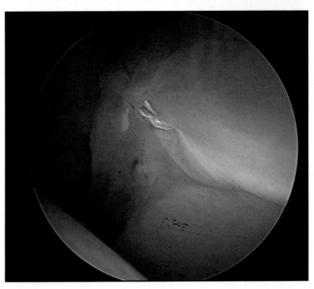

Matrix-Induced Autologous Chondrocyte Transplantation

Because the authors have not performed arthroscopic MACI in the hip, they present the technique described by Fontana.[22] The first step encompasses diagnostic arthroscopy and obtaining a cartilage biopsy specimen from the area surrounding the pulvinar. The cells are then sent to a cell-processing facility for chondrocyte culture expansion. Details of cell culture techniques and their durations, as well as matrices and scaffolds, vary by manufacturer.

The second step is arthroscopic implantation of the culture-expanded chondrocytes in the scaffold after approximately 30 days. First, the FCD is debrided using angled curettes or motorized shavers to the level of subchondral bone. Clear margins with vertical walls are created.

The scaffold membrane with the chondrocytes is cut to exactly fit the chondral defect after this has been prepared and is then rolled to pass through a cannula. The transplant is inserted directly into the joint through an arthroscopic cannula and is applied to the chondral defect. After the implant has been positioned, traction is released and the hip taken through ROM 5 times. Traction is then reapplied to verify arthroscopically under dry conditions that the transplant has not been dislodged.

Postoperatively, patients follow a standard rehabilitation program. Exercises begin the first postoperative day with the goal of quickly regaining full active and passive ROM. Continuous passive motion (CPM) devices are typically not used. Patients are kept nonweight bearing for 4 weeks and are then transitioned to partial weight bearing with the goal of full weight bearing without crutches at 7 weeks. The use of a stationary bike and swimming are recommended after 4 weeks. Running is allowed only after 6 months, whereas a typical complete return to sports is only recommended 1 year postoperatively.

POSTOPERATIVE PROTOCOLS

Microfracture

For postoperative rehabilitation after microfracture, the authors typically apply the following standard protocol, including the use of CPM:

Weeks 0 to 6

- ► Strict touch-down weight bearing with crutches
- ► No brace
- ► CPM 6 to 8 hours/day: Set at 1 cycle/minute. Begin at comfortable flexion and advance 10 degrees daily to full ROM
- ► Quadriceps strengthening, patellar mobilization

Weeks 6 to 8

- ► Advance to full weight bearing as tolerated (WBAT) by 8 weeks
- ► Discontinue crutches when gait normalizes
- ► Begin active ROM exercises as tolerated
- ► Straight-leg raise exercises, closed-chain quadriceps strengthening

Weeks 8 to 12

- ► Full WBAT
- ► Progressive strengthening
- ► Begin stationary bike

Weeks 12+

- ► Begin jogging and advance to running
- ► Progressive active strengthening
- ► Begin sports-specific exercises

Week 16

- ► Return to all activities, including cutting/pivoting sports

Chondroplasty and Cartilage Repair

For postoperative rehabilitation after chondroplasty or incorporation of the delaminated cartilage into the labral repair, the authors use the following standard rehabilitation protocol after labral repair. In cases in which microfracture was also performed, the authors apply the rehabilitation protocol previously described.

Weeks 0 to 3

- ► Foot-flat weight bearing, ROM (flexion limited to 90 degrees and abduction limited to 30 degrees for 2 weeks), and manual therapy
- ► CPM for 4 hours/day
- ► Gait training foot-flat weight bearing with bilateral crutches
- ► Bike (20-minute intervals, up to 2 times daily)
- ► Decrease CPM time by 1 hour for every 20 minutes biked
- ► Soft tissue mobilization
- ► Hip passive ROM within postoperative restrictions
- ► Modalities as indicated
- ► Muscle activation

Weeks 3 to 6

Weight Bearing and Range of Motion

- ▶ Progress weight bearing to WBAT (if no microfracture)
  - ▷ Wean off crutches (2 to 1 to 0)
- ▶ Progress with hip ROM as tolerated (maintain postoperative restrictions)
- ▶ Manual therapy
  - ▷ Deep tissue mobilization
- ▶ Muscle activation and neuromuscular reeducation
- ▶ Progress core strengthening (avoid hip flexor tendonitis)
- ▶ Progress with hip strengthening
- ▶ Bike progress time 5 minutes/week
- ▶ Aquatherapy (at week 3: 25% of body weight)

Weeks 6 to 9

Weight Bearing and Range of Motion

- ▶ Restore symmetrical ROM
- ▶ Restore normal reciprocal gait pattern
- ▶ Hip flexor and iliotibial band stretching (manual and self)
- ▶ Manual therapy:
  - ▷ Advance soft tissue mobilization as indicated to hip/pelvis and lumbar spine
  - ▷ Restore normal hip/pelvis/lumbar spine kinematics
- ▶ Advanced neuromuscular reeducation
- ▶ Progress core strengthening as tolerated (avoid hip flexor tendonitis)
- ▶ Progress hip strengthening
  - ▷ Progress closed-chain hip and pelvic stability and strengthening
  - ▷ Avoid plyometric and impact activities
- ▶ Cardiovascular/aerobic training
  - ▷ Advance bike as tolerated
  - ▷ Begin elliptical trainer
  - ▷ Begin stair climbing (avoid anterior hip pain/irritation)
  - ▷ Begin treadmill walking program as tolerated

Weeks 9 to 12

- ▶ Restore symmetrical hip ROM and pelvic mobility
- ▶ Progressive hip ROM to restore symmetry
- ▶ End-range stretching
- ▶ Manual therapy
  - ▷ Restore normal kinematics of the hip, pelvis, and lumbar spine
  - ▷ Advanced neuromusclar reeducation
  - ▷ Progressive lower extremity and core strengthening as tolerated

- ▷ Sport-specific core and lower extremity strength training
- ▷ Advanced balance proprioceptive training as tolerated
- ► Cardiovascular/aerobic training
  - ▷ Bike as tolerated
  - ▷ Elliptical as tolerated
  - ▷ Stair climbing as tolerated
  - ▷ Swimming as tolerated

Weeks 12 to 16

Cardiovascular/Aerobic Training

- ► Advanced as tolerated within running and sport-specific restrictions

Sport-Specific Training/Advanced Functional Training

- ► Initiate plyometrics training
- ► Begin running progression
- ► Sport-specific agility drills

Matrix-Induced Autologous Chondrocyte Transplantation

Based on the technique described by Fontana,[22] patients follow a standard rehabilitation program.

- ► The goal is to quickly regain full active and passive ROM.
- ► CPM is typically not used.
- ► Patients are kept nonweight bearing for 4 weeks.
- ► Transition to partial weight bearing with the goal of full weight bearing without crutches at 7 weeks.
- ► Use of a stationary bike and swimming after 4 weeks.
- ► Running after 6 months.
- ► Typically, a complete return to sports is only recommended at 1 year.

POTENTIAL COMPLICATIONS

Apart from the general potential complications associated with hip arthroscopy, the potential complications specific to the mentioned cartilage procedures include progressive delamination after repair, lack of fibrocartilage healing response after microfracture, dislodging of the MACI scaffold, recurrent cartilage defects, and generalized degeneration of the hip joint progressing from an FCD.

Top Technical Pearls for the Procedure

1. The authors prefer to perform acetabular rim trimming and labral refixation before addressing FCDs.

2. For partial-thickness cartilage defects (ICRS grade 1 to 3) or loose flaps, the goal is to create a stable surface to minimize the likelihood of loose cartilage bodies.

3. The chondral surface is debrided with an arthroscopic shaver, and stable shoulders are created with a meniscal biter and ring curette. The authors prefer a curved shaver to assist in accessing areas of the chondral surface that may be difficult to reach.

4. Using the shaver through the mid-anterior portal allows access to the anteromedial portion of the acetabulum, whereas the anterolateral portal allows access to the posterolateral portion. The anterolateral or distal accessory anterolateral portals can be used to access the anterosuperior aspect of the acetabulum.

5. To access femoral head lesions, additional portals may need to be created using a spinal needle to facilitate localization of the exact location.

References

1. Jordan MA, Van Thiel GS, Chahal J, Nho SJ. Operative treatment of chondral defects in the hip joint: a systematic review. *Curr Rev Musculoskelet Med.* 22012;5(3):244-253.
2. El Bitar YF, Lindner D, Jackson TJ, Domb BG. Joint-preserving surgical options for management of chondral injuries of the hip. *J Am Acad Orthop Surg.* 2014;22(1):46-56.
3. Girard J, Roumazeille T, Sakr M, Migaud H. Osteochondral mosaicplasty of the femoral head. *Hip Int.* 2011;21(5):542-548.
4. Sampson TG. Arthroscopic treatment for chondral lesions of the hip. *Clin Sports Med.* 2011;30(2):331-348.
5. Ilizaliturri VM Jr, Byrd JW, Sampson TG, et al. A geographic zone method to describe intra-articular pathology in hip arthroscopy: cadaveric study and preliminary report. *Arthroscopy.* 2008;24(5):534-539.
6. Philippon MJ, Stubbs AJ, Schenker ML, Maxwell RB, Ganz R, Leunig M. Arthroscopic management of femoroacetabular impingement: osteoplasty technique and literature review. *Am J Sports Med.* 2007;35(9):1571-1580.
7. Beck M, Leunig M, Parvizi J, Boutier V, Wyss D, Ganz R. Anterior femoroacetabular impingement: part II. Midterm results of surgical treatment. *Clin Orthop Relat Res.* 2004;(418):67-73.
8. McCarthy JC, Lee JA. Arthroscopic intervention in early hip disease. *Clin Orthop Relat Res.* 2004;(429):157-162.
9. Philippon MJ, Schenker ML, Briggs KK, Maxwell RB. Can microfracture produce repair tissue in acetabular chondral defects? *Arthroscopy.* 2008;24(1):46-50.
10. Guanche CA, Sikka RS. Acetabular labral tears with underlying chondromalacia: a possible association with high-level running. *Arthroscopy.* 2005;21(5):580-585.
11. Beck M, Kalhor M, Leunig M, Ganz R. Hip morphology influences the pattern of damage to the acetabular cartilage: femoroacetabular impingement as a cause of early osteoarthritis of the hip. *J Bone Joint Surg Br.* 2005;87(7):1012-1018.
12. Reijman M, Hazes JM, Pols HA, Koes BW, Bierma-Zeinstra SM. Acetabular dysplasia predicts incident osteoarthritis of the hip: the Rotterdam study. *Arthritis Rheum.* 2005;52(3):787-793.
13. Crawford K, Philippon MJ, Sekiya JK, Rodkey WG, Steadman JR. Microfracture of the hip in athletes. *Clin Sports Med.* 2006;25(2):327-335.
14. Ellis HB, Briggs KK, Philippon MJ. Innovation in hip arthroscopy: is hip arthritis preventable in the athlete? *Br J Sports Med.* 2011;45(4):253-258.
15. Stubbs AJ, Potter HG. Section VII: chondral lesions. *J Bone Joint Surg Am.* 2009;91 suppl 1:119.

16. Konan S, Rayan F, Meermans G, Witt J, Haddad FS. Validation of the classification system for acetabular chondral lesions identified at arthroscopy in patients with femoroacetabular impingement. *J Bone Joint Surg Br.* 2011;93(3):332-336.

17. Keeney JA, Peelle MW, Jackson J, Rubin D, Maloney WJ, Clohisy JC. Magnetic resonance arthrography versus arthroscopy in the evaluation of articular hip pathology. *Clin Orthop Relat Res.* 2004;(429):163-169.

18. Van Thiel GS, Harris JD, Kang RW, et al. Age-related differences in radiographic parameters for femoroacetabular impingement in hip arthroplasty patients. *Arthroscopy.* 2013;29(7):1182-1187.

19. Yen YM, Kocher MS. Chondral lesions of the hip: microfracture and chondroplasty. *Sports Med Arthrosc.* 2010;18:83-89.

20. Fontana A, Bistolfi A, Crova M, Rosso F, Massazza G. Arthroscopic treatment of hip chondral defects: autologous chondrocyte transplantation versus simple debridement—a pilot study. *Arthroscopy.* 2012;28(3):322-329.

21. Akimau P, Bhosale A, Harrison PE, et al. Autologous chondrocyte implantation with bone grafting for osteochondral defect due to posttraumatic osteonecrosis of the hip—a case report. *Acta Orthop.* 2006;77(2):333-336.

22. Fontana A. A novel technique for treating cartilage defects in the hip: a fully arthroscopic approach to using autologous matrix-induced chondrogenesis. *Arthrosc Tech.* 2012;1(1):e63-e68.

23. Nam D, Shindle MK, Buly RL, Kelly BT, Lorich DG. Traumatic osteochondral injury of the femoral head treated by mosaicplasty: a report of two cases. *HSS J.* 2010;6(2):228-234.

24. Hart R, Janecek M, Visna P, Bucek P, Kocis J. Mosaicplasty for the treatment of femoral head defect after incorrect resorbable screw insertion. *Arthroscopy.* 2003;19(10):E1-E5.

25. Sotereanos NG, DeMeo PJ, Hughes TB, Bargiotas K, Wohlrab D. Autogenous osteochondral transfer in the femoral head after osteonecrosis. *Orthopedics.* 2008;31(2):177.

26. Meyers MH. Resurfacing of the femoral head with fresh osteochondral allografts: long-term results. *Clin Orthop Relat Res.* 1985;(197):111-114.

27. Krych AJ, Lorich DG, Kelly BT. Treatment of focal osteochondral defects of the acetabulum with osteochondral allograft transplantation. *Orthopedics.* 2011;34(7):e307-e311.

28. Van Stralen RA, Haverkamp D, Van Bergen CJ, Eijer H. Partial resurfacing with varus osteotomy for an osteochondral defect of the femoral head. *Hip Int.* 2009;19(1):67-70.

29. Stafford GH, Bunn JR, Villar RN. Arthroscopic repair of delaminated acetabular articular cartilage using fibrin adhesive. Results at one to three years. *Hip Int.* 2011;21(6):744-750.

30. Tzaveas AP, Villar RN. Arthroscopic repair of acetabular chondral delamination with fibrin adhesive. *Hip Int.* 2010;20(1):115-119.

31. Knutsen G, Drogset JO, Engebretsen L, et al. A randomized trial comparing autologous chondrocyte implantation with microfracture. Findings at five years. *J Bone Joint Surg Am.* 2007;89(10):2105-2112.

32. Bartlett W, Skinner JA, Gooding CR, et al. Autologous chondrocyte implantation versus matrix-induced autologous chondrocyte implantation for osteochondral defects of the knee: a prospective, randomised study. *J Bone Joint Surg Br.* 2005;87(5):640-645.

33. Zeifang F, Oberle D, Nierhoff C, Richter W, Moradi B, Schmitt H. Autologous chondrocyte implantation using the original periosteum-cover technique versus matrix-associated autologous chondrocyte implantation: a randomized clinical trial. *Am J Sports Med.* 2010;38(5):924-933.

34. Beck M, Kalhor M, Leunig M, Ganz R. Hip morphology influences the pattern of damage to the acetabular cartilage: femoroacetabular impingement as a cause of early osteoarthritis of the hip. *J Bone Joint Surg Br.* 2005;87(7):1012-1018.

35. Haughom, BD, Erickson BJ, Rybalko D, Hellman M, Nho SJ. Arthroscopic acetabular microfracture with the use of flexible drills: a technique guide. *Arthrosc Tech.* 2014;3(4):e459-e463.

36. Steadman JR, Briggs KK, Rodrigo JJ, Kocher MS, Gill TJ, Rodkey WG. Outcomes of microfracture for traumatic chondral defects of the knee: average 11-year follow-up. *Arthroscopy.* 2003;19(5):477-484.

37. Gudas R, Gudaite A, Pocius A, et al. Ten-year follow-up of a prospective, randomized clinical study of mosaic osteochondral autologous transplantation versus microfracture for the treatment of osteochondral defects in the knee joint of athletes. *Am J Sports Med.* 2012;40(11):2499-2508.

38. Karthikeyan S, Roberts S, Griffin D. Microfracture for acetabular chondral defects in patients with femoroacetabular impingement: results at second-look arthroscopic surgery. *Am J Sports Med.* 2012;40(12):2725-2730.

39. Byrd JW, Jones KS. Osteoarthritis caused by an inverted acetabular labrum: radiographic diagnosis and arthroscopic treatment. *Arthroscopy.* 2002;18(7):741-747.
40. Haviv B, Singh PJ, Takla A, O'Donnell J. Arthroscopic femoral osteochondroplasty for cam lesions with isolated acetabular chondral damage. *J Bone Joint Surg Br.* 2010;92(5):629-633.
41. Byrd JW, Jones KS. Arthroscopic femoroplasty in the management of cam-type femoroacetabular impingement. *Clin Orthop Relat Res.* 2009;467(3):739-746.
42. Horisberger M, Brunner A, Herzog RF. Arthroscopic treatment of femoral acetabular impingement in patients with preoperative generalized degenerative changes. *Arthroscopy.* 2010;26(5):623-629.
43. Sekiya JK, Martin RL, Lesniak BP. Arthroscopic repair of delaminated acetabular articular cartilage in femoroacetabular impingement. *Orthopedics.* 2009;32(9).

Please see videos on the accompanying website at

www.ArthroscopicTechniques.com

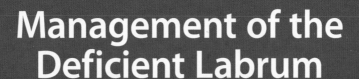

Management of the Deficient Labrum

Arthroscopic Labral Reconstruction— Indications and Technique

Christiano A. C. Trindade, MD and Marc J. Philippon, MD

INTRODUCTION

Recently, hip pathologies have become better understood. The hip labrum has a main role in joint biomechanics.[1] It is responsible for hip stability and synovial fluid hydrodynamics, as well as nociception and proprioception. The labrum is a triangular fibrocartilaginous structure with an inner two-thirds avascular portion.[2] The labrum increases acetabular contact surface area and, therefore, the acetabular volume.[3]

The hip fluid seal provided by the labrum is key to intra-articular fluid pressurization and stability through the suction effect.[4] The intra-articular fluid pressurization (IAFP) is responsible for protecting the cartilage matrix from loads passing through the joint and reducing friction between the articular surfaces. The stability during distraction and lateral translation of the femoral head are limited in part by the suction effect through negative intra-articular pressure.

In a recent biomechanical study,[5] the labrum was tested in various situations, and the IAFP was measured. Labral repair and labral reconstruction were simulated, and the IAFP was brought back to the level of the intact labrum. In the second part of this study,[6] it was determined that the labrum is a primary stabilizer to distractive forces at small displacements (1 to 2 mm).

Large unrepaired lesions of the labrum disrupt the seal and alter the biomechanics of the hip, leading to delamination of the cartilage and thus to early arthrosis of the joint.[3] Studies have demonstrated better outcomes in primary hip arthroscopy when labral repair is done instead of debridement of the labral tissue.[7]

This has led to a general consensus that labral tissue should be preserved whenever possible. If the repair is not feasible, reconstruction is indicated in an attempt to keep the biomechanical characteristics of the articulation. Several techniques have been described. Allografts and autograft can be used, and techniques have been described for open[8,9] or arthroscopic techiques.[10] The source of grafts include iliotibial band (ITB), gracilis tendon,[11] semitendinosus,[3] quadriceps tendon,[12]

Byrd JWT, Bedi A, Stubbs AJ, eds. *The Hip: AANA Advanced Arthroscopic Surgical Techniques* (pp 163-171). © 2016 AANA.

Figure 13-1. Complex tear of the labrum, unlikely to be reparable.

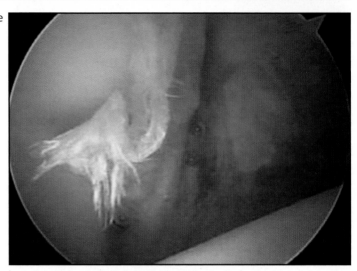

and ligamentum teres,[13] among others. Allograft techniques using tibialis anterior[14] and ITB and hamstring tendon[15] have also been described. The authors' preferred technqiue is arthroscopic ITB autograft. When a large graft is needed, allograft is used.

INDICATIONS

▶ The labrum cannot be repaired due to a complex tear (Figure 13-1) or if there is inadequate labral tissue (generally less than 5 mm in width), characterized by an anatomical variation or degeneration.

▶ Primary arthroscopies and revision cases.[1,8]

▶ In revisions, due to prior debridement or capsulolabral adhesions,[16] resulting in a thin or absent labrum. Preferably, the patient should be young and active, with a desire to return to sports.[17]

▶ Joint space should be at least 2 mm.

▶ More rarely, in cases of coxa profunda, labral reconstruction can also be indicated after circumferencial resection of acetabular bone.[15]

PERTINENT PHYSICAL FINDINGS

Physical examination should be thorough, including palpation, range of motion (ROM), and specific tests.

▶ Anterior groin pain and present positive tests for femoroacetabular impingement (flexion, adduction, and internal rotation) if any bony pathology is unaddressed.

▶ Flexion, abduction, and external rotation distance test[16] (Figure 13-2) can be positive in cases of unilateral pathology, indicating limitation of internal rotation.

▶ Possible signs of instability in the absence of generalized laxity; in those cases, the dial test and maneuvers for anterior apprehension can be positive.[18]

▶ Other symptoms may be clicking, locking, catching, giving way, and stiffness.

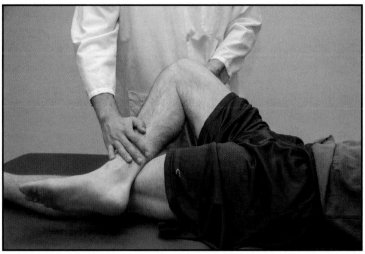

Figure 13-2. Flexion, abduction, and external rotation distance test in the supine position. The leg is flexed, and the heel of the affected leg is placed on the contralateral knee just above the patella. The distance from the lateral femoral epicondyle of the knee to the examination table is measured while stabilizing the pelvis. A positive test is defined as greater than 3-cm difference between the sides.[16]

PERTINENT IMAGING

An adequate preoperative radiographic evaluation is crucial. Bony morphological alterations, such as femoroacetabular impingement, are detected and must be addressed to protect the graft.

- ▶ X-rays
  - ▷ Supine anteroposterior pelvis view to determine the joint space and lateral center-edge angle.
  - ▷ Cross-table lateral view to evaluate the alpha angle.
  - ▷ False-profile view to determine acetabular overcoverage and compare with observations of the anteroposterior view, including the crossover sign and posterior wall sign.[19]
- ▶ Magnetic resonance imaging can be used to evaluate the alpha angle, cartilage surfaces, adhesions, and status of the labrum.
- ▶ Computed tomography scan can be useful to facilitate the detection of an incomplete femoral osteoplasty; however, these are performed on only select patients.

EQUIPMENT

For this procedure, the standard equipment for hip arthroscopy is used, including a 70-degree arthroscope. For graft preparation, absorbable and synthetic sutures are used, including #2 and 2-0 Vicryl (Ethicon) sutures. For easy handling, the graft is positioned on a Graftmaster table (Smith & Nephew).

POSITIONING

The patient is positioned in the modified supine position (10 degrees of flexion, 15 degrees of internal rotation, 10 degrees of lateral tilt, and neutral abduction).

STEP-BY-STEP DESCRIPTION OF THE PROCEDURE

The procedure is conducted under complete muscular paralysis, and the perineum is protected with a padded bolster. Manual table traction is applied to the operative hip, and countertraction is applied to the other side. Traction is carefully increased until the vacuum sign is evident.[8] The operative leg is adducted to neutral and the foot internally rotated so the femoral neck is parallel to the ground.

The anterolateral and mid-anterior arthroscopic portals are used. An interportal capsulotomy is performed to ensure good visualization in the joint and access to all areas of the joint. A detailed inspection of the central compartment is performed to look for labral tears and other conditions such as chondral defects, ligamentum teres injuries, and bony impingement. A dynamic examination is performed to determine if the labrum provides a seal with the femoral head. If an irreparable labrum is found, with an inadequate seal, the defect is measured using a 5.5-mm shaver to estimate the size of the graft. At this time, acetabular bony preparation is completed using a motorized shaver and burr. Pincer, cam, and subspinal impingements are resected as indicated. A bleeding cancellous bony bed along the acetabular rim is desired for proper integration of the graft.

Traction is released, and the lower extremity is extended and internally rotated. A longitudinal incision of approximately 8 cm is made just distal to the anterolateral portal. It is located over the greater trochanter at the junction of the anterior two-thirds and posterior one-third of the ITB. The ITB is cleaned of any fat tissue in situ using a Cobb elevator, and a rectangle section of tissue is cut. The length of the autograft is adjusted to the defect size, and an additional 30% to 40% of tissue is harvested to ensure the graft will not be too small. The typical width of the graft is between 15 and 20 mm. The defect created in the ITB is closed using #0 Vicryl, and the remaining harvest site incision is closed in layers.

On the back table, the graft is cleared of any soft tissue and kept moist. The ends of the graft are captured with hanging sutures using #2 Vicryl that are attached to the Graftmaster (Figure 13-3). These sutures at the end of the graft must be durable to diminish the risk of suture pullout from the graft ends during fixation. The graft is tubularized with 2-0 Vicryl. The thickest part of the graft is considered its lateral end and, at this part, a loop of suture (Figure 13-4) is placed with a #2 Vicryl suture. The loop will help to facilitate intra-articular control of the graft and its fixation. The graft is measured again to reassure that it is appropriately sized. It should provide a tubular structure with an about 7-mm width and enough length to replace the deficient labrum. The graft is then filled with 4 mL of platelet-rich plasma to enhance cellular healing.

When the graft is ready, traction is reestablished. A suture anchor is placed in the medialmost aspect and in the lateralmost aspect of the labral defect. While drilling the path of the anchor, it is critical to visualize the articular surface of the acetabulum to ensure that the articular surface is not being compromised. The anchor should be placed close to the acetabular rim. The graft is transfixed at its medial portion with one of the suture limbs of the medial anchor and is advanced into the joint through the mid-anterior portal. The other limb of the suture should join the native reminiscent anterior labrum if existent. The graft is then placed into position by a sliding knot and fixed. The procedure is repeated to fix the lateral end of the graft, using the suture loop to aid in control. Sequentially, additional anchors are placed separated by 1.0 to 1.5 cm to fix the graft to the acetabular rim, as is routinely done to repair labral tears (Figure 13-5). After an adequate fixation of the graft, it should simulate the native labrum. If coexisting chondral injury must be addressed, microfracture should be performed on completion of labral reconstruction.

Traction is released, and the reconstruction is evaluated dynamically in all planes of motion to assess the fixation and position of the graft. The reconstructed labrum must provide a seal with the femoral head. Additional femoral osteoplasty and suture anchor fixation may be necessary. A flexible radiofrequency probe can be used to remove frayed edges of the native labrum and the graft itself to ensure a smooth movement in the hip joint (Figure 13-6).

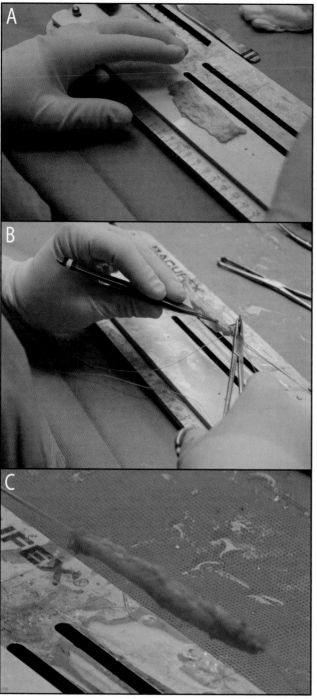

Figure 13-3. Iliotibial band graft preparation. (A) Following harvest of the graft, fat and other tissue is removed and is cut to size based on the defect. (B) The graft is tubularized using 2-0 absorbable synthetic suture. (C) Tubularized graft.

At the end of the procedure, the capsule is closed to maintain the stability of the hip joint. In cases of capsular laxity, a capsular plication is preferred. More rarely, severe capsular defects may exist due to capsulotomies not properly closed previously, and capsular reconstruction can be performed at this time.

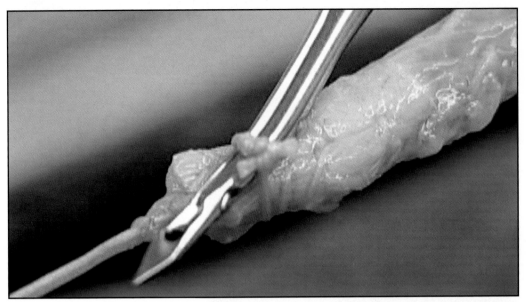

Figure 13-4. Loop made at the lateral end of the tubularized graft using a #2 absorbable synthetic suture.

Figure 13-5. Adequate positioning of the graft on the acetabular rim.

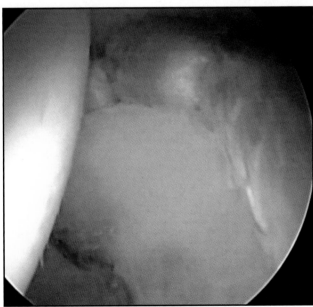

POSTOPERATIVE PROTOCOL

After labral reconstruction, a postoperative protocol similar to the labral repair protocol is initiated. The rehabilitation is divided into 3 phases. The first involves ROM and protection. The objectives are to protect surgical repair, diminish pain and swelling, restore ROM within restrictions, and relearn muscle activation. Patients are encouraged to begin no-resistance stationary biking within 4 hours postoperatively.

In the second phase, the patient should return to walking normally and restore the ability to ascend and descend stairs. The patient is advised to be 20-lb partial weight bearing and use 4 to

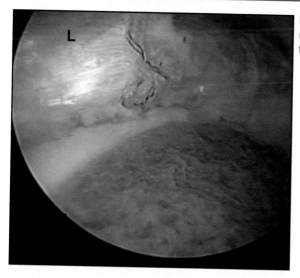

Figure 13-6. View of the completed labral reconstruction (L) providing a seal with the femoral head.

6 hours per day of continuous passive motion (CPM) for 2 weeks. A brace is used to restrict extension and abduction, and an antirotation cushion is used for hip external rotation control. Both are used for 14 to 21 days postoperatively.

To prevent hip flexor contractures while using CPM machines, patients are recommended to lay prone for 2 hours per day. When microfracture is performed to treat associated chondral lesions, patients are kept partial weight bearing and using CPM machines for a longer period, usually about 8 weeks.

In the last phase, the patient begins to gain strength and muscular endurance. The goals are to restore full ROM in all planes, build muscle strength and endurance, improve core and pelvic stability, and incorporate functional strengthening as cleared by the senior author.

In summary, the first goal of physical therapy is to restore passive followed by active motion and then strength. It is essential for the patients to perform passive circumduction motions (Figure 13-7) of the hip as soon after arthroscopy as possible to prevent capsular adhesions. Each patient is prescribed an individual protocol based on the other procedures done at arthroscopy and the patient's goals.

POTENTIAL COMPLICATIONS

Complications are rare and can include adhesions, infection, muscle hernia, and pain at the donor site.[9] These complications can be avoided with proper aseptic techniques, accurate closure of the defect in the fascia, and an appropriate rehabilitation process, including circumduction exercises.

Figure 13-7. Circumduction exercises are key to prevent adhesions.

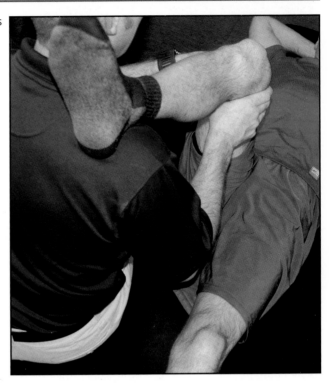

TOP TECHNICAL PEARLS FOR THE PROCEDURE

1. Adequate treatment of underlying pathologies of the joint is required to protect the graft from injury.
2. Precise measurement of the graft and precise positioning on the rim are critical for recovering the seal effect.
3. Start fixation of the graft medial on the acetabular rim and then go lateral.
4. Make a loop at the lateral side of the graft with a #2 Vicryl suture.
5. An appropriate rehabilitation process with circumduction exercises is necessary to prevent adhesions.

REFERENCES

1. Ayeni OR, Alradwan H, de Sa D, Philippon MJ. The hip labrum reconstruction: indications and outcomes—a systematic review. *Knee Surg Sports Traumatol Arthrosc.* 2014;22(4):737-743.
2. Ejnisman L, Philippon MJ, Lertwanich P. Acetabular labral tears: diagnosis, repair, and a method for labral reconstruction. *Clin Sports Med.* 2011;30(2):317-329.
3. Domb BG, El Bitar YF, Stake CE, Trenga AP, Jackson TJ, Lindner D. Arthroscopic labral reconstruction is superior to segmental resection for irreparable labral tears in the hip: a matched-pair controlled study with minimum 2-year follow-up. *Am J Sports Med.* 2014;42(1):122-130.
4. Dwyer MK, Jones HL, Hogan MG, Field RE, McCarthy JC, Noble PC. The acetabular labrum regulates fluid circulation of the hip joint during functional activities. *Am J Sports Med.* 2014;42(4):812-819.

5. Philippon MJ, Nepple JJ, Campbell KJ, et al. The hip fluid seal—part I: the effect of an acetabular labral tear, repair, resection, and reconstruction on hip fluid pressurization. *Knee Surg Sports Traumatol Arthrosc.* 2014;22(4):722-729.

6. Nepple JJ, Philippon MJ, Campbell KJ, et al. The hip fluid seal—part II: the effect of an acetabular labral tear, repair, resection, and reconstruction on hip stability to distraction. *Knee Surg Sports Traumatol Arthrosc.* 2014;22(4):730-736.

7. Skendzel JG, Philippon MJ. Management of labral tears of the hip in young patients. *Orthop Clin North Am.* 2013;44(4):477-487.

8. Ejnisman L, Philippon MJ. Arthroscopic labral reconstruction in the hip using iliotibial band autograft. *Oper Tech Sports Med.* 2011;19:134-139.

9. Philippon MJ, Briggs KK, Hay CJ, Kuppersmith DA, Dewing CB, Huang MJ. Arthroscopic labral reconstruction in the hip using iliotibial band autograft: technique and early outcomes. *Arthroscopy.* 2010;26(6):750-756.

10. Deshmane PP, Kahlenberg CA, Patel RM, Han B, Terry MA. All-arthroscopic iliotibial band autograft harvesting and labral reconstruction technique. *Arthrosc Tech.* 2012;2(1):e15-e19.

11. Matsuda DK. Arthroscopic labral reconstruction with gracilis autograft. *Arthrosc Tech.* 2012;1(1):e15-e21.

12. Park SE, Ko Y. Use of the quadriceps tendon in arthroscopic acetabular labral reconstruction: potential and benefits as an autograft option. *Arthrosc Tech.* 2013;2(3):e217-e219.

13. Sierra RJ, Trousdale RT. Labral reconstruction using the ligamentum teres capitis: report of a new technique. *Clin Orthop Relat Res.* 2009;467(3):753-759.

14. Larson CM, Giveans MR, Samuelson KM, Stone RM, Bedi A. Arthroscopic hip revision surgery for residual femoroacetabular impingement (FAI): surgical outcomes compared with a matched cohort after primary arthroscopic FAI correction. *Am J Sports Med.* 2014;42(8):1785-1790.

15. Costa Rocha P, Klingenstein G, Ganz R, Kelly BT, Leunig M. Circumferential reconstruction of severe acetabular labral damage using hamstring allograft: surgical technique and case series. *Hip Int.* 2013;23 suppl 9:S42-S53.

16. Geyer MR, Philippon MJ, Fagrelius TS, Briggs KK. Acetabular labral reconstruction with an iliotibial band autograft: outcome and survivorship analysis at minimum 3-year follow-up. *Am J Sports Med.* 2013;41(8):1750-1756.

17. Boykin RE, Patterson D, Briggs KK, Dee A, Philippon MJ. Results of arthroscopic labral reconstruction of the hip in elite athletes. *Am J Sports Med.* 2013;41(10):2296-2301.

18. Domb BG, Stake CE, Lindner D, El-Bitar Y, Jackson TJ. Revision hip preservation surgery with hip arthroscopy: clinical outcomes. *Arthroscopy.* 2014;30(5):581-587.

19. Clohisy J, Carlisle JC, Beaulé P, et al. A systematic approach to the plain radiographic evaluation of the young adult hip. *J Bone Joint Surg Am.* 2008;90(suppl 4):47-66.

Please see videos on the accompanying website at

www.ArthroscopicTechniques.com

14

Arthroscopic Treatment of Rim Impingement

Focal Retroversion, Global Retroversion, and Extra-Articular Impingement

Ryan M. Degen, MD; Eilish O'Sullivan, PT, DPT, OCS, SCS; and Bryan T. Kelly, MD

INTRODUCTION

Rim impingement patterns have historically been reported to be more common in women, although increasing evidence suggests that this impingement pattern rarely occurs in isolation and is frequently associated with mixed patterns with an associated cam lesion.[1,2] Regardless of its demographics, various anatomical factors may contribute to producing acetabular overcoverage. Focal overcoverage may result from a prominent segment of the acetabular rim, often anterosuperiorly, or an unhealed stress fracture or os acetabuli.[1,3] Relative overcoverage can result from true acetabular retroversion that could be idiopathic or iatrogenic following a periacetabular osteotomy, creating increased anterior coverage and deficient posterior coverage.[1] In addition, extra-articular pathology may contribute to a relative overcoverage of the femoral head, often in the form of a prominent anterior inferior iliac spine (AIIS), which is often the result of an apophyseal traction injury from the direct head of the rectus femoris before skeletal maturity. This results in an elongated AIIS that may reach, or extend beyond, the rim of the acetabulum, creating impingement between the inferior femoral head-neck junction and AIIS with hip flexion.[4] Finally, global overcoverage may result from a deepened acetabulum with coxa profunda or protrusio, which is often seen in conjunction with coxa vara, leading to impingement within a physiologic range of motion (ROM) and more extensive, circumferential labral pathology.[1,5]

Historically thought of as a contraindication to hip arthroscopy, acetabular protrusio has primarily been managed conservatively until joint replacement once arthritic symptoms become unmanageable. This notion was initially challenged by Leunig et al,[6] who reviewed the utility of surgical hip dislocation and acetabuloplasty with labral refixation or labral transplantation in these patients, with good results. Subsequently, Matsuda[7] indicated that select patients with acetabular protrusio may respond well to arthroscopic acetabuloplasty with labral repair or debridement, shifting protrusio from the list of contraindications to possible indications for hip arthroscopy, although still controversial.

Byrd JWT, Bedi A, Stubbs AJ, eds. *The Hip: AANA Advanced Arthroscopic Surgical Techniques* (pp 173-182). © 2016 AANA.

Although multiple anatomical factors contribute to this process, the concerning end result is a labral injury, most commonly identified in the anterosuperior region. Rather than the shearing injury noted with cam impingement, which usually produces separation at the chondrolabral junction, rim impingement causes an impaction injury with complex tearing with multiple cleavage planes of varying depth within the substance of the labrum.[8] In addition, impingement alters the kinematics of the hip, causing posterior translation as the impingement occurs with hip flexion, creating a shearing force on the posterior chondral surface, resulting in a contrecoup injury.[5] This combination of injuries to the labrum and chondral surface predisposes the hip to development of osteoarthritis and may warrant surgical intervention in the form of labral repair or debridement with acetabular rim resection in symptomatic patients.

Intra-articular injections may also help to define patients who would benefit from hip arthroscopy because they would be expected to have improvement in symptoms following the injection to indicate intra-articular pathology as the source of pain. Injections have been found to have a sensitivity of 90% for intra-articular pathology, although specificity is significantly lower and these results should be used in conjunction with physical examination and imaging findings to decide on surgical intervention.[9] In the setting of AIIS impingement, patients may not have full relief of symptoms with an intra-articular injection. Targeted extra-articular injections may also be useful in this scenario to confirm the diagnosis.

For each patient, it is imperative to begin with a systematic approach to the examination of the hip. There are several potential pain generators, and unless a systematic approach is used, one risks missing potential pathology that could be contributing to the patient's discomfort and decreased physical function. Although a review of all relevant physical examination tests for the hip is beyond the scope of this chapter, the authors focus on specific tests used for identifying rim impingement patterns. Rim impingement often exists in conjunction with cam-type impingement; thus, positive physical examination findings may not be exclusively indicative of either pattern.

INDICATIONS

▶ Refractory hip pain that fails to improve with a trial of nonsurgical management, with reproducible clinical examination findings and imaging studies to support intra-articular pathology (ie, labral injury, impingement)[5]

▶ Patients with extra-articular impingement with prominent AIIS morphology and reproducible pain with hip flexion

▶ Impingement-induced rim fractures with associated labral injury

Controversial Indications

▶ Acetabular profunda or protrusion

PERTINENT PHYSICAL FINDINGS

▶ With focal overcoverage, only specific movements will be limited.

  ▷ Anterior overcoverage may be indicated with limited/painful internal rotation with the hip in flexion.

  ▷ Forward flexion may also be limited/painful with anterosuperior overcoverage or subspine deformity extending to or caudal to the acetabular margin.

  ▷ Posterior overcoverage may cause decreased external rotation with flexion and abduction.

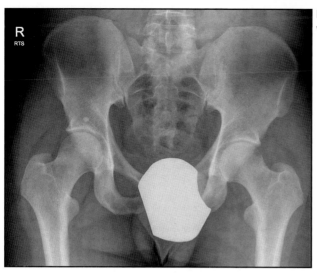

Figure 14-1. AP pelvis x-ray of a patient with coxa profunda.

▷ With global overcoverage, as in acetabular profunda or protrusio, a more global loss of motion may be observed.[5]

► For anterosuperior impingement, the hip is taken into flexion, adduction, and internal rotation.[10]

► For posterior impingement, the leg is lowered off of the edge of the examination table, bringing the hip into extension, while adding abduction and external rotation. This test is known as the posterior rim impingement test, and a positive result is indicative of posterior impingement.[10]

► Lateral rim impingement may be assessed for with pure abduction; a positive test is indicated with lateral pain with the superolateral femur and acetabular rim at the 12-o'clock position.

► Subspine impingement may be assessed with terminal hip flexion, with a positive test indicated with anterior/groin pain with this maneuver, along with restriction of motion.

PERTINENT IMAGING

► Imaging of the hip to assess for pincer impingement should begin with plain x-rays, including well-centered anteroposterior (AP) pelvis, Dunn lateral, and false-profile views.[11]

   ▷ The AP pelvis x-ray is reviewed for findings of acetabular retroversion, including a cross-over sign, ischial spine sign, and posterior wall sign.[12]

   ▷ The lateral center-edge angle and Tönnis angle can be calculated, with respective values of greater than 40 degrees (Figure 14-1) and less than 0 degrees being indicative of overcoverage.[11,12] Findings of coxa profunda or protrusio may also be identified, with the cotyloid fossa or femoral head extending medial to the ilioischial line, respectively.[5]

   ▷ The Dunn lateral view is largely used for identification of concomitant cam lesions, with an alpha angle greater than 50 to 55 degrees suggestive of this pathology (Figure 14-2).

   ▷ The false-profile view is used to identify the anterior center-edge angle and any potential posterior acetabular rim impingement or joint space narrowing.

► Magnetic resonance imaging may help to delineate the extent of labral pathology present (Figure 14-3). In addition, more cartilage-sensitive imaging sequences (eg, delayed gadolinium-enhanced magnetic resonance imaging of cartilage or T2 mapping with T1rho) may help to identify associated injury to the articular cartilage.

Figure 14-2. Lateral x-ray depicting a cam lesion and acetabular rim fracture.

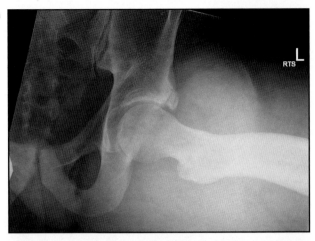

Figure 14-3. Rim fracture and labral injury on magnetic resonance imaging.

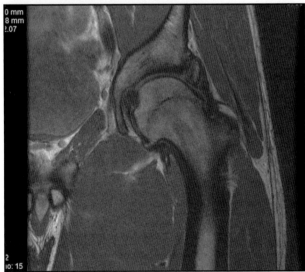

▶ Computed tomography scanning will provide better visualization of the acetabular rim, allowing for calculation of acetabular version, typically done at the 1-, 2-, and 3-o'clock positions to look for focal overcoverage or true retroversion, as well as classification of the AIIS based on morphology. In addition, it allows better characterization of the cam-type lesion and femoral version while also revealing any associated rim fractures or os acetabuli lesions (Figure 14-4).[5]

   ▷ Quantification of the size of these rim lesions or os acetabuli fragments is important because it can affect whether they are simply resected or whether they are too large and resection would introduce iatrogenic instability, fixation is required.[3]

EQUIPMENT

For safe completion of hip arthroscopy, the following equipment is required:

▶ Fracture table or traction table

▶ C-arm fluoroscopy

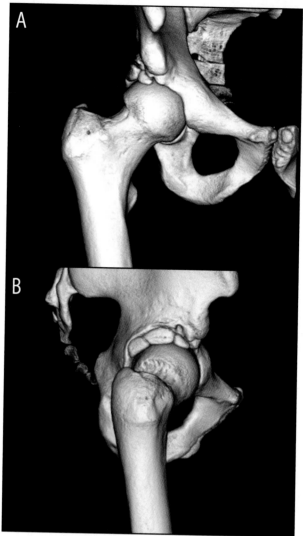

Figure 14-4. (A) Anterior- and (B) lateral-view computed tomography scans with 3-dimensional reconstruction of a 3-part acetabular rim fracture in a 19-year-old basketball player.

- ▶ A dedicated hip arthroscopy instrumentation set, including the following:
  - ▷ Long spinal needles for percutaneous portal placement using the Seldinger technique
  - ▷ Long nitinol wires
  - ▷ Percutaneous, long cannulas with blunt, cannulated obturators to allow placement over the nitinol guidewires
  - ▷ 70-degree arthroscope for visualization, and optional use of a 30-arthroscope in some cases
  - ▷ Intra-articular scalpel for creation of the interportal capsulotomy
  - ▷ Long straight and curved motorized shavers and burrs
  - ▷ Radiofrequency ablation device
  - ▷ Anchor system (including drill guide and drill)
  - ▷ Suture-passing device/suture penetrator
- ▶ Arthroscopic fluid management system

Positioning

Supine and lateral decubitus positioning have been described for performing hip arthroscopy. Supine positioning is generally a more familiar approach because this position is commonly used with hip fracture management. It can be performed on a standard fracture table or a dedicated hip arthroscopy traction table. Advantages include familiarity with positioning, more expeditious setup, and improved orientation for management of intra-articular pathology. Disadvantages include its use in obese patients, with the pannus limiting instrument maneuverability, as well as limited access for posterior portal placement or access to the posterior aspect of the joint.[13]

For both positions, the operative side is prepared by wrapping the foot with padding to prevent pressure ulcer formation while in traction. This foot is placed into a boot that allows traction to be applied to the leg to distract the joint. The contralateral foot is also wrapped in padding and placed into a boot for countertraction, with the limb slightly abducted. Care should be taken to pad bony prominences. A perineal post is used to provide countertraction and should be well-padded to reduce the incidence of pudendal neuropraxia. A combination of traction and adduction are applied to the limb, using the perineal post as a lever to help distract and lateralize the hip. Approximately 10 mm of distraction is required for safe access to the joint without injuring the labrum or femoral head cartilage, which should be confirmed fluoroscopically prior to proceeding with portal placement.[13,14] Careful observation of traction time should be performed, noting the time that traction was applied to the limb and aiming to limit traction time to less than 60 minutes but absolutely no more than 120 minutes.

Step-by-Step Description of the Procedure

Using fluoroscopic guidance, the anterolateral portal is established just anterior and proximal to the greater trochanter with needle localization and use of the Seldinger technique to introduce the cannula. Under direct arthroscopic visualization, the mid-anterior portal is then established, again using spinal needle localization. This portal starts approximately 2 cm distal and lateral to the intersection point of a horizontal line from the anterior superior iliac spine and a vertical line from the tip of the greater trochanter. Often, these 2 portals are sufficient for management of rim pathology; however, occasionally a distal accessory portal, known as the distal anterolateral portal, is placed to assist with anchor insertion. In addition, a posterolateral portal, just posterior and proximal to the greater trochanter, may be needed if there is any posterior impingement or posterior extension of the labral tear.[5] Portal placement may have to be adjusted based on the degree of acetabular retroversion or bony overhang of pincer lesions. Portals may have to be moved slightly distal to their original descriptions to gain access to the joint as a result.[15]

After establishing the anterolateral and mid-anterior portals, an intra-articular curved blade is used to create an interportal capsulotomy to improve instrument maneuverability and visualization of the extra-articular side of the labrum and the acetabular rim. At this point, there should be complete access to the central compartment, allowing for a brief diagnostic arthroscopy prior to management of the rim lesion and labral pathology.[16] The goal of the procedure is then to perform adequate rim resection and preservation or repair of viable labral tissue. Depending on the pathology present, typically one of the following 3 treatment techniques is used: acetabular rim resection with labral debridement, acetabular rim resection with labral preservation and repair, or acetabular rim resection with labral takedown and repair.[5,15]

Acetabular rim resection and labral debridement are performed when the labrum is found to have extensive damage, with multiple cleavage planes and calcification that precludes repair. Debridement should involve as small a segment of the labrum as possible and should be tapered out to the adjacent normal labrum to preserve as much labral tissue as possible.[15] Appropriate rim resection can be gauged fluoroscopically, as described by Larson and Wulf.[17] This technique involves obtaining a proper AP pelvis view intraoperatively to visualize the crossover sign where present and then using a burr to resect 5 to 8 mm of the anterior wall to eliminate the crossover sign and create a smooth transition from the anterior to posterior wall.[15,17] Care should be taken to avoid overresection and introduction of iatrogenic instability.

When the labrum looks viable and remains attached to the acetabular rim, the adjacent rim lesion should be inspected to determine if it can be appropriately resected with labral attachments preserved. If so, a burr can be used adjacent to the extra-articular margin of the labrum to debride the rim lesion, taking care to minimize the amount of capsular tissue resected. The same technique as previously described can be used to gauge appropriate acetabular resection. Following debridement, the labrum should be reassessed. If there is intrasubstance tearing or increased mobility following rim resection with disruption of the labral attachments, anchors should be placed immediately adjacent to the labrum and sutures passed to secure the labrum and prevent further hypermobility and associated tearing.[5]

If it is felt that the acetabular rim resection cannot be adequately performed while leaving the labrum attached, such as in large profunda deformities, it can be liberated at the chondrolabral junction with an intra-articular blade to expose the acetabular rim for resection with a burr, followed by refixation using suture anchors.[5] Fluoroscopy should be used to gauge the adequacy of rim resection. After labral repair or refixation and upon completion of central compartment treatment, traction should be released to ensure appropriate restoration of the suction-seal effect of the labrum.

With a rim fracture or unfused os acetabuli, consideration should be given to its size and contribution to hip stability. If it is contributing to impingement and resection would not sufficiently decrease the lateral center-edge angle, it can often be managed with resection and labral refixation (Figure 14-5). However, if it is a large fragment that may predispose the hip to instability if resected, it can be repaired as described by Epstein and Safran,[3] with arthroscopic debridement of the fibrous junction between the fragment and acetabular rim and percutaneous, interfragmentary screw fixation. Larson et al[18] described a partial resection and internal fixation of the fragment in the case where larger fragments contributed to a pincer-type impingement but were of such a size that removal would create iatrogenic instability (Figure 14-6).

Finally, if subspine impingement is a contributing factor, following interportal capsulotomy, a motorized shaver can be used to resect fibrous tissue from the capsulolabral recess and a minimal amount of capsular tissue to expose the AIIS. A burr is then used to debride this region, while preserving as much of the insertion of the direct head of rectus as possible. Further rim resection and labral repair or debridement can then also be performed after addressing the subspine region. After completion of all central compartment work, the traction can be released and a dynamic examination performed to ensure sufficient resection of the subspine region to prevent further impingement under direct visualization. Fluoroscopy can also be used to ensure sufficient decompression.[4]

Following the management of rim pathology, cam pathology should be addressed in the peripheral compartment if present. At the completion of the case, the capsulotomy can be repaired prior to skin closure, although the need for capsular repair is somewhat controversial and beyond the scope of this chapter.

POSTOPERATIVE PROTOCOL

Patients are placed on heterotopic ossification prophylaxis consisting of 4 days of 75 mg of indomethacin, followed by 4 weeks of 500 mg of naproxen twice a day. They are provided with a pneumatic cooling device and a continuous passive motion machine to be used for 3 to 4 weeks to decrease inflammation and promote mobility. Patients are protected weight bearing for 2 to 4 weeks with bilateral crutches. A progressive physical therapy program is initiated on postoperative day 1 for ROM, isometric strengthening, and functional mobility. Patients may begin on a

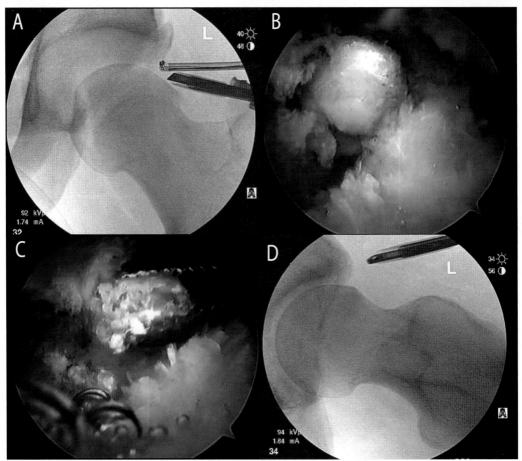

Figure 14-5. Excision of an acetabular fragment that was not required for stability. (A) Fluoroscopic view prior to excision. (B) Exposure of fragment. (C) Extraction of fragment. (D) Fluoroscopic view following removal.

stationary bike as early as postoperative day 1. The first 6 weeks of the rehabilitative process focus on increasing ROM and regaining functional mobility. In weeks 6 through 12, patients begin to build functional strength in preparation for initiation of a progressive return to recreational/sport activities at approximately 12 weeks postoperatively. Patients are progressed based on soft tissue healing time frames and the achievement of functional milestones.

POTENTIAL COMPLICATIONS

Complications associated with this procedure include general complications associated with hip arthroscopy, including infection, potential traction neuropraxia (most commonly involving the pudendal nerves), neurovascular injury with portal placement, or iatrogenic chondral or labral injuries.[13]

Specific to rim resection with labral debridement or repair, complications can include inaccurate resection, inadequate resection leaving residual impinging lesions, and overresection, which may predispose the hip to postoperative iatrogenic instability.[17] Many of these complications can be avoided with careful attention to the preoperative diagnosis and location of pathology and the use of intraoperative fluoroscopy to guide acetabular resection.[5]

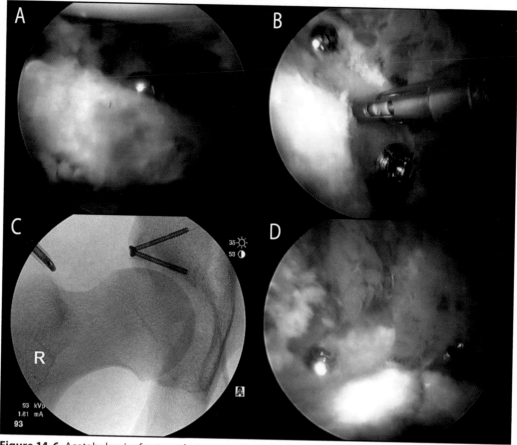

Figure 14-6. Acetabular rim fracture that required stabilization. (A) Exposure. (B) Screw fixation. (C) Labral repair. (D) Fluoroscopic view.

TOP TECHNICAL PEARLS FOR THE PROCEDURE

1. Ensure appropriate distraction of 8 to 10 mm or greater in pincer-type deformity cases to avoid iatrogenic injury to the labrum.

2. Consider altering the placement and number of portals required for rim resection based on the location of rim lesions on preoperative imaging studies.

3. Use fluoroscopy to guide the amount and location of acetabular rim resection.

4. Avoid overresection of the rim.

5. Attempt to preserve labral attachments during acetabular rim resection where feasible.

REFERENCES

1. Bedi A, Kelly BT. Femoroacetabular impingement. *J Bone Joint Surg Am.* 2013;95(1):82-92.
2. Nepple JJ, Riggs CN, Ross JR, Clohisy JC. Clinical presentation and disease characteristics of femoroacetabular impingement are sex-dependent. *J Bone Joint Surg Am.* 2014;96(20):1683-1689.

3. Epstein NJ, Safran MR. Stress fracture of the acetabular rim: arthroscopic reduction and internal fixation. A case report. *J Bone Joint Surg Am.* 2009;91(6):1480-1486.

4. Hetsroni I, Larson CM, Dela Torre K, Zbeda RM, Magennis E, Kelly BT. Anterior inferior iliac spine deformity as an extra-articular source for hip impingement: a series of 10 patients treated with arthroscopic decompression. *Arthroscopy.* 2012;28(11):1644-1653.

5. Larson CM. Arthroscopic management of pincer-type impingement. *Sports Med Arthrosc.* 2010;18(2):100-107.

6. Leunig M, Nho SJ, Turchetto L, Ganz R. Protrusio acetabuli: new insights and experience with joint preservation. *Clin Orthop Relat Res.* 2009;467(9):2241-2250.

7. Matsuda DK. Protrusio acetabuli: contraindication or indication for hip arthroscopy? And the case for arthroscopic treatment of global pincer impingement. *Arthroscopy.* 2012;28(6):882-888.

8. Seldes RM, Tan V, Hunt J, Katz M, Winiarsky R, Fitzgerald RH Jr. Anatomy, histologic features, and vascularity of the adult acetabular labrum. *Clin Orthop Relat Res.* 2001;(382):232-240.

9. Skendzel JG, Weber AE, Ross JR, et al. The approach to the evaluation and surgical treatment of mechanical hip pain in the young patient: AAOS exhibit selection. *J Bone Joint Surg Am.* 2013;95(18):e133.

10. Martin HD, Kelly BT, Leunig M, et al. The pattern and technique in the clinical evaluation of the adult hip: the common physical examination tests of hip specialists. *Arthroscopy.* 2010;26(2):161-172.

11. Clohisy JC, Carlisle JC, Beaulé PE, et al. A systematic approach to the plain radiographic evaluation of the young adult hip. *J Bone Joint Surg Am.* 2008;90 suppl 4:47-66.

12. Tannast M, Siebenrock KA, Anderson SE. Femoroacetabular impingement: radiographic diagnosis—what the radiologist should know. *AJR Am J Roentgenol.* 2007;188(6):1540-1552.

13. Smart LR, Oetgen M, Noonan B, Medvecky M. Beginning hip arthroscopy: indications, positioning, portals, basic techniques, and complications. *Arthroscopy.* 2007;23(12):1348-1353.

14. Lynch TS, Terry MA, Bedi A, Kelly BT. Hip arthroscopic surgery: patient evaluation, current indications, and outcomes. *Am J Sports Med.* 2013;41(5):1174-1189.

15. Ayeni OR, Pruett A, Kelly BT. Arthroscopic management of pincer impingement. In: Kelly BT, Philippon MJ, eds. *Arthroscopic Techniques in the Hip: A Visual Guide.* Thorofare, NJ: SLACK Incorporated; 2010:69-88.

16. Bedi A, Kelly BT, Khanduja V. Arthroscopic hip preservation surgery: current concepts and perspective. *Bone Joint J.* 2013;95(1):10-19.

17. Larson CM, Wulf CA. Intraoperative fluoroscopy for evaluation of bony resection during arthroscopic management of femoroacetabular impingement in the supine position. *Arthroscopy.* 2009;25(10):1183-1192.

18. Larson CM, Kelly BT, Stone RM. Making a case for anterior inferior iliac spine/subspine hip impingement: three representative case reports and proposed concept. *Arthroscopy.* 2011;27(12):1732-1737.

Please see videos on the accompanying website at

www.ArthroscopicTechniques.com

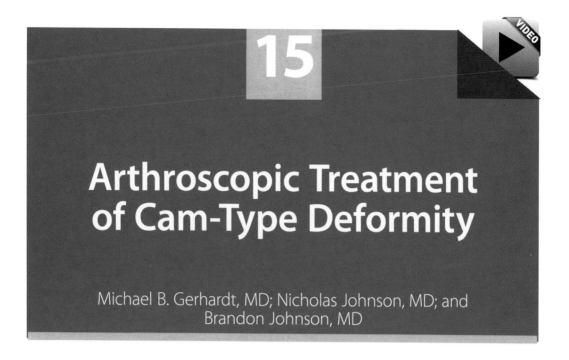

Arthroscopic Treatment of Cam-Type Deformity

Michael B. Gerhardt, MD; Nicholas Johnson, MD; and
Brandon Johnson, MD

INTRODUCTION

The concept of hip impingement has been described for nearly 100 years in the orthopedic literature.[1,2] However, its significance in the development of pain in the adult hip was only recently more clearly defined by Ganz et al.[3] Femoroacetabular impingement (FAI) has been an area of interest and intense research in recent years due to an increased understanding of its pathological process and its potential implications in the development of hip osteoarthritis (OA).[4]

Occult hip and groin pain was a common complaint in athletic individuals over the past several decades. In the not-too-distant past, athletes who experienced hip and/or groin pain with no obvious fracture or arthritis were often told to play through the pain. In retrospect, it is now understood that many of these individuals were suffering from unrecognized hip impingement. This was particularly devastating to elite athletes, who often developed more debilitating hip and groin pain that then led to ongoing symptoms and, in some cases, premature termination of their career. A growing understanding of FAI has led to the ability of orthopedists to recognize subtle impingement and offer previously unavailable remedies. Early and appropriate arthroscopic treatment has led to promising outcomes in athletes and nonathletes. Although the classical description of FAI includes cam, pincer, and mixed types, the focus of this chapter is restricted to the arthroscopic treatment of cam-type FAI.

Cam-type FAI in the simplest form refers to a nonspherical femoral head rotating inside the acetabulum (Figure 15-1).[5] With flexion, the prominent portion of the head rotates into the acetabulum, generating a shear force on the anterolateral edge of the acetabular articular surface (Figure 15-2). With repeated motion, this edge shearing leads to articular delamination. Initially, the labrum is spared as it is pushed out of the way; however, as the disease progresses, labral pathology often follows (Figure 15-3). In a pure cam impingement scenario, the classic intra-articular pathology can be described as undersurface fraying of the labrum and carpet delamination of the

Byrd JWT, Bedi A, Stubbs AJ, eds. *The Hip:*
AANA Advanced Arthroscopic Surgical Techniques (pp 183-196).
© 2016 AANA.

Figure 15-1. Representation of cam-type impingement bump at the femoral head-neck junction.

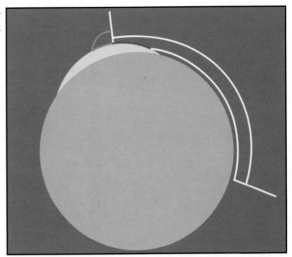

Figure 15-2. Focal prominence of bone cam-type FAI.

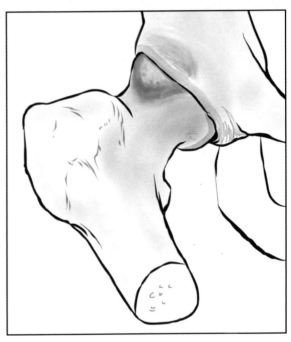

adjacent acetabular articular cartilage. The degree of pathology varies greatly, largely depending on the severity of the cam deformity and chronicity of the problem, as well as other variables, such as the type and intensity of exposure to a certain sport or activity. Initially, the articular cartilage simply appears soft and spongy, but it progressively deteriorates, leading to a partial delamination, or wave sign. The end stage is ultimately full-thickness delamination of the cartilage with areas of underlying exposed subchondral bone.

Although cam impingement is seen in both sexes, the overall prevalence of cam impingement appears to be approximately 3 times more common in males than females.[5] In addition, there appears to be a bimodal age predilection as to when cam impingement presents with symptoms, the first occurring in the 20s and the second in the 40s. It has been reported that there is a markedly increased prevalence of cam deformities in asymptomatic adolescents involved in high-impact sports, such as basketball and soccer, as compared with nonathlete controls.[6-8]

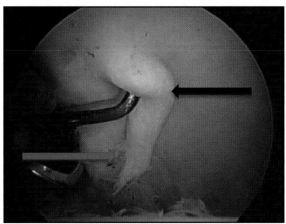

Figure 15-3. Typical appearance of chondrolabral disruption caused by longstanding cam-type impingement. The probe is demonstrating the precise area of chondrolabral damage, which includes undersurface labral fraying (red arrow) and focal delamination of the adjacent articular cartilage (black arrow).

The etiology of cam-type FAI is uncertain. Recent studies seem to implicate intense athletic activity during adolescence in the accentuation of cam deformity. This theory suggests that the exercise creates a stress phenomenon at the lateral epiphysis of the femoral head that results in asymmetric growth of the hip during these formative years. The end result of this deformity may ultimately be what is described as the cam bump. Although this is current theory, no definitive proof of this phenomenon has yet been offered.[6] A better understanding of this developmental phenomenon would be valuable to the clinician because it may lead to the development of preventive measures, which, if successful, could potentially affect the development of OA in the adult hip joint.

The evolutionary progression of hip impingement leading to the eventual development of OA is variable and poorly understood. Current consensus suggests that cam-type FAI is a risk factor for OA; however, recent reports have shown that not all patients with FAI ultimately develop OA.[9-11] Therefore, imaging studies demonstrating morphological abnormalities, such as cam deformity, must be interpreted carefully because many of these patients may never show signs of intra-articular pain and may not develop OA of the hip. Although many athletic individuals with impingement morphology will ultimately go on and develop symptoms and some of those will go on to develop OA, the risk stratification has not yet been clearly established. Until a direct association and quantification between deformity and disease has been determined, prophylactic surgery in the asymptomatic impinging hip is not widely accepted.

In symptomatic patients, hip arthroscopy for cam-type FAI represents a minimally invasive procedure with consistently good to excellent results in patients with minimal or no OA.[11-14] Arthroscopic femoroplasty of the cam-type deformity is the essential step in alleviating hip impingement, improving the biomechanics of the hip, and effectively reducing the risk of recurrent labral and chondral injury. The arthroscopic technique illustrated in this chapter is a joint-preserving procedure that may delay or diminish the need for early arthroplasty in afflicted patients.

INDICATIONS

Hip specialists should look for favorable prognostic factors when choosing appropriate surgical candidates for hip arthroscopy. In general, the younger the patient, the less likely it is that significant arthritic changes have set in. This is why younger patients generally have better outcomes than their elder counterparts. In addition, patients who demonstrate more mechanical symptoms, such as catching, clicking, and apprehension, tend to be better candidates than patients who

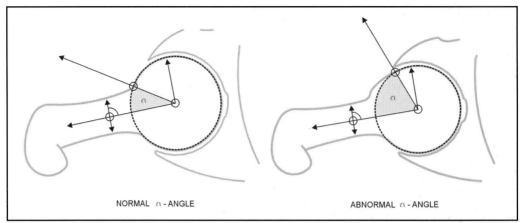

NORMAL α - ANGLE   ABNORMAL α - ANGLE

Figure 15-4. The alpha angle can be calculated by first drawing a line down the longitudinal axis of the femoral neck to the center of the femoral head. A second line is created from the center of the femoral head to the point at which the normal sphericity of the head is lost. The angle between these 2 lines is considered the alpha angle. Alpha angles greater than 55 degrees are considered abnormal and suggest the presence of a cam-type of deformity.

demonstrate more ambiguous complaints, such as generalized night pain or global pelvic soreness in a distribution that does not suggest intra-articular hip pathology.

Other common features include sitting intolerance, difficulty with low-lying chairs, and increasing intolerance to exercise, particularly sports requiring change of direction, such as soccer and hockey. Cam-type impingement tends to be more common and pronounced in males and is notable for internal rotation deficits that are slightly more significant on the symptomatic side.

By identifying these types of favorable prognostic factors, surgeons can then more appropriately interpret patients' imaging studies, which will then increase the ability to choose appropriate candidates for arthroscopic femoroplasty. Although many imaging studies can give clues as to potential causes of hip pain, only one objective measurement has been described that can quantify the degree of cam-type deformity in the hip: the alpha angle, which remains one of the few unambiguous measurable signs of morphological abnormality in the hip and should be routinely measured in all patients with FAI (Figure 15-4).[15]

Identifying appropriate candidates for hip arthroscopy remains one of the most challenging parts of treating patients with hip pain. It is only after a thorough review of the history, physical examination, and available ancillary data that correct identification of hip arthroscopy candidates can be done. If one of these areas is considered in isolation, inappropriate candidates may be selected for surgery.

This is illustrated in a common scenario in which a patient presents to the surgeon's office with magnetic resonance imaging (MRI) suggesting a labral tear. However, upon examination, this patient demonstrates no signs of true hip irritability. If the orthopedic surgeon does not take the time to properly examine the patient's hip, it would be easy to make an inappropriate surgical indication based on the MRI only. This is a critical point when considering candidates for arthroscopic femoroplasty because the literature clearly demonstrates a high prevalence of asymptomatic cam-type deformity in the general population.[16]

Although arthroscopic femoroplasty of cam deformities has proven to be effective in the treatment of patients with cam-type impingement, surgery should be reserved for individuals who clearly demonstrate refractory hip symptoms and for whom conservative treatment has failed.[17,18]

Conservative treatment should be part of the initial algorithm for all patients; however, physicians should also appreciate the limits of nonsurgical treatment. It is important to establish a timeline, especially in elite athletes for whom return to play pressures loom large. In general, patients for whom conservative treatment has failed for 6 to 8 weeks and who meet the diagnostic criteria for hip impingement can be indicated for surgery. It is not uncommon for patients with FAI to have waited many months before the correct diagnosis is discovered and they are ultimately referred to the hip surgeon. In these situations, a much longer time period has already elapsed prior to presentation to the hip specialist, in which case the decision to proceed with surgery may be expedited.

INDICATIONS

- Patient characteristics
  - Young athletic patients (the younger the age, the more favorable the outcomes)
  - Minimal OA
  - Pain present for longer than 6 weeks
  - Reproducible symptoms on examination (positive provocative tests)
  - Failure of conservative treatment
  - Failure of pain test (intra-articular injection)
- Bony deformity
  - Demonstrable deformity on imaging studies (alpha angle > 55 degrees)
  - Pistol-grip deformity
  - Deformity confined mainly to the anterolateral zones of the femoral head-neck junction (posterior femoral pathology may require open surgical dislocation of the hip)
- Overall condition of hip joint
  - Minimal or no OA
  - More than 2 mm of joint space remaining on x-rays
  - Minimal subchondral edema/cysts on MRI

Controversial Indications

- Patient characteristics
  - Older athletic patients (use caution in patients > 60 years)
    - Osteopenia
    - Higher likelihood of OA
    - Higher likelihood of failure
  - Dysplasia: Cam bump may be present in these patients, but use caution if the center-edge angle is less than 25 degrees (recommend capsular closure/plication and avoidance of ilio-psoas release).
  - Long-standing symptoms with atypical complaints
    - Night pain, gluteal pain with radicular nature
    - Failed pain test
    - Severe obesity: access and maneuverability can be difficult

PERTINENT PHYSICAL FINDINGS

A thorough physical examination is of utmost importance in the diagnosis and treatment of hip impingement. A complete physical examination allows for evaluation of the dynamic and static sources of hip pain and, perhaps most importantly, allows for the differentiation of intra- and extra-articular sources of pain. An experienced clinician should be able to effectively differentiate between true intra-articular hip pathology and nonhip-related problems.[17]

A proper physical examination of the hip should begin with a systematic evaluation of the hip, pelvis, and lower back. Notation should be made of any obvious abnormalities in the gait or any obvious movement dysfunction. Next, a circumferential palpation of the hip and its periarticular soft tissues should be performed and documented. This includes palpation of the proximal hip adductors, the inguinal region, the hip flexors and iliopsoas, the trochanteric bursae and abductors, and the posterior structures, such as the sacroiliac joint and piriformis and lower back. A cursory low back examination should be documented, particularly if posterior hip pain is the primary complaint.[16] Next, a side-to-side assessment of hip range of motion should be performed, focusing particularly on rotational differences between the normal and symptomatic hips.

Following this initial assessment, the examiner can enlist a variety of specialized tests in an effort to pinpoint the specific pathology present. The impingement test is considered a so-called best test for evaluating patients with symptomatic FAI. The impingement test is a nonspecific test for hip pathology and is not exclusive for cam-type impingement; however, if the impingement test is negative, the likelihood of that patient having cam-type impingement is low.

The impingement test has been described as the following 2 separate maneuvers: the flexion, adduction, internal rotation (FADDIR) test and the flexion, abduction, external rotation test (FABER) test. The FADDIR test, as described by Klaue et al,[20] is performed by flexing the hip to 90 degrees or more and then maneuvering the hip into adduction and internal rotation. This is regarded as the most sensitive test for traditional FAI and is present in 99% of the affected population.[21,22] Two important points should be made about the FADDIR test. First, if this maneuver is performed aggressively with extreme flexion and internal rotation, the examiner can elicit pain in nearly every person if pushed hard enough. Therefore, it is important that this test be performed with a minimal to moderate amount of force and should be interpreted in relationship to the test performed on the contralateral side. Second, although the test is highly sensitive, it is not highly specific and does not necessarily confirm the presence of hip impingement because many intra-articular disorders elicit a positive FADDIR test. Conversely, if this test is negative, it is highly unlikely that hip impingement is present; for this reason, it is considered a best test for ruling out hip impingement.

The FABER test, also considered an impingement test, is performed by flexing the hip beyond 90 degrees and forcefully abducting and externally rotating the hip.[10] This maneuver is also highly sensitive for eliciting pain in an impinging hip and should be documented as part of every hip examination. In addition, with the hip in this figure-4 position, the examiner can also measure the vertical distance between the lateral femoral epicondyle and the examination table while stabilizing the pelvis. This distance is typically greater than the contralateral noninvolved hip and can be an indication of articular irritability. An abnormal FABER test has been reported to be present in as many as 97% of patients with FAI.[21,22]

If uncertainty of diagnosis exists after a thorough history, physical examination, and appropriate imaging studies, selective intra-articular injection may prove helpful in confirmation of intra-articular pathology. A pain test is performed by introducing a small dose of 1% lidocaine without epinephrine into the joint. This is another best test technique and represents a rapid way to confirm an intra-articular source of pain in ambiguous cases. Pain relief following an intra-articular injection of local anesthetic is as high as 90% in some series. Previously, this test was most commonly performed under fluoroscopic guidance, usually in conjunction with the pre-MRI arthrogram. However, ultrasound guidance has recently been shown to be as accurate as, less painful than, and more convenient than the fluoroscopic technique and is currently the preferred method for delivering intra-articular hip injections in the clinician's office.[19,23] Some examiners take this opportunity to include a small dose of corticosteroid as an adjunct to the pain test injection, but this is at the discretion of the physician.

The physician should carefully examine or perform each of the following in order to deduce the pathology present in the patient's hip:

► Gait analysis and functional movement screen

► Low back examination (brief): further workup for lumbosacral pathology if indicated

► Palpation of painful hip anatomy: anterior, lateral, and posterior structures

► Hip range of motion: side-to-side documentation is critical (limited internal rotation is common in cam-type impingement and pronounced in symptomatic hips)

► Impingement tests (high sensitivity, low specificity): best test to rule out FAI

  ▷ FADDIR

  ▷ FABER

► Intra-articular diagnostic injection (pain test): best test to confirm intra-articular source of hip pain

Pertinent Imaging

Plain radiographic imaging is an essential part of evaluating and understanding the pathoanatomy leading to potential causes of hip pain. An anteroposterior (AP) view of the pelvis and a lateral view of the proximal femur and hip are the standard views that should be obtained in every patient. Other more specific views can be obtained should further information be needed depending on the problem at hand.

The AP view should be used to assess the condition of the acetabulum and, most importantly, to give a side-to-side comparison of both hips. Basic information can be gleaned from the AP pelvis view, including measurements of remaining joint space and assessment of overall morphologic abnormalities of the acetabular and femoral aspects of the joint.[13,24]

The lateral view of the proximal femur and hip is the most important view for identifying abnormalities suggestive of cam-type impingement. The lateral view of the hip can be obtained using several radiographic techniques, including, but not limited to, the frog lateral view, the 45-degree modified Dunn view, the 90-degree modified Dunn view, and a cross-table lateral view. Although one of these views is generally adequate in most cases, in more subtle situations it may be beneficial to include more than one of these views to obtain maximal data at varying points along the head-neck junction. Advances in MRI have allowed physicians to make more accurate diagnosis of various types of intra-articular hip pathology, including subtle cases of cam-type impingement. MRI is considered an essential part of the evaluation for all patients with suspected FAI or intra-articular pathology in general. Historically, MR arthrogram was considered the gold standard because it provided the most sensitive way to detect labral tears and chondral defects; however, recent reports using higher-resolution scanners suggest that these nonarthrogram studies may be approaching the utility of the previous arthrogram studies. Although recent advancements in MRI imagery and sequencing have allowed us to better detect labral lesions, the ability to detect articular cartilage damage in these FAI patients remains largely unreliable. Recent studies have shown a directly proportional correlation between hips with high alpha angles and increasing prevalence of acetabular articular cartilage damage. Therefore, it is important for surgeons to maintain a healthy sense of suspicion at the time of arthroscopy, particularly in patients with large alpha angle measurements.[25-27]

Recent advancements in computed tomography (CT) imaging and sequencing have established this modality as a powerful tool for better evaluating patients with hip pain. If presented with a complex patient whose findings are equivocal, one may use a 3-dimensional (3D) CT scan to further assess hip architecture. This is thought to be the most accurate imaging technique and is useful in determining the bony morphology of the hip joint.[27]

Pertinent imaging includes the following:

- X-rays
  - AP pelvis view
  - Lateral view of the proximal femur: critical for diagnosis of cam-type impingement
    - Positive cam-type FAI if alpha angle is > 55 degrees
    - Frog-lateral, modified Dunn, or cross-table lateral view
- MRI with or without gadolinium
  - High sensitivity for labral pathology
  - Low specificity for chondral pathology
  - Accurate calculation of α angle (radial plane images)
- CT scan with 3D reconstruction
  - Precise topographic representation of proximal femoral anatomy
  - Proprietary software programs available for virtual recreation of dynamic hip impingement

EQUIPMENT

The following equipment is needed:

- C-arm fluoroscopy unit
- Portable hip distractor
  - Hip arthroscopic traction device (preferable to standard fracture table)
  - Attaches to radiolucent Amsco operating table
  - Overpadded perineal post (critical to prevent pudendal nerve problems)
- Arthroscopy tower
  - Light source
  - Monitor and recording device
  - 70-degree arthroscope (30-degree arthroscope can be used effectively in viewing certain parts of the joint, including the fovea and peripheral compartment)
- Irrigation system
  - Inflow variable pressure pump system with preference for low pressures
  - Outflow to suction/pump
- Sterile arthroscopy pack
  - Drapes (prefer Ioban shower curtain drape [3M])
  - Inflow/outflow tubing
- Instruments
  - Basic hip-specific arthroscopy tray
    - Including arthroscopic probe; switching sticks; sharp and blunt slotted cannulas; arthroscopic curettes; arthroscopic liberators; various angled meniscal biters/graspers; long-handled, hip-specific suture graspers and retrievers; and arthroscopic cannulas

- Handheld motorized instruments: minimum requirement includes 4.5-mm, full-radius, hip-specific shaver; 5.5-mm arthroscopic round burr with low-profile hood (burr is work-horse instrument for arthroscopic femoroplasty)
- Radiofrequency (RF) ablation device: prefer standard, rigid, hip-specific RF probe (flexible RF probes available)

POSITIONING

The authors' preferred technique for positioning hip arthroscopy patients involves the use of a detachable hip distractor device. The hip distractor is attached to a standard Amsco table (Steris Corporation). Although hip arthroscopy can be performed on a standard fracture table, the authors have found that using the portable hip distractor is less cumbersome, more versatile, and more efficient. Also, most outpatient surgery centers are not equipped with traditional fracture tables, and the portable hip distractor offers a cost-effective alternative.

The patient is positioned in the supine position on the table with both feet overly padded and secured to traction boots. A well-padded perineal post is critical, regardless of the type of traction device being used. Without an adequately padded perineal post, the risk of pudendal nerve palsy increases significantly. The post is firmly situated against the perineum and lateralized toward the operative hip, with care taken to protect the genitalia and ensure that the testicles of the male patient in particular are positioned up away from the post before any traction is applied.

The arm on the nonoperative side is abducted on an arm board and the arm on the operative side is padded and secured across the body. The operative leg is positioned in neutral abduction or slight adduction, neutral flexion-extension, and neutral or slight internal rotation. To start the case, gentle traction is applied to the nonoperative leg, which will counterbalance the nonoperative leg when gross traction is applied to that side. Once the patient is positioned properly, traction is applied to the operative limb. First, gross traction is applied manually. Then, fine traction using the turn-handle can be applied as needed. This should be done in increments and monitored with serial images from the fluoroscopic image intensifier. Gentle progressive distraction should be applied until a minimum of 8 to 10 mm of femoroacetabular joint space is created to provide ample working space for the arthroscope within the joint. The circulating nurse should document the time that traction was placed, and this should be monitored throughout the case and limited to less than 2 hours of consecutive traction time, similar to the use of a tourniquet. If more than 2 hours of traction is required, a brief 10- to 15-minute break without traction should be allowed before traction is reapplied.

Most surgeons prefer to start the hip arthroscopy with the patient's hip in traction, which allows the central compartment part of the procedure to be completed. This includes management of any chondral and labral pathology and completion of any acetabular rim reduction that may need to be addressed in pincer-type FAI. Once the central compartment work is complete, the surgeon prepares for the peripheral compartment aspect of the case. The peripheral compartment is accessed without hip distraction. Therefore, at this point, under the hip traction is let down and the femoral head is reduced into the acetabulum under direct arthroscopic visualization. The circulating nurse then unlocks the gross traction and rotation and assists the surgeon in placing the operative leg in a flexed and slightly externally rotated position. In this position, the surgeon can adequately access the cam lesion, which resides in the peripheral compartment, and can perform the arthroscopic femoroplasty.

STEP-BY-STEP DESCRIPTION OF THE PROCEDURE

Standard hip arthroscopy is performed using the anterolateral and distal anterior portals (Video). Central compartment arthroscopy is performed first. Although femoroplasty can be performed without significant capsulotomy in some hips, maneuverability and visualization can prove challenging unless a generous capsulotomy is performed. An arthroscopic knife blade is used to perform a horizontal capsultomy—basically, a portal-to-portal cut. The authors do not routinely T the capsule unless it is absolutely necessary to access parts of the cam lesion that are proving difficult to address. Although the authors advocate capsular closure routinely following hip arthroscopy, many surgeons do not perform this routinely. However, most would agree that if extensive vertical extension of the capsulotomy, or the so-called T cut, of the capsule is performed, then the surgeon should at a minimum close this part of the capsulotomy. Once the central compartment work has been completed, the traction is released, and the hip is flexed up to about 45 to 50 degrees. Slight external rotation often allows for the capsule to relax such that diagnostic arthroscopy of the peripheral compartment can be performed.

Prior to preparation for the femoroplasty, one important landmark is identified and documented: the lateral synovial fold. This is important to protect and respect throughout the femoroplasty procedure because inadvertent ablation of this landmark could potentially create avascular necrosis of the femoral head. This lateral retinacular fold contains the terminal branches of the medial circumflex femoral artery, which are located posterolaterally on the femoral neck.

Next, the cam lesion is identified. The authors prefer to start with the arthroscope in the anterolateral portal and use the anterior portal as the working portal. The cam lesion can be identified via direct visualization and is usually obvious. The surface area of the cam lesion often shows signs of inflammation and excoriation secondary to the long-standing bony conflict due to the impingement. However, if the location of the cam lesion is not obvious on direct visualization, fluoroscopy can help to identify the topographical abnormalities of the head-neck junction. In essence, the surgeon is able to map the dimensions of the cam bump using fluoroscopy.

Next, the thin synovial lining over the cam lesion is removed. This allows the motorized burr to work more efficiently during bony resection of the cam lesion. In this case, a 50-degree RF ablation device is used to remove the soft tissue; however, some surgeons prefer to use a curette. Once thorough soft tissue ablation has been completed, the next step is performing the actual femoroplasty using a motorized burr. The authors prefer to start proximally and work distally (ie, work from the femoral head down toward the femoral neck). The goals are to obliterate the cam lesion and recreate the sphericity of the normal head-neck junction. This takes time to do correctly and involves a combination of fluoroscopic visualization as the femoroplasty proceeds and dynamic positioning of the hip in varying degrees of flexion, extension, and rotation.

Some technical pearls may help at this stage. First, one should remember that each hip capsule is different, and if the surgeon finds himself fighting against the capsule as the femoroplasty is attempted, a couple things can be done to help. The authors have had some success in establishing an accessory portal proximally through which a switching stick can serve as a capsular retractor. Another option is to vertically T the capsule, which effectively opens up the working space and allows the femoroplasty to proceed in a less cumbersome manner.

Second, the most common zone for the surgeon to underresect the cam lesion is laterally and proximally. One technique that the authors have used in this hard-to-access lateral extension of the bump is to place the hip into nearly full or full extension. This relaxes the lateral part of the hip just enough that these lateral cam extensions can be accessed more easily.

The next step in the femoroplasty is switching portals so that the surgeon is viewing via the anterior portal and working via the more lateral portal. This simple change allows the surgeon to visualize the head-neck junction from a different perspective and, invariably, areas of unresected bony prominences become obvious. It also allows the motorized burr to reach laterally and posterolaterally more easily. The surgeon must always remember what lurks laterally: the lateral synovial fold. It is wise to visualize this landmark at the completion of the femoroplasty to document that this structure has not been violated. Once the bony resection is complete, a final check of the femoroplasty is performed using a dynamic range of motion check and live fluoroscopy. It is helpful to disengage the boot from the distractor device and to remove the perineal post, which will allow the hip many more degrees of freedom. If obvious areas of residual impingement are found, the motorized burr is reinserted and the bone is touched up accordingly.

This marks the end of the femoroplasty. The authors prefer to close the capsule at the end of the case. The sutures can be passed using standard arthroscopic penetrators or handheld injector devices. Arthroscopic knots are placed to complete the capsular stitch. One should note how the repaired capsule lifts the capsular tissue away from the freshly resected bone and the labrum, which is thought to be preventive in scarring between these structures.

POSTOPERATIVE PROTOCOL

The approach to rehabilitation is highly dependent on coexistent pathologies in association with cam impingement. Any rehabilitation protocol should aim to establish functional use of the joint and correct muscle imbalances that may have developed due to the pathological process of the impingement and the rigors of the surgical procedure itself.

For procedures involving isolated cam impingement that were treated with femoral neck osteoplasty, it is recommended that the patient be protected with foot-flat partial weight bearing for 1 to 2 weeks. This is to avoid the feared and serious complication of fracturing the femoral neck. In postmenopausal women and any patient older than 55 years, these precautions should be strictly adhered to in order to avoid this potential complication.

The rehabilitation protocol may vary depending on the constellation of pathologies and procedures required intraoperatively. The most common scenario includes a femoroplasty with some combination of labral work and rim trimming. In these cases, partially protected crutch weight bearing is recommended for 1 to 2 weeks. Consideration for extending this restriction is recommended in certain cases, such as in patients with osteopenia (eg, postmenopausal females). Also, in cases in which microfracture is required, it is generally accepted that touch-down weight bearing be implemented for a minimum of 6 weeks.

A few other specific restrictions are recommended following arthroscopic femoroplasty in the early phase of rehabilitation. The patients are counseled to avoid impact activities so as not to expose the remodeling bone to high-caliber stress. Also, patients are instructed to be cautious in the first 4 weeks following osteoplasty if they are exposed to high-risk environments, such as icy or wet, slippery surfaces. A fall during this period could prove devastating to the compromised bone, and femoral neck fractures have been described following early postoperative trauma.

Generally, these patients should be allowed to gradually increase their activities under the care of their physical therapist and surgeon. Return to play varies widely depending on the rigors and demands of each athlete's particular sport. The goal for patients undergoing standard hip arthroscopy involving a femoroplasty with or without labral repair is approximately 3 to 5 months.

POTENTIAL COMPLICATIONS

Recent literature suggests that the overall complication rate associated with hip arthroscopy is low (range, 0.5% to 6.3%).[28-30] However, some of the more serious complications were directly related to the femoroplasty portion of the procedure. These include femoral neck fracture, incomplete resection of the cam lesion, overcorrection of the cam lesion, capsular disruption, and fluid extravasation.

Excessive resection of bone during arthroscopic femoroplasty has several potential risks. Perhaps the most devastating of these is femoral neck fracture. Femoral neck fracture following hip arthroscopy was first reported by Sampson et al[31] and was determined to be due to several potential factors, including excessive resection of bone, excessive early weight bearing, and osteopenia. Cadaveric studies have shown that up to 30% of the diameter of the femoral neck can be resected safely.[32] However, surgeons should exercise caution when performing arthroscopic femoroplasty, particularly in patients with any propensity for osteopenia (eg, elderly patients, peri- or postmenopausal females, and young females with exercise-induced osteopenia).

Another potential risk of excessive femoral neck resection is the possibility of losing the suction-seal of the labrum at the interface of the femoral head-neck junction. One of the main biomechanical functions of the labrum has been shown to confer this suction-seal, thus creating an inherent stabilizer of the femoral head into the acetabulum. When this suction-seal is disrupted, a theoretical potential for microinstability is created. Therefore, if the resection at the head-neck junction is excessive, the patient is effectively left with a shark-bite type of contour. When the hip is flexed, the labrum loses direct contact with the bone surface, which is thought to result in loss of the suction-seal and potentially cause microinstability symptoms.

Perhaps the most common complication of arthroscopic femoroplasty is related to underresection of bone at the head-neck junction. This has been cited as a common cause of failed hip arthroscopy requiring revision femoroplasty.[33] In the authors' experience, the most common areas that are underresected tend to be in the proximal lateral and posterolateral aspect of the identified cam lesion. These tend to be the zones that are technically harder to visualize and access. Diligent use of intraoperative fluoroscopy and meticulous technique usually allow the surgeon access to these areas. One technical pearl to reach these far lateral regions is to work with the hip in near full or full extension. This allows easier access to these zones, particularly when working through the anterolateral portal. As the surgeon gains experience, the risk of underresection and other potential complications diminishes. Judicious use of intraoperative fluoroscopy can also help ensure that these hard-to-access areas are adequately addressed.

Top Technical Pearls for the Procedure

1. Have a preoperative plan. Try to match the intraoperative fluoroscopic views to the preoperative x-rays, which will provide consistent imaging according to the preoperative plan and femoral resection template. This will give accurate real-time intraoperative information when resecting bone. Preoperative 3D reconstruction studies can also be helpful in preoperative planning.

2. Viewing and working from multiple portals is critical to adequately view and access all areas necessary for osteoplasty at the anterolateral head-neck junction of the hip. Use each established portal for viewing and working to optimize success. The proximal anterior portal is a valuable accessory portal for capsular management and bony resection.

3. Capsulotomy is critical for adequate exposure of the cam deformity during femoroplasty. Make a generous capsulotomy as necessary to visualize adequately.

(continued)

4. Judicious use of the fluoroscope is critical to accurately define the lesion before, during, and after resection. Fluoroscopy will ensure that adequate recontouring has been performed (particularly over the proximal and lateral extent of the cam lesion) and, conversely, to help the surgeon avoid overresecting the bone, thus creating a shark-bite lesion, which is an irreparable situation.

5. Respect and protect the lateral synovial fold. It is located over the posterolateral aspect of the head-neck junction and should be identified and documented before and after femoroplasty. Indiscriminate resection of the lateral synovial fold and the retinacular vessels can put the patient at risk for osteonecrosis of the femoral head.

REFERENCES

1. Smith-Petersen MN. The classic: treatment of malum coxae senilis, old slipped upper femoral epiphysis, intrapelvic protrusion of the acetabulum, and coxa plana by means of acetabuloplasty. *J Bone Joint Surg Am.* 1936;18:869-880.
2. Vulpius O, Stöffel A. *Orthopädische Operationslehre.* Stuttgart, Germany: F. Enke; 1913.
3. Ganz R, Parvizi J, Beck M, Leunig M, Nötzli H, Siebenrock KA. Femoroacetabular impingement: a cause for osteoarthritis of the hip. *Clin Orthop Relat Res.* 2003;(417):112-120.
4. Stulberg SD, Cordell LD, Harris WH, Ramsey PL, MacEwen GD. Unrecognized childhood hip disease: a major cause of idiopathic osteoarthritis of the hip. In: H*ip Society, Scientific Meeting.* The Hip: Proceedings of the Third Open Scientific Meeting of the Hip Society. St. Louis, MO: CV Mosby; 1975:212-228.
5. Byrd JW, Jones KS. Arthroscopic femoroplasty in the management of cam-type femoroacetabular impingement. *Clin Orthop Relat Res.* 2009;467(3):739-746.
6. Agricola R, Bessems JH, Ginai AZ, et al. The development of cam-type deformity in adolescent and young male soccer players. *Am J Sports Med.* 2012;40(5):1099-1106.
7. Siebenrock KA, Ferner F, Noble PC, Santore RF, Werlen S, Mamisch TC. The cam-type deformity of the proximal femur arises in childhood in response to vigorous sporting activity. *Clin Orthop Relat Res.* 2011;469(11):3229-3240.
8. Mirtz TA, Chandler JP, Eyers CM. The effects of physical activity on the epiphyseal growth plates: a review of the literature on normal physiology and clinical implications. *J Clin Med Res.* 2011;3(1):1-7.
9. Bardakos NV, Villar RN. Predictors of progression of osteoarthritis in femoroacetabular impingement: a radiological study with a minimum of ten years follow-up. *J Bone Joint Surg Br.* 2009;91(2):162-169.
10. Audenaert EA, Peeters I, Van Onsem S, Pattyn C. Can we predict the natural course of femoroacetabular impingement? *Acta Orthop Belg.* 2011;77(2):188-196.
11. Hartofilakidis G, Bardakos NV, Babis GC, Georgiades G. An examination of the association between different morphotypes of FAI in asymptomatic subjects and the development of osteoarthritis of the hip. *J Bone Joint Surg Br.* 2011;93(5):580-586.
12. Philippon MJ, Briggs KK, Yen YM, Kuppersmith DA. Outcomes following hip arthroscopy for femoroacetabular impingement with associated chondrolabral dysfunction: minimum two-year follow-up. *J Bone Joint Surg Br.* 2009;91(1):16-23.
13. Byrd JW, Jones KS. Arthroscopic management of femoroacetabular impingement: minimum two-year follow-up. *Arthroscopy.* 2011;27(10):1379-1388.
14. Botser IB, Smith TW Jr, Nasser R, Domb BG. Open surgical dislocation versus arthroscopy for femoroacetabular impingement: a comparison of clinical outcomes. *Arthroscopy.* 2011;27(2):270-278.
15. Nötzli HP, Wyss TF, Stoecklin CH, Schmid MR, Treiber K, Hodler J. The contour of the femoral head-neck junction as a predictor for the risk of anterior impingement. *J Bone Joint Surg Br.* 2002;84(4):556-560.
16. Tibor LM, Sekiya JK. Differential diagnosis of pain around the hip joint. *Arthroscopy.* 2008;24(12):1407-1421.
17. Philippon MJ, Maxwell RB, Johnston TL, Schenker M, Briggs KK. Clinical presentation of femoroacetabular impingement. *Knee Surg Sports Traumatol Arthrosc.* 2007;15(8):1041-1047.

18. Martin RL, Irrgang JJ, Sekiya JK. The diagnostic accuracy of a clinical examination in determining intra-articular hip pain for potential hip arthroscopy candidates. *Arthroscopy*. 2008;24(9):1013-1018.
19. Byrd JW, Potts EA, Allison RK, Jones KS. Ultrasound-guided hip injections: a comparative study with fluoroscopy-guided injections. *Arthroscopy*. 2014;30(1):42-46.
20. Klaue K, Durnin CW, Ganz R. The acetabular rim syndrome. A clinical presentation of dysplasia of the hip. *J Bone Joint Surg Br*. 1991;73(3):423-429.
21. Martin HD, Kelly BT, Leunig M, et al. The pattern and technique in the clinical evaluation of the adult hip: the common physical examination tests of hip specialists. *Arthroscopy*. 2010;26(2):161-172.
22. Maslowski E, Sullivan W, Forster Harwood J, et al. The diagnostic validity of hip provocation maneuvers to detect intra-articular hip pathology. *PM R*. 2010;2(3):174-181.
23. Byrd JW, Jones KS. Diagnostic accuracy of clinical assessment, magnetic resonance imaging, magnetic resonance arthrography, and intra-articular injection in hip arthroscopy patients. *Am J Sports Med*. 2004;32(7):1668-1674.
24. Parvizi J, Bican O, Bender B, et al. Arthroscopy for labral tears in patients with developmental dysplasia of the hip: a cautionary note. *J Arthroplasty*. 2009;24(6 suppl):110-113.
25. Johnston TL, Schenker ML, Briggs KK, Philippon MJ. Relationship between offset angle alpha and hip chondral injury in femoroacetabular impingement. *Arthroscopy*. 2008;24(6):669-675.
26. Ganz R, Parvizi J, Beck M, Leunig M, Nötzli H, Siebenrock KA. Femoroacetabular impingement: a cause for osteoarthritis of the hip. *Clin Orthop Relat Res*. 2003;(417):112-120.
27. Larson CM, Sikka RS, Sardelli MC, et al. Increasing alpha angle is predictive of athletic-related "hip" and "groin" pain in collegiate National Football League prospects. *Arthroscopy*. 2013;29(3):405-410.
28. Gupta A, Redmond JM, Hammarstedt JE, Schwindel L, Domb BG. Safety measures in hip arthroscopy and their efficacy in minimizing complications: a systematic review of the evidence. *Arthroscopy*. 2014;30(10):1342-1348.
29. Möckel G, Labs K. Complications in hip arthroscopy and follow-up therapy: analysis over a 5-year time period with a total of 13,000 cases [in German]. *Orthopade*. 2014;43(1):6-15.
30. Oak N, Mendez-Zfass M, Lesniak BP, Larson CM, Kelly BT, Bedi A. Complications in hip arthroscopy. *Sports Med Arthrosc*. 2013;21(2):97-105.
31. Sampson TG. Complications of hip arthroscopy. *Clin Sports Med*. 2001;20(4):831-835.
32. Mardones RM, Gonzalez C, Chen Q, Zobitz M, Kaufman KR, Trousdale RT. Surgical treatment of femoroacetabular impingement: evaluation of the effect of the size of the resection. *J Bone Joint Surg Am*. 2005;87(2):273-279.
33. Philippon MJ, Schenker ML, Briggs KK, Kuppersmith DA, Maxwell RB, Stubbs AJ. Revision hip arthroscopy. *Am J Sports Med*. 2007;35(11):1918-1921.

Please see videos on the accompanying website at

www.ArthroscopicTechniques.com

SECTION IV

Extracapsular Management

16

Treatment of the Iliopsoas Tendon

Indications and Arthroscopic Approaches for Lengthening and Release

Allston J. Stubbs, MD, MBA and Elizabeth A. Howse, MD

INTRODUCTION

Coxa saltans interna, also known as internal snapping hip, presents as groin pain associated with a catching sensation when bringing the hip from a position of flexed abduction to extended adduction. First described by Nunziata and Blumenfeld in 1951,[1] it is attributed to movement of the iliopsoas tendon. It is postulated that the tendon typically becomes caught when traveling over the iliopectineal eminence at the pelvic brim, the anterior inferior iliac spine, or the anterior femoral head. Although there is debate as to what exactly obstructs the path of the iliopsoas tendon, it is generally agreed upon that it is due to anatomic factors that result in a tight musculotendinous unit. Whereas a painless, internal snapping hip is a normal population variant in up to 10% of the population, a painful internal snapping hip is due to intrinsic iliopsoas tendon pathology or is secondary to other factors, such as native or arthroplasty hip joint pathology, instability, or high femoral antetorsion. In the setting of primary intrinsic tendon pathology and some secondary pathologies, surgical lengthening or release may be considered.[2]

INDICATIONS

- ► Coxa saltans interna
- ► Iliopsoas impingement across anterior acetabulum
- ► Iliopsoas irritation after total hip arthroplasty (Figure 16-1)
- ► Refractory iliopsoas tendonitis

Byrd JWT, Bedi A, Stubbs AJ, eds. *The Hip:*
AANA Advanced Arthroscopic Surgical Techniques (pp 199-206).
© 2016 AANA.

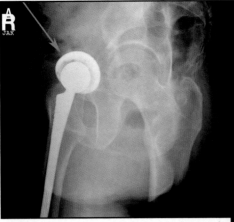
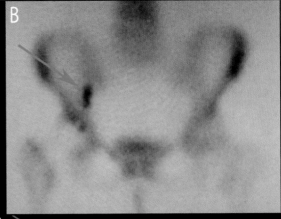
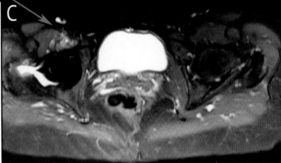

Figure 16-1. (A) Plain film false-profile view showing a prominent acetabular cup. (B) Technetium Tc-99 scintigraphy and (C) T2-weighted noncontrasted magnetic resonance image of a patient with iliopsoas tendinitis 15 months after right total hip arthroplasty.

Controversial Indications

- ▶ Asymptomatic snapping hip
- ▶ Femoral antetorsion > 25 degrees
- ▶ Acetabular dysplasia
- ▶ Skeletally immature pelvis
- ▶ High-performance athlete

PERTINENT PHYSICAL FINDINGS

- ▶ Iliopsoas dynamic stress test
- ▶ Modified Stinchfield test
- ▶ Thomas test

PERTINENT IMAGING

- ▶ Dynamic ultrasound visualization/local anesthetic (Figure 16-2)
- ▶ Plain x-rays
- ▶ Magnetic resonance imaging

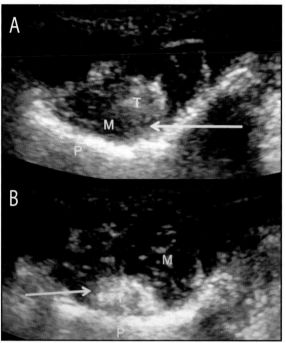

Figure 16-2. (A) Normal sonographic anatomy displaying the muscle (M) between the tendon (T) and pelvis (P). (B) Tendon overlying the bone after the snap. (Reprinted with permission from Dr. Maha Torabi, Wake Forest University School of Medicine.)

EQUIPMENT

The following equipment is needed:

▶ Arthroscope
▶ Arthroscopic blade
▶ Blunt switching stick
▶ Radiofrequency device
▶ Nitinol guidewire
▶ Shavers
▶ Slotted cannula

POSITIONING

Once in the operating room, a surgical timeout should be performed to confirm the patient, surgical side, and availability of the necessary equipment. The patient is then placed in the modified supine or lateral decubitus position on the operating table, depending on surgeon preference. While positioning the patient, care should be taken to appropriately pad all dependent bony prominences. The pelvis is stabilized with the use of a lateral hip positioner or beanbag (in the lateral decubitus position) or a padded perineal post lateralized toward the operative side (supine position). The operative hip must retain the ability to be mobilized throughout the procedure and is placed in a commercially available distraction system.

STEP-BY-STEP DESCRIPTION OF THE PROCEDURE

Endoscopic release of the iliopsoas tendon can be performed from the central or peripheral compartment or extra-articularly at the lesser trochanter. All techniques yield favorable outcomes, and surgical technique is largely due to surgeon preference.[3,4] The level of release determines the percentage of tendon to muscle of the iliopsoas unit. The central compartment release is approximately 40% tendon,[4] the peripheral compartment release is approximately 50% tendon,[4] and the lesser trochanter release is approximately 60% tendon.[4] For native hips, the authors prefer the central compartment technique (Video) to avoid potential iatrogenic injury to the zona orbicularis in the peripheral compartment. Conversely for prosthetic joints, release of iliopsoas impingement at the lesser trochanter away from the prosthesis is preferable to minimize the possibility of an iatrogenic infection. The goal of the release is to lengthen the musculotendinous unit while leaving the muscle fibers intact; clinical judgment determines whether a partial or complete release is needed for each patient.[5] A complete release may be necessary based on the patient's anatomy (bifid or trifid appearance of the iliopsoas tendon), and additional pathology, such as a spur located at the lesser trochanter resulting in continued snapping if only a partial release is performed.[5,6] Most patients with coxa saltans interna have additional forms of hip pathology; therefore, regardless of which technique the surgeon prefers, he or she may also perform a full diagnostic and therapeutic arthroscopy to yield the best possible results.[3]

Central Compartment

Using a standard operative technique, anterolateral and modified anterior portals are established. The surgeon then performs a diagnostic hip arthroscopy in which he or she can determine whether there is any concomitant pathology that needs to be addressed. With the hip in traction, the hip is placed in neutral rotation with approximately 20 degrees of flexion and neutral abduction.[2] Visualization of the synovial reflection of the psoas tendon is achieved by directing the arthroscope anteromedially from the anterolateral portal.[2] Prominence of the iliopsoas tendon across the anterosuperior rim with associated labral ecchymosis and chondrolabral dysfunction is consistent with iliopsoas impingement (Figure 16-3A). Anterior to the hip joint, capsular tissue forms a thin veil that is lateral to the tendon and iliopsoas bursa, which is gently resected.[2] This part of the capsule adjacent to the iliopsoas tendon may be inflamed; furthermore, bruising or tearing of the adjacent labrum may be seen in patients with coxa saltans interna (Figure 16-3B).[2] A transcapsular window of 5 mm is formed with the arthroscopic blade, and the tendinous portion of the iliopsoas is identified (Figure 16-3C). Under direct visualization using the medial protection technique, the tendinous aspect of the iliopsoas is transected, leaving the iliacus muscle fibers intact (Figures 16-3D and E).[7] Following tendon transection, the musculotendinous unit and bursa are reassessed for additional pathology. The femoral nerve, artery, and vein lie directly anterior to the iliopsoas at this level; therefore, care must be taken to avoid iatrogenic injury.[2,8]

Peripheral Compartment

Using a standard operative technique, anterolateral and modified anterior portals are established as described for the central compartment. With the hip out of traction, the hip is placed in neutral rotation/abduction and approximately 40 degrees of flexion. The camera is placed in the anterolateral portal, and the medial synovial fold is visualized along the inferior femoral neck. An arthroscopic blade is introduced via the modified anterior portal, and a 5- to 10-mm capsulotomy is made medial to the zona orbicularis and inferior to the medial synovial fold. The tendon portion of the iliopsoas is identified. Under direct visualization, the tendon portion is cut with a radiofrequency device or an arthroscopic knife. Similar precautions to the central compartment release are followed to avoid iatrogenic injury to the surrounding anatomy.

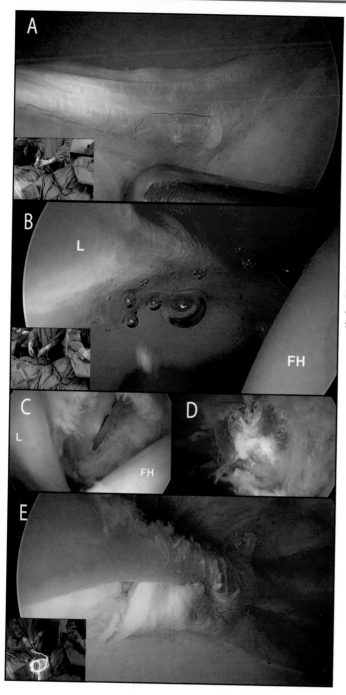

Figure 16-3. (A) Ecchymosis differential across the anterosuperior acetabulum from the perspective of the capsulolabral interface. (B) Iliopsoas impingement triad: prominent iliopsoas tendon across the anterior acetabulum with focal capsulolabral synovitis/labral ecchymosis, labral tear, and thin rim of chondromalacia. (C) Small fenestration of the anterior capsule with an arthroscopic knife to cut the tendon. Note the avoidance of the labrum and femoral head. (D) Status post released iliopsoas tendon at level of central compartment with arthroscopic knife. Note the yellow discoloration of the tendon associated with chronic tendinopathy. (E) Status post release of iliopsoas from central compartment. Also, status post labral repair anterosuperior acetabulum.

Extra-Articular Release

Peripheral endoscopic iliopsoas release is performed with the hip out of traction, using 2 distal anterolateral accessory portals. These portals are approximately 5 cm apart from each other. The hip is externally rotated and placed in approximately 15 to 20 degrees of flexion.[2] Under fluoroscopic guidance, the lesser trochanter is identified. The proximal accessory portal serves as the primary camera portal, and the distal accessory portal serves as the instrumentation portal. The

Figure 16-4. Iliopsoas release status post total hip arthroplasty. Proximal camera and radio-frequency wand distal at the level of the lesser trochanter.

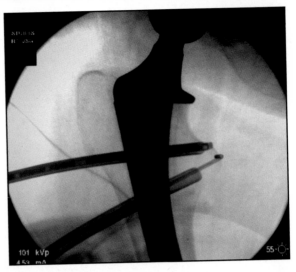

tendinous portion of the iliopsoas muscle-tendon insertion is identified in the iliopsoas bursa as a bright white structure. Using the arthroscopic blade and radiofrequency device, the tendinous portion is released off the lesser trochanter without excising any muscle (Figure 16-4). The surgeon should take care to keep the release distal, at the level of the lesser trochanter, to avoid damage to the medial and lateral femoral circumflex arteries, which wrap around the tendon approximately 2 to 3 cm proximal to its insertion.[2,9] Hemostasis is achieved with the radiofrequency device.

POSTOPERATIVE PROTOCOL

Postoperatively, patients are protected by ambulating with crutches and are limited to approximately 20 lb of foot-flat weight bearing as tolerated until limping resolves. Generally, patients are maintained on crutches for 2 weeks or until gait normalizes. Duration of crutch use is dependent on additional hip pathology and intervention, as well as preoperative peripelvic condition and activity level. Adjunctive use of an abduction hip orthosis may provide support during early stages of rehabilitation. Physical therapy is started on postoperative day 1, with an emphasis on gait education and gentle hip range of motion exercises. Prior to surgical intervention, patients are counseled to expect weakness of the hip flexors for 2 to 4 weeks that typically normalizes over 6 months.[2,10] Hip flexor–strengthening exercises should not begin until postoperative week 6 to avoid inflammation of the hip flexor area.[2,10] Finally, a nonsteroidal anti-inflammatory drug is prescribed for 3 to 6 weeks to minimize the risk for potential heterotopic ossification.

POTENTIAL COMPLICATIONS

Numerous complications have been reported after iliopsoas tenotomy, including hip flexor weakness, heterotopic ossification, anterolateral numbness of the thigh, persistent pain, infection, hematoma, and recurrent snapping.[2,5,6,11-16] Complication rates after endoscopic release are lower than those after open approaches. In a systematic review evaluating outcomes of open and arthroscopic approaches for the surgical treatment of coxa saltans interna, Khan et al[16] showed that arthroscopic treatment had significantly fewer complications compared with open techniques. Three (2.3%) patients of 129 treated arthroscopically reported continued pain; no patients reported continued snapping. Furthermore, patients who were treated via the central compartment had a lower risk of complications (2%) compared with patients treated through the peripheral approach.[4,16] In addition to having a higher risk of continued pain in the peripheral compartment group, 1 of the 37 patients had greater trochanteric bursitis and 2 had ischial bursitis compared with none in the central compartment group. In the study by Khan et al,[16] there was almost a ten-fold increase in complication rate for the 119 patients who underwent an open surgical procedure (21%); however, complication rates have been reported in up to 50%.[12,16,18]

Presumptively, continued pain and hip flexor weakness are some of the most worrisome potential complications in high-functioning athletes. One surgeon reported a 2.8% (1 patient) complication rate of hip flexor weakness after performing 35 releases at the level of the lesser trochanter.[5] Although hip flexor weakness is to be expected in the immediate postoperative period, most patients will regain their strength with time. Philippon et al[15] demonstrated preservation of hip flexion and torque at 4.3 months postoperatively in a study of 50 patients who underwent arthroscopic fractional lengthening of the iliopsoas tendon at the musculotendinous junction. Furthermore, they showed that patients who required iliopsoas release had significantly less strength and torque preoperatively compared with a similar cohort of patients who did not have coxa saltans interna. In a comparative study of the central vs lesser trochanter release, Ilizaliturri et al[4] hypothesized that the reason hip flexor weakness is more common when using the lesser trochanter approach is because the muscular portion is preserved in the central approach.

Risk of hip flexor weakness may be less in the central approach; however, in contrast to the peripheral approach, there is a greater risk of anterior thigh paresthesias due to femoral nerve branches lying directly over the iliopsoas muscle and a branch of the lateral femoral cutaneous nerve, which lies in close proximity to the location of the anterior portal.[2,4,8,14] In the authors' approach, they minimize this risk through the use of the modified anterior portal, which is typically 2 cm away from any nerve branches, instead of the anterior portal, which is typically within 2 to 4 mm of branches of the lateral femoral cutaneous nerve and 32 mm away from the femoral nerve.[19]

Top Technical Pearls and Pitfalls for the Procedure

Pearls

1. Consider concomitant central compartment arthroscopy to address associated intra-articular pathology.
2. Use the medial protection technique to protect the surrounding anatomy.
3. For release at the level of the lesser trochanter, externally rotate the femur.
4. Maintain meticulous hemostasis after release to avoid bursal hematoma.

Pitfalls

1. Failure to prevent heterotopic ossification with postoperative chemoprophylaxis.
2. Neurovascular injury can be caused by not resecting the iliopsoas tendon at the muscular portion.
3. Bifid or trifid tendons can result in incomplete release due to not fully visualizing the tendon.
4. Weakness of hip flexion when more than the necessary amount of the iliopsoas tendon is released, or the rehabilitation program is too vigorous.

REFERENCES

1. Nunziata A, Blumenfeld I. Snapping hip; note on a variety. *Prensa Med Argent*. 1951;38(32):1997-2001.
2. Jani S, Safran MR. Internal snapping hip syndrome. In Byrd JW, Guanche CA, eds. *AANA Advanced Arthroscopy: The Hip*. Philadelphia, PA: Elsevier; 2010:125-132.
3. Ilizaliturri VM, Ugalde HG, Camacho-Galindo J. Iliopsoas tendon release. In: Byrd JW, ed. *Operative Hip Arthroscopy*. 3rd ed. New York, NY: Springer; 2013:279-290.
4. Ilizaliturri VM, Buganza-Tepole M, Olivos-Meza A, Acuna M, Acosta-Rodriquez E. Central compartment release versus lesser trochanter release of the iliopsoas tendon for the treatment of internal snapping hip: a comparative study. *Arthroscopy*. 2014;30(7):790-795.
5. Sampson TG. Arthroscopic iliopsoas release for coxa saltans interna (snapping hip syndrome). In: Byrd JW, ed. *Operative Hip Arthroscopy*. 2nd ed. New York, NY: Springer; 2005:189-194.
6. Shu B, Safran MR. Case report: bifid iliopsoas tendon causing refractory internal snapping hip. *Clin Orthop Relat Res*. 2011;469(1):289-293.
7. Stubbs AJ. Intraarticular Arthroscopic Recession of the Iliopsoas Tendon: Medial Protection Technique. AAOS Video [DVD]. Rosemont, IL: American Academy of Orthopaedic Surgeons; 2011..
8. Kelly BT, Williams RJ III, Philippon MJ. Hip arthroscopy: current indications, treatment options, and management issues. *Am J Sports Med*. 2003;31(6):1020-1037.
9. Flanum ME, Keene JS, Blankenbaker DG, DeSmet AA. Arthroscopic treatment of the painful "internal" snapping hip: results of a new endoscopic technique and imaging protocol. *Am J Sports Med*. 2007;35(5):770-779.
10. Ilizaliturri VM Jr, Chaidez PA, Villegas P, Briseño A, Camacho-Galindo J. Prospective randomized study of 2 different techniques for endoscopic iliopsoas tendon release in the treatment of internal snapping hip syndrome. *Arthroscopy*. 2009;25(2):159-163.
11. Dobbs MB, Gordon JE, Luhmann SJ, Szymanski DA, Schoenecker PL. Surgical correction of the snapping iliopsoas tendon in adolescents. *J Bone Joint Surg Am*. 2002;84(3):420-424.
12. McCulloch PC, Bush-Joseph CA. Massive heterotopic ossification complicating iliopsoas tendon lengthening: a case report. *Am J Sports Med*. 2006;34(12):2022-2025.
13. Fabricant PD, Bedi A, De La Torre K, Kelly BT. Clinical outcomes after arthroscopic psoas lengthening: the effect of femoral version. *Arthroscopy*. 2012;28(7):965-971.
14. Wettstein M, Jung J, Dienst M. Arthroscopic psoas tenotomy. *Arthroscopy*. 2006;22(8):907.e1-907.e4.
15. Philippon MJ, Boykin RE, Patterson D, Briggs KK. Hip flexion strength and torque after arthroscopic fractional lengthening of the iliopsoas tendon. *Arthroscopy*. 2013;19(10):e165-e166.
16. Khan M, Adamich J, Simunovic N, Philippon MJ, Bhandari M, Ayeni OR. Surgical management of internal snapping hip syndrome: a systemic review evaluating open and arthroscopic approaches. *Arthroscopy*. 2013;29(5):942-948.
17. Deslandes M, Guillin R, Cardinal E, Hobden R, Bureau NJ. The snapping iliopsoas tendon: new mechanisms using dynamic sonography. *AJR Am J Roentgenol*. 2008;190(3):576-581.
18. Hoskins JS, Burd TA, Allen WC. Surgical correction of internal coxa saltans: a 20-year consecutive study. *Am J Sports Med*. 2004;32(4):998-1001.
19. Byrd JW, Pappas JN, Pedley MJ. Hip arthroscopy: an anatomic study of portal placement and relationship to the extra-articular structures. *Arthroscopy*. 1995;11(4):418-423.

Please see videos on the accompanying website at

www.ArthroscopicTechniques.com

17

Greater Trochanteric Pain Syndrome and Endoscopy of the Peritrochanteric Space

Víctor M. Ilizaliturri Jr, MD; Marco Acuna-Tovar, MD;
Eduardo Acosta-Rodriguez, MD; and Pedro Joachin-Hernandez, MD

INTRODUCTION

Greater trochanteric pain syndrome (GTPS) is a regional pain syndrome characterized by chronic, intermittent pain accompanied by tenderness of the lateral proximal thigh, involving the greater trochanter (GT) area and the buttock.[1,2] It was first known as *trochanteric bursitis* because it was believed that only the bursa caused the symptoms. It is now known that there are many causes of this syndrome. The syndrome encompasses a wide spectrum of etiologies, including tendinosis, muscle tears, trigger points, iliotibial band (ITB) disorders, and surrounding soft tissue pathology.[1,3]

The first description of trochanteric bursitis was in 1923 by Stegeman[4] for symptoms of lateral hip pain. The term *GTPS* was first used by Leonard,[5] who proposed using the phrase *trochanteric syndrome* to refer to the symptoms in the proximity of the trochanter major. GTPS has been referred to as the great mimicker because it is frequently mistaken for other conditions, including, but not limited to, myofascial pain, degenerative joint disease, and spinal pathology.[1,6] Recent advances in the understanding of hip pathology—thanks to better magnetic resonance imaging (MRI), arthroscopic hip instrumentation, and surgical techniques—have enabled orthopedic surgeons to expand arthroscopic principles to the treatment of extra-articular pathology in the peritrochanteric space.

Byrd JWT, Bedi A, Stubbs AJ, eds. *The Hip:*
AANA Advanced Arthroscopic Surgical Techniques (pp 207-220).
© 2016 AANA.

Figure 17-1. (A) Illustration showing the 3 main bursae, including the (1) subgluteus maximus bursa, (2) subgluteus minimus bursa, and (3) subgluteus media bursa. (Reprinted with permission from Dr. Angélica Martínez Ramos Méndez.) (B) Anatomy of the gluteus muscle insertions, including the (1) gluteus medius, (2) piriformis, (3) gluteus minimus, and (4) long head gluteus minimus.

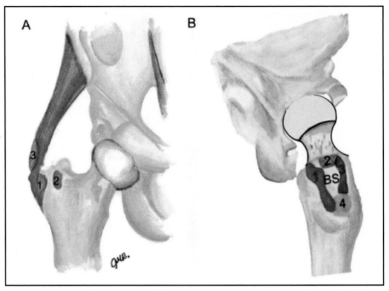

Anatomy

Bursa

Bursae are fluid-filled sacs between bony prominences and surrounding soft tissues.[3] Twenty-one bursae have been described around the GT, but only 3 of these are present in most individuals.[3] These include the subgluteus medius bursa, found deep to the gluteus medius tendon; the gluteus minimus bursa, located anterosuperior to the GT; and the subgluteus maximus bursa, located between the gluteus medius tendon and the gluteus maximus muscle (Figure 17-1).[1] They provide cushioning for the gluteus tendons, ITB, and tensor fascia latae. The subgluteus maximus bursa is the largest of the GT bursae and is most frequently incriminated in GTPS.

Many secondary bursae can be present, and this, together with variable locations of the bursae, add to the misdiagnosis and varied response to steroid injections.[3]

Iliotibial Tract

The iliotibial tract has 2 musculotendinous attachments proximally: the tensor fascia lata anteriorly and the gluteus maximus posteriorly. The gluteus medius is indirectly attached through its overlying aponeurosis. These muscles pull on the iliotibial tract, making it tense whether the hip is flexed or extended. The iliotibial tract is firmly attached on its deep surface to the linea aspera and the posterior femur. In the distal portion, the thickened posterior border of the iliotibial tract inserts on the lateral tibia at Gerdy's tubercle. Because the iliotibial tract remains tense throughout motion of the hip, not only does it act as a tension band on the lateral thigh, but any small anatomic change or swelling may precipitate snapping over the GT. The GT bursa lies between the iliotibial tract and the GT, and it may become inflamed and cause pain when snapping occurs.

Gluteus Muscles

Efforts to accurately describe and repair persistently symptomatic tears require an improved understanding of the gluteus medius and minimus footprint anatomy. Robertson et al[7] accurately described the anatomy of the gluteus muscles (see Figure 17-1). The gluteus medius tendon inserts into the GT in 2 sites: the superoposterior facet and the lateral facet. The superoposterior insertion is wide and square (196.5 ± 48.4 mm^2). The lateral insertion is more rectangular, with a surface area of 438 ± 48.4 mm^2. The capsular insertion of the gluteus minimus is separated from the proximal portion of the lateral facet footprint by the trochanteric bald spot. Distal to this, the long head of the gluteus minimus begins.

EPIDEMIOLOGY

GTPS is estimated to affect between 10% and 20% of the population in industrialized societies, especially between the fourth and sixth decades of life.[1] The incidence of GT pain is reported to be approximately 1.8 patients per 1000 per year.[1] Of all sports-related injuries, 2.5% involve the hip.[1] Segal et al[6] found the prevalence of GTPS to be 17.6%; it was higher in women and patients with coexisting low back pain, osteoarthritis, ITB tenderness, and obesity. The increased prevalence in women may be attributed to altered biomechanics associated with differences in the size, shape, and orientation of the pelvis (gynecoid vs android) and its relationship with the ITB. Obesity was significantly associated with GTPS (body mass index > 30 kg/m^2). The presence of low back pain seems to predispose patients to hip pain. The prevalence of GTPS in adults with musculoskeletal low back pain is between 20% and 35%.[1,2]

PHYSIOPATHOLOGY

Disorders of the peritrochanteric space include 3 well-described entities: external coxa saltans, GT bursitis, and gluteus medius and/or minimus tears. True bursitis could be secondary to direct trauma, muscle dysfunction, or overuse.[1,3,8] The origin of the pain could be the bursae, the ITB, or the gluteal muscle insertions. Anteriorly, it was believed that the most common cause of pain was bursal inflammation, but in recent histopathologic and MRI studies, it was shown that this condition (inflammation) is uncommon.[8-10]

Altered lower limb biomechanics predispose to muscle abnormalities, which is the major cause of GTPS. Also, tendinoses, inflammation, and tears of the gluteus medius and minimus can be originated by overuse mechanisms or an increase in the tension of the ITB. Contrary to expectations, Silva et al[10] could not find histological evidence of acute or chronic inflammation in patients with criteria for GTPS. Most of the tears of the muscle insertions are on the undersurface (similar to a shoulder partial articular supraspinatus tendon avulsion lesion).[11]

INDICATIONS

The most common indications for endoscopic surgery of the peritrochanteric space include the following:
- External snapping hip syndrome
- GTPS with or without associated tears of the abductor muscles

Controversial Indications

- Revision surgery of external snapping hip syndromes (In these cases, surgeons may prefer to perform open revisions.)
- Gluteus minimus tears that may require opening tendon of the gluteus medius for access, which some surgeons may prefer not to do[11]

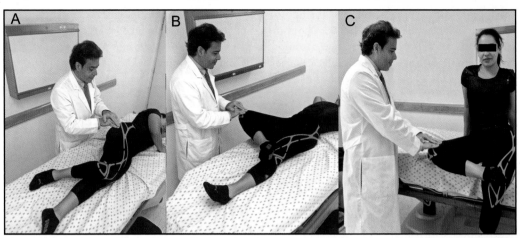

Figure 17-2. (A) A tender spot is usually found in the posterosuperior corner of the greater trochanter. (B) FABER (flexion, abduction, and external rotation) test. The examiner must comparatively measure the distance between the table and the knee on the examined side. With a thigh ITB, hip osteoarthritis, and sacroiliac pathology, a difference may be found in the comparative distances. The location of the pain or discomfort may orient the examiner to the origin of the pathology. Increased motion may be related to hip instability. (C) A modification of the FABERE test with patient in sitting position. Tightness of the ITB usually generates discomfort when performing this test.

► Massive tears too difficult to fix using endoscopic techniques that may be more adequate for an open type of repair or muscle transfer[12]

PERTINENT PHYSICAL FINDINGS

The diagnosis of trochanteric bursitis is clinical. Ege Rasmussen and Fanø[13] proposed the following clinical criteria for the diagnosis of trochanteric bursitis: lateral hip pain and GT tenderness with pain at the extreme of hip rotation, a positive Patrick-FABERE (flexion, abduction, external rotation, and extension; Figure 17-2) test, pseudoradiculopathy (extending to the lateral thigh), or pain on forced hip abduction. These criteria are frequently used but have not been validated. Pain extending to the groin or down the lateral thigh that mimics lumbar disk herniation may be reported by some individuals. Usually, the irradiation pattern produces a misdiagnosis because of the overlapping with the iliotibial tract and the mid-lumbar dermatomes (L2-L4).[2]

Regional pain syndromes are also in the differential diagnosis, such as lesions to the nerve supply of structures such as the gluteus maximus (inferior gluteal nerve), tensor fascia lata, and gluteus medius and minimus (superior gluteal nerve).[14]

Clinical tests include the Jump sign, or palpation of the affected area that reveals tenderness on the GT (the patient pulls away forcefully on contact of the area) at the site of the gluteus medius tendon insertion.[15] Pain can be reproducible by active resistance to abduction and external rotation but rarely in hip extension. Trendelenburg's test (Figure 17-3) was the most accurate test in detecting a tendon tear, with a sensitivity of 73% and a specificity of 77% in a study conducted by Bird et al.[8] Ober's test may differentiate between an ITB problem and GTPS (Figure 17-4). Pain from GTPS does not radiate beyond the proximal thigh, ITB pain has a positive Ober's test, and true nerve root compression causes symptoms in the lower leg.[2]

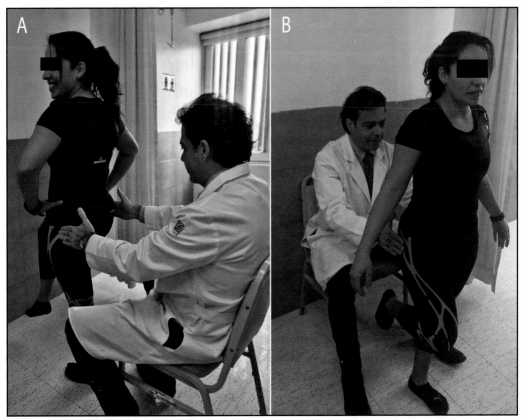

Figure 17-3. (A, B) Trendelenburg's test. The examiner sits behind the patient and asks the patient to elevate one of the legs. The pelvis must remain stable. A drop on the elevated side means abductor power deficiency of the supported leg. The test can be comparative over time, producing a fatigue Trendelenburg, typically with 10-second increments.

PERTINENT IMAGING

▶ Plain x-rays of the pelvis are used to make the differential diagnosis (hip osteoarthritis, femoral neck fractures, and avascular necrosis of the femoral head). Pathologies such as protrusion acetabula and femoroacetabular impingement may be implicated in gluteal muscle pathology.[8]

▶ Ultrasound is able to distinguish gluteus tendinopathy from trochanteric bursitis and assess snapping hip related to the ITB in real time. It is superior to MRI for identification of calcific tendinosis (Figure 17-5)[9]; however, the primary indications for ultrasound are external snapping hip tendinopathy and bursitis in this region.[16]

▶ MRI is the gold standard study for recalcitrant lateral hip pain. The most important advantage is the ability to observe the soft tissue structures (signals of peritendinitis, tendinosis, and partial or complete tears of the gluteus medius) and indirect signs of lesions (fatty atrophy, calcification of the tendon, and bursal fluid; Figure 17-6).[8,9]

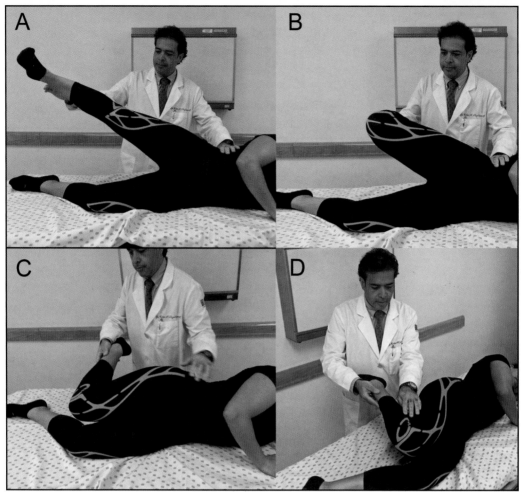

Figure 17-4. Ober's test. The patient is in the lateral decubitus position. Her right side is examined. (A) The patient is asked to actively elevate the right lower limb. (B) While in active abduction, the knee is bent by the examiner. (C) The patient is asked to relax, and the knee should fall on the opposite knee resting on the table. (D) If the test is positive, the knee may not fall all the way down, and the examiner may find a spring effect if pressure is applied on the upper knee.

EQUIPMENT

Endoscopic examination of the iliopsoas bursa is typically performed using standard hip arthroscopy instruments. A 70- and a 30-degree arthroscope are commonly used. An extra-long arthroscope may also be an option for obese patients. Standard arthroscopy hand instrument shavers and radiofrequency (RF) probes are also used for tissue resection and ablation. Suture management equipment and disposable cannulas are used for abductor muscle repair, as well as suture anchors.

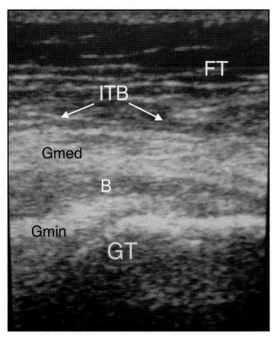

Figure 17-5. Ultrasound image of the peritrochanteric space in a right hip. At the top of the photograph, the fatty tissue (FT) and the ITB are observed. The gluteus medius (Gmed) tendon can be identified directly under the ITB because the cut proximal the subgluteus maximus bursa is not observed. Deep to the gluteus medius is the gluteus minimus (Gmin) tendon. Between them is the subgluteus medius bursa (B). The GT is observed at the bottom of the image.

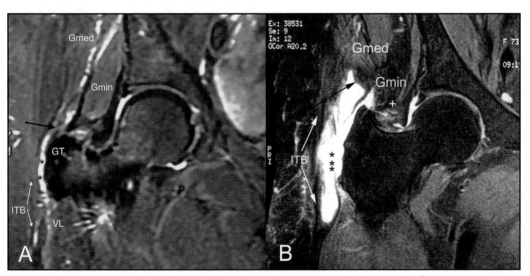

Figure 17-6. (A) T2-weighted coronal MRI of a right hip. The ITB is observed. A tear of the gluteus medius (Gmed) tendon is seen (black arrow). Note the fluid (*) in the GT bursa. The origin of the vastus lateralis (VL) is observed distal to the fluid accumulation. Insertion of the gluteus minimus (Gmin) is observed in the GT. (B) T2-weighted coronal MRI of a right hip. The ITB is demonstrated (white arrows). A massive retractive Gmed tear is seen (black arrow). The Gmin is observed with a small tear (+) at its tendon. A massive amount of fluid is in the bursa (***).

POSITIONING

Endoscopic access to the peritrochanteric space can be obtained with the patient in the supine and lateral positions. The patient may also be prepared for traction when arthroscopic surgery of the hip will be performed in conjunction with endoscopy of the peritrochanteric space.

STEP-BY-STEP DESCRIPTION OF THE PROCEDURE

GTPS is a self-limiting condition and usually resolves with conservative measures, such as nonsteroidal anti-inflammatory drugs, ice, weight loss, and physical therapy aimed to improve flexibility, muscle strengthening, and joint mechanics.[17] If these options fail, bursa or lateral hip injections are performed with corticosteroids, with a success rate of 60% to 100%.[3,13] No studies have compared the effect with placebo, but an epidemiology study has shown a recovery rate 2.7 times higher with patients treated with steroid injections.[17] According to Cohen et al,[18] there is no difference between the use of anatomic landmarks and fluoroscopy.

In patients in whom conservative treatment fails, surgical intervention has been advocated. This recalcitrant trochanteric bursitis can sometimes be addressed with arthroscopic bursectomy and/or ITB release. There are 3 main causes of GTPS that can be treated surgically and are discussed separately.

Endoscopic Access to the Peritrochanteric Space

Before focusing on the peritrochanteric pathology, it is important to discard the presence of hip joint pathology; this can be by preoperative studies or by performing an arthroscopic evaluation of the hip joint before peritrochanteric space endoscopy. The peritrochanteric endoscopy can be managed in the supine[19] or lateral[20,21] position. No traction is necessary to access the peritrochanteric space.

The GT is the main landmark for portal placement and is always marked on the skin. The senior author (VMI) uses 2 portals: a proximal trochanteric and a distal trochanteric portal (Figure 17-7). When treating a snapping hip, the area of snapping should be between both portals to ensure that ITB release will include the area of the problem. Other authors have described the use of a mid-anterior portal and other portals to access the peritrochanteric space and as a primary viewing portal.[19] Endoscopic access to the peritrochanteric space can be obtained with the outside-in technique, which involves placing endoscopic instruments inside the peritrochanteric space through a window or a defect on the ITB lateral to the GT, or the inside-out technique, which places portals through the ITB into the peritrochanteric space without creating a window.[22,23] The pump pressure is often set at 50 mm Hg to avoid overdistension of the space and prevent excessive fluid. The authors favor the use of a 30-degree endoscope for the peritrochanteric space, but it is always better to have a 70-degree arthroscope available also.

Trochanteric Bursectomy

Trochanteric bursitis is associated with low back pain, external coxa saltans, and long-distance runners, and it is usually described as an overuse injury that most commonly presents in women.[2,24] The clinical onset is an intermittent pain on the lateral aspect of the hip characterized for point tenderness over the GT. The treatment is mostly conservative, with physiotherapy accompanied by a local corticosteroid shot in the concerned area.

Bursitis refractory to conservative treatment requires a surgical procedure. The usual endoscopic exploration of the peritrochanteric space requires resection of the GT bursa for adequate examination of the tendinous insertion of the gluteus medius through which bursectomy is performed with an arthroscopic shaver and RF instruments. In order to perform a methodological bursectomy, the authors prefer to remove it from distal to proximal (Figure 17-8). RF is used because the bursa is highly vascularized. One prospective study treated 25 patients with endoscopic bursectomy with a follow-up of 25.1 months. General improvements in Harris Hip Scores and Short Form 36 scores were observed after 1 to 3 months, and only one patient required an open procedure for a failed endoscopy.[23]

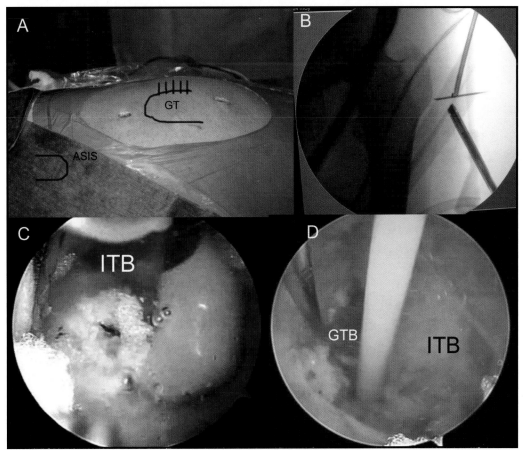

Figure 17-7. (A) Clinical photograph demonstrating portal positions to access the peritrochanteric space of a left hip. The GT and the anterior-superior iliac spine (ASIS) had been marked on the skin. In this case of an external snapping hip, the transverse lines indicate the area of snapping. Note how the portals are placed around the area of the snapping. (B) Fluoroscopic image of a left hip demonstrating instruments in position to access the peritrochanteric space. The arthroscope is in the distal trochanteric portal, and the ablation RF probe is in the proximal peritrochanteric portal. A needle is in position pointing to the GT to guide the instruments endoscopically. (C) Endoscopic image of the ITB as observed in the subcutaneous space. The needle points to the GT to guide the endoscopic cuts and RF ablation device is used for hemostasia. (D) A cut is performed on the ITB to create a defect for access to the peritrochanteric space. The needle points to the GT. The GT bursa (GTB) is observed to the defect of the ITB.

Iliotibial Band Lengthening

External snapping hip syndrome, or coxa saltans, is the clearest indication for lengthening or decompression of the ITB. Decompression of the ITB has also been used in the treatment of GTPS to release pressure from the ITB on the GT bursa and the gluteus medius tendon. External snapping hip syndrome is produced by a posterior thickening of the ITB and an anterior thickening of fibers of the gluteus maximus. These fibers lie posterior to the GT. The thickened fibers snap over the GT with flexion and extension of the hip, and in more severe cases, the phenomenon may be also reproduced with hip rotations.[21,25] Asymptomatic snapping must be considered a normal occurrence. The clinical diagnosis is evident. The phenomenon is always voluntary, and the patient often volunteers to show it. The snapping will occur when flexing and extending the hip. The authors prefer to examine this with the patient in the lateral decubitus position by passively flexing and extending the hip. A different form of the external snapping hip is also described by

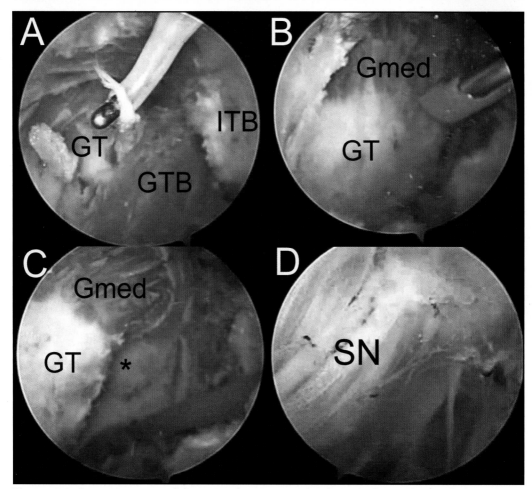

Figure 17-8. Anatomic aspects of the peritrochanteric space endoscopically. (A) The greater trochanteric bursa (GTB) has been resected with a RF hook. GT is observed through a defect in the GTB. The posterior aspect of the released ITB is seen. (B) GT is observed. The gluteus medius (Gmed) and its insertion in GT are seen. An RF ablation device points to the posterior margin of the Gmed. (C) The Gmed, GT, and piriformis tendon (*) are seen. An RF ablation points to the area of the sciatic nerve. (D) As the 30-degree arthroscope is pushed deep behind the peritrochanteric space, subgluteal space is accessed. The sciatic nerve (SN) is seen.

some patients as the ability to dislocate the hip. This is often shown by rotating the affected hip while tilting the pelvis in the standing position. The voluntary dislocators are more frequently painless and should only be treated with stretching exercises of the ITB. A positive Ober's test may also be found at physical examination (see Figure 17-3).[21] Symptomatic external snapping hip syndrome is always accompanied by pain in the GT region. The pain is secondary to GT bursitis or abductor tendon pathology.

Symptomatic cases can be treated conservatively with stretching physical therapy, nonsteroidal anti-inflammatory drugs, and corticosteroid infiltration of the GT bursa.[18] When surgical lengthening of the ITB is performed, a thorough bursectomy should be performed to ensure adequate examination of the gluteus medius tendon. The pathology is the thickened posterior third of the ITB. An associated erythematous zone of injury can sometimes be seen on the lateral prominence of the trochanter, corresponding to the site of ITB snapping. After the endoscopic exploration, an RF hook probe is introduced through the proximal trochanteric portal, and a 4- to 6-cm vertical retrograde cut is performed on the ITB. After that, a 2-cm-long cut is performed at the middle of the vertical cut. The flap created is resected with the shaver. A posterior cut is made at the same level of the anterior cut, and the flap is resected with the shaver. Different types of ITB procedures exist. Brignall and Stainsby[25] popularized a technique with the use of a Z-plasty. Zoltar et al[26] used an ellipsoid-shaped segment of the ITB. It is accepted that the common goal, regardless of the method, is to eliminate the snapping with some type of relaxing procedure of the ITB. Ilizaliturri et al[20] reported results with the use of a diamond-shaped release in 11 patients (9 female, 1 bilateral, and 1 male) with an average age of 26 years at an average 2-year follow-up. One patient reported persistent nonpainful snapping, whereas the remainder of the patients had no complaints and returned to their previous level of activity.

Gluteus Medius Repair

Gluteus medius and minimus tears have been recently recognized as a cause of GTPS resistant to conservative treatment. The etiology of these tears remains unknown. Their natural history appears to be degenerative. Conservative treatment includes physical therapy, rest, and nonsteroidal anti-inflammatory drugs. If conservative treatment fails and there is evidence of significant gluteus medius pathology, an endoscopic repair may be performed (Figure 17-9).

Dishkin-Paset et al[27] recently reported the results of a cadaveric biomechanical study comparing double-row massive cuff stitch constructs to double-row knotless anchor constructs. The biomechanical stability of the 2 constructs for gluteus medius tendon repair was similar.

Gluteus Minimus

The gluteus minimus may be also a source of lateral hip pain. However, these tears are often missed or misdiagnosed as bursitis. Partial-thickness tears of the gluteus medius and minimus may go unnoticed because they are covered by an intact tendon and are not directly visible through an open or endoscopic approach.

POSTOPERATIVE PROTOCOL

Rehabilitation for patients after bursectomy or ITB release limits weight bearing to 20 lb of foot-flat weight bearing as tolerated with crutches for 2 weeks. Full weight bearing is advanced without crutches thereafter per the patient's pain tolerance when a normal gait is established. Range of motion and hip strengthening without restrictions begin as soon as the patient's pain allows. It is important to avoid overaggressive therapy to avoid persistent inflammation of the lateral hip. Patients undergoing repair of gluteus medius and minimus tears are treated for 6 weeks with 20 lb of foot-flat weight bearing with crutches. The patient uses a hip abduction brace that blocks active abduction. No limitation of hip flexion or extension is necessary. Isometric strengthening of the hip abductors is initiated at 6 weeks. At 12 weeks, plyometric and progressive strengthening activities are introduced. Running is not allowed until the patient displays equal abductor strength bilaterally.

POTENTIAL COMPLICATIONS

No specific studies in the literature have reported the incidence of complications in surgical endoscopy of the peritrochanteric space. The complications that may occur include hematoma and fluid extravasations into the soft tissue. Recurrence of trochanteric bursitis; persistent, painful external coxa saltans; and retearing of gluteus medius tendon repairs are all potential complications.

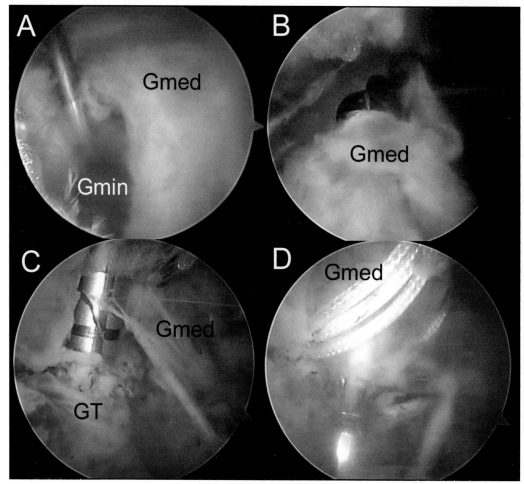

Figure 17-9. Endoscopic sequence of photographs demonstrating a gluteus medius (Gmed) tear repair in a left hip. (A) Gmed tear at the junction of the inferior and middle-third fibers. A probe is inside the tear, and the gluteus minimus (Gmin) is visible through the defect. (B) In the proximal aspect of the Gmed, the tear has been reduced with side-to-side polydioxanone stitches. (C) A suture anchor is placed on the footprint of the Gmed on the GT. A polydioxanone suture is observed behind the anchor impactor. (D) Sutures are passed to both sides of the tear.

TOP TECHNICAL PEARLS FOR THE PROCEDURE

1. The GT is the main landmark for portal establishment.

2. Placing a needle using fluoroscopy outside onto the GT facilitates creating the cut on the ITB in the correct position above the GT when using an outside-in technique.

3. The GT, vastus lateralis, and gluteus medius are the main anatomical landmarks once inside the peritrochanteric space.

4. Disposable closed cannulas are useful for suture management inside the peritrochanteric space.

5. Instruct the use of a walker in the postoperative period to protect abductor muscle repair.

REFERENCES

1. Williams BS, Cohen SP. Greater trochanteric pain syndrome: a review of anatomy, diagnosis and treatment. *Anesth Analg.* 2009;108(5):1662-1670.
2. Tortolani PJ, Carbone JJ, Quartararo LG. Greater trochanteric pain syndrome in patients referred to orthopedic spine specialists. *Spine J.* 2002;2(4):251-254.
3. Shbeeb MI, Matteson EL. Trochanteric bursitis (greater trochanter pain syndrome). *Mayo Clin Proc.* 1996;71(6):565-569.
4. Stegeman H. Die chirurgische Bedeutung paratkularer Kalkablagerungen. *Arch Klin Chir.* 1923;125:718-738.
5. Leonard MH. Trochanteric syndrome; calcareous and noncalcareous tendonitis and bursitis about the trochanter major. *J Am Med Assoc.* 1958;168(2):175-177.
6. Segal NA, Felson DT, Torner JC, et al. Greater trochanteric pain syndrome: epidemiology and associated factors. *Arch Phys Med Rehabil.* 2007;88(8):988-992.
7. Robertson WJ, Gardner MJ, Barker JU, Boraiah S, Lorich DG, Kelly BT. Anatomy and dimensions of the gluteus medius tendon insertion. *Arthroscopy.* 2008;24(2):130-136.
8. Bird PA, Oakley SP, Shnier R, Kirkham BW. Prospective evaluation of magnetic resonance imaging and physical examination findings in patients with greater trochanteric pain syndrome. *Arthritis Rheum.* 2001;44(9):2138-2145.
9. Kong A, Van der Vliet A, Zadow S. MRI and US of gluteal tendinopathy in greater trochanteric pain syndrome. *Eur Radiol.* 2007;17(7):1772-1783.
10. Silva F, Adams T, Feinstein J, Arroyo RA. Trochanteric bursitis: refuting the myth of inflammation. *J Clin Rheumatol.* 2008;14(2):82-86.
11. Domb BG, Nasser RM, Botser IB. Partial-thickness tears of the gluteus medius: rationale and technique for transtendinous endoscopic repair. *Arthroscopy.* 2010;26(12):1697-1705.
12. Whiteside LA. Surgical technique: transfer of the anterior portion of the gluteus maximus muscle for abductor deficiency of the hip. *Clin Orthop Relat Res.* 2012;470(2):503-510.
13. Ege Rasmussen KJ, Fanø N. Trochanteric bursitis. Treatment by corticosteroid injection. *Scand J Rheumatol.* 1985;14(4):417-420.
14. Dunn T, Heller CA, McCarthy SW, Dos Remedios C. Anatomical study of the "trochanteric bursa." *Clin Anat.* 2003;16(3):233-240.
15. Anderson TP. Trochanteric bursitis: diagnostic criteria and clinical significance. *Arch Phys Med Rehabil.* 1958;39(10):617-622.
16. Bancroft LW, Merinbaum DJ, Zaleski CG, Peterson JJ, Kransdorf MJ, Berquist TH. Hip ultrasound. *Semin Musculoskelet Radiol.* 2007;11(2):126-136.
17. Lievense A, Bierma-Zeinstra S, Schouten B, Bohnen A, Verhaar J, Koes B. Prognosis of trochanteric pain in primary care. *Br J Gen Pract.* 2005;55(512):199-204.
18. Cohen SP, Strassels SA, Foster L, et al. Comparison of fluoroscopically guided and blind corticosteroid injections for greater trochanteric pain syndrome: multicentre randomized controlled trial. *BMJ.* 2009;338:b1088.
19. Voos JE, Shindle MK, Pruett A, Asnis PD, Kelly BT. Endoscopic repair of gluteus medius tendon tears of the hip. *Am J Sports Med.* 2009;37(4):743-747.
20. Ilizaliturri VM Jr, Martinez-Escalante FA, Chaidez PA, Camacho-Galindo J. Endoscopic iliotibial band release for external snapping hip syndrome. *Arthroscopy.* 2006;22(5):505-510.
21. Ilizaliturri VM Jr, Camacho-Galindo J. Endoscopic treatment of snapping hips, iliotibial band, and iliopsoas tendon. *Sports Med Arthrosc.* 2010;18(2):120-127.
22. Barnthouse NC, Wente TM, Voos JE. Greater trochanteric pain syndrome: endoscopic treatment options. *Oper Tech Sports Med.* 2012;20(4):320-324.
23. Baker CL Jr, Massie RV, Hurt WG, Savory CG. Arthroscopic bursectomy for recalcitrant trochanteric bursitis. *Arthroscopy.* 2007;23(8):827-832.
24. Karpinski MR, Piggott H. Greater trochanteric pain syndrome. A report of 15 cases. *J Bone Joint Surg Br.* 1985;67(5):762-763.
25. Brignall CG, Stainsby GD. The snapping hip, treatment by Z-plasty. *J Bone Joint Surg Br.* 1991;73(2):253-254.

26. Zoltan DJ, Clancy WG Jr, Keene JS. A new operative approach to snapping hip and refractory trochanteric bursitis in athletes. *Am J Sports Med.* 1986;14(3):201-204.
27. Dishkin-Paset JG, Salata MJ, Gross CE, et al. A biomechanical comparison of repair techniques for complete gluteus medius tears. *Arthroscopy.* 2012;28(10):1410-1416.

Please see videos on the accompanying website at

www.ArthroscopicTechniques.com

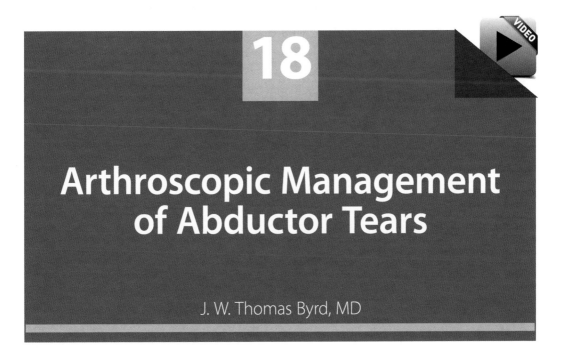

Arthroscopic Management of Abductor Tears

J. W. Thomas Byrd, MD

INTRODUCTION

Lesions of the gluteus medius and minimus are increasingly recognized as a source of laterally based hip pain and dysfunction, and there is a growing body of evidence to support the role of arthroscopy to address this pathology.[1-4] Magnetic resonance imaging (MRI) findings of signal changes within these structures may be an incidental finding and a normal consequence of aging.[5] Clinical relevance is established by the history and physical examination and is further supported by ultrasound (US)-guided injections.

INDICATIONS

Indications include symptomatic abductor tears that have failed conservative treatment, including the following:

► Activity modification
► Oral nonsteroidal anti-inflammatory drugs
► Supervised physical therapy
► Judicious use of corticosteroid injections

Controversial Indications

► Large tears with retraction
  ▷ Technically challenging to mobilize the tendon to accomplish a relatively tension-free repair.
  ▷ Alternatively appropriately indicated for open repair.

Byrd JWT, Bedi A, Stubbs AJ, eds. *The Hip:*
AANA Advanced Arthroscopic Surgical Techniques (pp 221-230).
© 2016 AANA.

▶ It is contraindicated for massive tears with fatty infiltration that may benefit from tendon transfer techniques.[6]

PERTINENT PHYSICAL FINDINGS

History

▶ Laterally based pain
▶ Pain with ambulation, especially painful for first few steps
▶ Pain worsens with distance
▶ Pain exacerbated with stairs and inclines
▶ Pain when lying on the affected side
▶ Night pain

Examination

▶ A significant antalgic gait is often present, including an abductor lurch.
▶ The Trendelenburg test exacerbates lateral pain, but it may only be positive with severe lesions.
▶ Pain with palpation over the greater trochanter.
▶ Abductor strength on manual testing is sometimes surprisingly well preserved, even in the presence of substantial structural deficit. Conversely, weakness can be as much a consequence of reflex inhibition as a structural deficiency.

In thin people, it can be possible to differentiate the various lateral structures. Manual testing of abductor strength with the knee flexed isolates for the gluteus medius, whereas checking with the knee extended recruits the iliotibial band (ITB).

Impingement testing and other maneuvers to assess for intra-articular pathology are a normal part of the examination but usually do little to exacerbate lateral symptoms. External rotation of the hip in a flexed position is often painful, presumably from stressing the anterior portion of the gluteus medius.

PERTINENT IMAGING

X-rays are essential to assessing any hip joint disorder but are usually unrevealing for signs of abductor pathology.[7] In chronic cases, ossification may be present around the insertion on the lateral and anterior facets.

MRI is generally sensitive at detecting lesions of the abductors. High-resolution images with small field of view sequences of the affected hip are best at assessing the pattern of pathology.

US demonstrates good sensitivity in detecting abductor lesions. This may be an appropriate substitute in patients for whom MRI is contraindicated or in cases where a prosthesis or other hardware may create significant artifact.

A US-guided injection of anesthetic is the most conclusive test to substantiate the clinical relevance of an abductor lesion. Concomitant use of cortisone can often be a useful therapeutic tool.

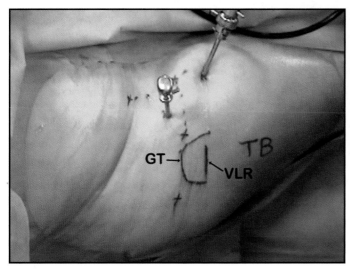

Figure 18-1. On this right hip, 2 anteriorly based portals have been established into the peritrochanteric space, lateral to the greater trochanter (GT), deep to the ITB. Surface markings for the GT and vastus lateralis ridge (VLR) are noted, as well as routine markings that would be used for arthroscopy of the central compartment. (© J. W. Thomas Byrd, MD.)

EQUIPMENT

Standard hip arthroscopy instruments are needed. Additional instruments are necessary for the tendon repair, including various suture-passing devices and implants. Double- and triple-loaded suture anchors are most commonly used with knotless fixation devices for the distal row when double-row fixation is performed.

POSITIONING

The patient is positioned supine on a fracture table or conventional table that incorporates an extremity positioner for hip arthroscopy.

STEP-BY-STEP DESCRIPTION OF THE PROCEDURE

Peritrochanteric Access With Gluteus Medius Repair

Endoscopy of the peritrochanteric space is usually preceded by arthroscopy of the hip joint to assess and address any potential intra-articular pathology (Video 18-1).[8,9] After that is completed, all instruments are removed, and particular attention is given to make sure that all traction has been released, alleviating any pressure on the perineum. The hip is in extension with neutral rotation and slight abduction.

The peritrochanteric space is initially accessed via 2 anteriorly based portals: one proximal and one distal to the vastus lateralis ridge, which is identified by fluoroscopy (Figure 18-1).[10] Typically, these portals are 6 to 8 cm apart, although this varies depending on the depth of the soft tissues. The purpose is to have them converge at the vastus ridge without being too crowded by each other. By convention, the distal portal is placed first. It should pass deep to the ITB, targeting a point just lateral to the vastus lateralis ridge. This helps to avoid inadvertently perforating the insertion of the gluteus medius above the ridge or the origin of the vastus lateralis below. Palpating the ridge with the cannula under fluoroscopy helps to determine the proper anterior-to-posterior depth of

Figure 18-2. Three laterally based portals have been established for gluteal repair. A viewing portal for the 30-degree arthroscope is just posterior to the vastus lateralis ridge. A working portal with an 8.5-mm disposable cannula is just posterior to the ridge. Anchors are inserted from a proximal portal, allowing placement perpendicular to the trochanteric cortex. (© J. W. Thomas Byrd, MD.)

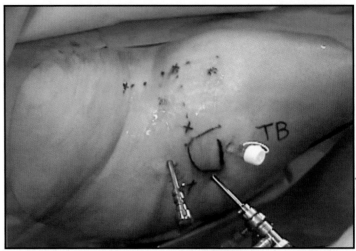

the cannula. A proximal-to-distal sweeping motion may help clear some of the bursal tissue. The 30-degree arthroscope is placed.

The proximal portal is placed under direct arthroscopic visualization. Prepositioning is performed with a spinal needle. If the view is obscured by adhesions, a cannulated system can be used with a guidewire through the spinal needle. If the view is clear, it is a simple process to place the cannula adjacent to the prepositioned needle. Bursal tissue and debris can then be cleared, identifying the normal structures within the peritrochanteric space, including the myotendinous insertion of the abductors above the vastus lateralis ridge, the ridge itself, the origin of the vastus lateralis below the ridge covered in a glistening tendon, the deep surface of the ITB, and the insertional portion of the gluteus maximus coursing diagonally to its insertion on the posterior aspect of the proximal femur. Once the space has been fully cleared and the pathology identified, preparation is made for repair of the gluteus medius.

A new viewing portal is established at the posterior margin of the vastus lateralis ridge, and the anterior portals are removed (Figure 18-2). Compared to rotator cuff repair in the shoulder, this is comparable to the posterior subacromial portal. A working portal is established just distal to the ridge for preparing the tendon and managing the repair. This is comparable with the lateral subacromial portal in the shoulder. The torn tendon edges are identified and mobilized. The exposed bony footprint, usually involving the anterior and some of the lateral trochanteric facets, is lightly freshened with a burr, creating a healthy bed for the repair site. An 8.5-mm cannula facilitates managing the repair.

The anchors are placed from a site proximal to the ridge, entering roughly perpendicular to the cortical bone surface. The exact number, size, and distribution pattern of the anchors is influenced by the principal tear pattern of the tendon. In the provided example, the tendon disruption is mostly vertically oriented (Figure 18-3). Thus, 2 vertically oriented, triple-loaded anchors are used. The more proximal anchor is inserted first (Figure 18-4). With the hollow core of this anchor device, marrow products can exude up through its open center (Figure 18-5).

Once the anchor is seated, mattress sutures are created by passing one limb of the suture through the posterior leaf and one through the anterior leaf of the tendon tear. Various suture-passing devices and shuttle techniques aid in properly placing the sutures. As sutures are passed, it is convenient to retrieve them through the previous anterior portal site where they can be docked and out of the way during subsequent suture management. The distal anchor is then placed in an identical fashion (Figure 18-6).

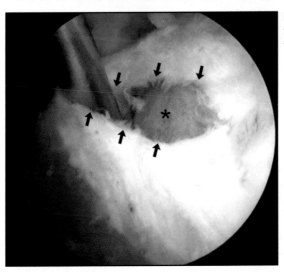

Figure 18-3. A vertically oriented tear of the gluteus medius (arrows) reveals the underlying bony footprint (asterisk). (© J. W. Thomas Byrd, MD.)

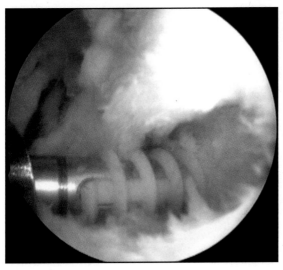

Figure 18-4. A triple-loaded anchor is inserted at the proximal aspect of the repair site. (© J. W. Thomas Byrd, MD.)

Once all sutures have been passed, they are then tied, working from distal to proximal (Figure 18-7). The final construct of the repair is carefully inspected (Figure 18-8). Assessment of the security of the fixation is important in guiding the postoperative rehabilitation process.

DOUBLE-ROW FIXATION (GLUTEUS MEDIUS REPAIR WITH DOUBLE-ROW FIXATION)

Double-row fixation is best suited for large full-thickness lesions (Video 18-2).[11] The bony footprint of the repair site, typically including the anterior and part of the lateral trochanteric facet, is lightly prepared with a burr to provide a fresh surface, potentiating healing of the restored tendon. The tendon is mobilized and cleared of adhesions on its deep and superficial surfaces (Figure 18-9). Proximal fixation is accomplished with 2 to 3 transverse or horizontally oriented double-loaded anchors. The most anterior anchor is placed first (Figure 18-10). A tendon-penetrating device is used to pass the sutures in a mattress fashion through the proximal portion of the

Figure 18-5. Viewing down the anchor, the open center reveals a conduit from where the tendon will be approximated over the anchor to the underlying marrow products. (© J. W. Thomas Byrd, MD.)

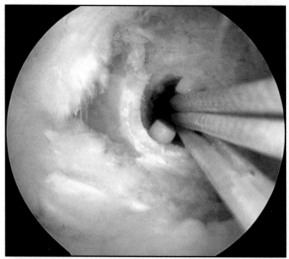

Figure 18-6. A more distal anchor is being seated. The 3 sutures from the proximal anchor are passed through the posterior and anterior leaves of the torn tendon. (© J. W. Thomas Byrd, MD.)

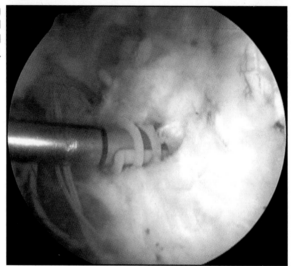

Figure 18-7. All 6 suture pairs have been passed and are ready to be tied, restoring the tendinous insertion site of the gluteus medius. (© J. W. Thomas Byrd, MD.)

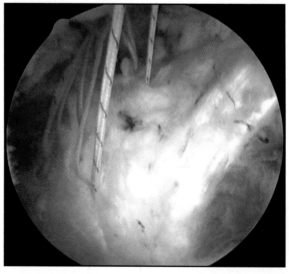

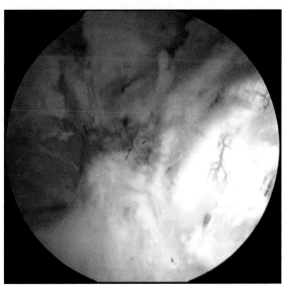

Figure 18-8. The final repair construct is inspected, with secure approximation of the tendon back to its bony footprint. (© J. W. Thomas Byrd, MD.)

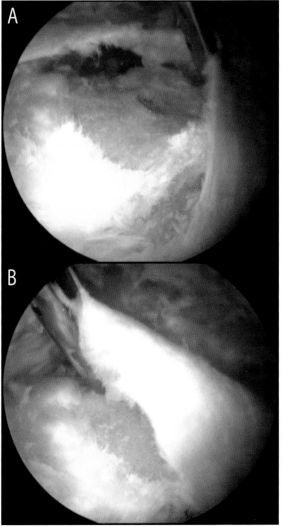

Figure 18-9. A grasper assesses the mobility of the tendon. (A) Moving the tendon proximally exposes the bony footprint. (B) The tendon is mobilized distally over its insertion site. (© J. W. Thomas Byrd, MD.)

Figure 18-10. The anterior of 2 double-loaded anchors is being inserted in the proximal portion of the bony footprint. (© J. W. Thomas Byrd, MD.)

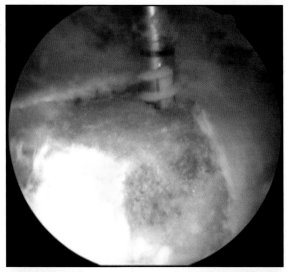

Figure 18-11. The posterior of the 2 anchors is being inserted. The colored sutures of the anterior anchor are seen emerging from the anchor hole (arrows) that have already been passed in a mattress fashion through the proximal tendon. (© J. W. Thomas Byrd, MD.)

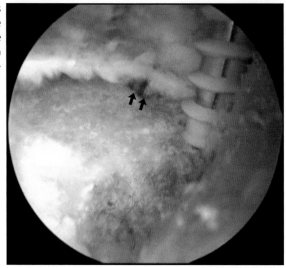

tendon. Once passed, the sutures can then be retrieved through an anterior portal site and docked out of the way during subsequent suture management. One or 2 more Healicoil anchors (Smith & Nephew) are then placed from anterior to posterior, as needed, to provide broad-based coverage of the damaged tendon (Figure 18-11).

Once all sutures have been passed, each pair is tied, beginning from posterior to anterior. With each knot, one suture limb is retained to be incorporated into the distal fixation (Figure 18-12).

After assuring the structural integrity of the proximal row, attention is then turned to the distal row. Fixation is achieved with knotless anchors. One knotless anchor is used per proximal anchor. The pair of suture limbs, one from each knot accompanying the doubly loaded proximal anchor, is incorporated with the distal knotless anchor (Figure 18-13).

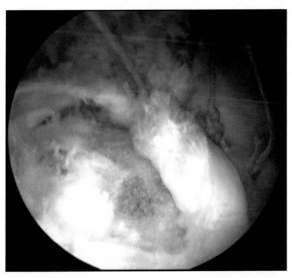

Figure 18-12. The 4 sutures from the 2 double-loaded anchors have been tied, leaving one suture limb from each knot to be incorporated into the distal fixation. (© J. W. Thomas Byrd, MD.)

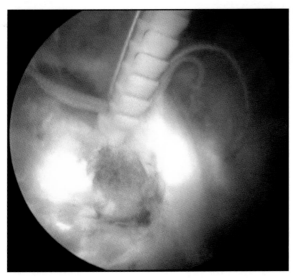

Figure 18-13. The distal knotless anchor is driven into place, incorporating 2 suture limbs from the proximal knots. (© J. W. Thomas Byrd, MD.)

POSTOPERATIVE PROTOCOL

Protected weight bearing is maintained for 6 to 8 weeks depending on the security of the repair.[12] During this time, active abduction and internal rotation and passive adduction and external rotation are avoided. Functional progression as tolerated may begin at 3 months, with some precautions for at least the first 4 months postoperatively.

POTENTIAL COMPLICATIONS

Complications associated with this procedure are unusual other than general complications described in conjunction with routine hip arthroscopy.[13] Working in the peritrochanteric space, the surgeon must be mindful of potential concerns for fluid extravasation and instrument or implant breakage.

TOP TECHNICAL PEARLS FOR THE PROCEDURE

1. Properly access and develop the peritrochanteric space, identifying the pertinent anatomic structures and preserving the ITB.

2. Properly position the viewing and working portals for the abductor repair.

3. Properly prepare the bony footprint.

4. Properly prepare the torn tendon edges, especially clearing the superficial surface of adhesions and fibrous or fatty tissue that might hinder visualization during suture passage.

5. Docking sutures through the anterior portal help in suture management and keep the strands organized.

REFERENCES

1. Kingzett-Taylor A, Tirman PF, Feller J, et al. Tendinosis and tears of gluteus medius and minimus muscles as a cause of hip pain: MR imaging findings. *AJR Am J Roentgenol.* 1999;173(4):1123-1126.
2. Voos JE, Shindle MK, Pruett A, Asnis PD, Kelly BT. Endoscopic repair of gluteus medius tendon tears of the hip. *Am J Sports Med.* 2009;37(4):743-747.
3. Domb BG, Botser I, Giordano BD. Outcomes of endoscopic gluteus medius repair with minimum 2-year follow-up. *Am J Sports Med.* 2013;41(5):988-997.
4. McCormick F, Alpaugh K, Nwachukwu BU, Yanke AB, Martin SD. Endoscopic repair of full-thickness abductor tendon tears: surgical technique and outcome at minimum of 1-year follow-up. *Arthroscopy.* 2013;29(12):1941-1947.
5. Haliloglu N, Inceoglu D, Sahin G. Assessment of peritrochanteric high T2 signal depending on the age and gender of the patients. *Eur J Radiol.* 2010;75(1):64-66.
6. Davies JF, Stiehl JB, Davies JA, Geiger PB. Surgical treatment of hip abductor tendon tears. *J Bone Joint Surg Am.* 2013;95(15):1420-1425.
7. Jones KS, Potts EA, Byrd JW. Perioperative care. In: Byrd JW, ed. *Operative Hip Arthroscopy.* 3rd ed. New York, NY: Springer; 2013:441-454.
8. Byrd JW. Hip arthroscopy utilizing the supine position. *Arthroscopy.* 1994;10(3):275-280.
9. Byrd JW. Routine arthroscopy and access: central and peripheral compartments, iliopsoas bursa, peritrochanteric, and subgluteal spaces. In: Byrd JW, ed. *Operative Hip Arthroscopy.* 3rd ed. New York, NY: Springer; 2013:131-160.
10. Byrd JW. Peritrochanteric access and gluteus medius repair. *Arthrosc Tech.* 2013;2(3):e243-e246.
11. Byrd JW. Gluteus medius repair with double-row fixation. *Arthrosc Tech.* 2013;2(3):e247-e250.
12. Coplen EM, Voight ML. Rehabilitation of the hip. In: Byrd JW, ed. *Operative Hip Arthroscopy.* 3rd ed. New York, NY: Springer; 2013:411-440.
13. Mather RC III, Reddy A, Nho SJ. Complications of hip arthroscopy. In: Byrd JW, ed. *Operative Hip Arthroscopy.* 3rd ed. New York, NY: Springer; 2013:403-410.

Please see videos on the accompanying website at

www.ArthroscopicTechniques.com

Arthroscopic Management of Traumatic Hip Instability

Indications and Approach

G. Peter Maiers II, MD and Emily Cha, MD

INTRODUCTION

Hip instability can be divided into traumatic or atraumatic etiologies. Traumatic hip instability is ill defined and represents a spectrum of injury that ranges from major trauma, such as dislocations with osseous injury, to minor trauma, such as simple dislocations (no associated fracture) or subluxation. Although a substantial amount of force is required to dislocate the hip joint, the incidences of hip dislocations and hip fracture-dislocations are increasing. The majority of these injuries occur in the young adult population due to high-energy injuries, such as motor vehicle accidents. Although motor vehicle accident dashboard injuries are the most common mechanism of injury, hip dislocations have been reported with lower-energy mechanisms, such as football, soccer, skiing, gymnastics, rugby, jogging, and basketball.[1] Regardless of the mechanism, hip dislocations and associated fractures increase the risk of hip instability, which may be missed as a diagnosis if a high index of suspicion is not upheld.

The hip joint is considered one of the most stable diarthrodial joints, which relies on a combination of its bony and soft tissue anatomy. The soft tissue stabilizers of the hip joint comprise the extra-capsular ligaments, labrum, and local soft tissue musculature. The joint capsule has 3 fibrous thickenings that compose the main capsular ligaments: the iliofemoral ligament (Y ligament of Bigelow), the pubofemoral ligament, and the ischiofemoral ligament. The Y ligament is the strongest of the 3 and protects against anterior translation in extension and external rotation. The terminal fibers of the Y ligament also insert onto the femoral neck in a circumferential orientation, forming the zona orbicularis. The labrum is a fibrocartilaginous structure that runs circumferentially around the acetabulum. The labrum acts to stabilize the hip joint in extremes of motion, especially flexion. In addition, the labrum acts as an important seal to the hip joint by preventing excessive joint fluid expression during periods of weight bearing. The synovial fluid allows for even distribution of the loads; thus, by maintaining the fluid volume during periods

Byrd JWT, Bedi A, Stubbs AJ, eds. *The Hip:*
AANA Advanced Arthroscopic Surgical Techniques (pp 231-240).
© 2016 AANA.

Table 19-1. Classification Systems for Hip Dislocation[18]

Classification	Type	Description
Thompson and Epstein	I	Dislocation with or without minor fracture
	II	Posterior fracture-dislocation with a single significant fragment
	III	Dislocation in which the posterior wall contains comminuted fragments with or without a major fragment
	IV	Dislocation with a large segment of posterior wall that extends into the acetabular floor
	V	Dislocation with fracture of the femoral head
Steward and Millford	I	Simple dislocation with no fracture or with an insignificant fracture
	II	Dislocation in a stable hip that has a significant single or comminuted element of the posterior wall
	III	Dislocation with a grossly unstable hip resulting from loss of bony support
	IV	Dislocation associated with femoral head fracture

of weight bearing, the labrum indirectly plays a critical role in even contact pressures along the articular surfaces.[2]

Upadhyay and Moulton[3] reported the long-term outcomes of traumatic posterior dislocations, which revealed a rate of posttraumatic osteoarthritis of 24% for simple hip dislocations and 88% for those with an associated acetabular fracture. In simple hip dislocations, traumatic instability is attributed to capsular laxity. Despite the increased incidence of traumatic hip dislocations, the rate of traumatic instability is thought to be low.[4]

Hip injury is classified based on the direction of the femoral head displacement, whether it is anterior or posterior. Anterior hip dislocations represent less than 10% of all dislocations. The most widely used systems are the Thompson and Epstein[5] or the Steward and Millford[6] classification systems (Table 19-1).

INDICATIONS

1. Nonconcentric reduction secondary to retained loose bodies

2. Persistent mechanical symptoms after 6 to 12 weeks of rest and physical rehabilitation

3. A sense of instability despite 6 to 12 weeks after initial injury

4. Continued hip pain for 6 to 12 weeks after dislocation. Common findings include loose bodies, posterior labral tears, bony Bankart lesions, articular cartilage damage, ligamentum teres tears, anterior labral tears, and concomitant femoroacetabular impingement.

The clearest indication for arthroscopic surgery in the setting of treatment for traumatic hip instability is nonconcentric reduction of the hip joint with retained loose bodies blocking the reduction.[1,7-9] In these situations, urgent arthroscopic intervention is necessary for the removal of the loose bodies to allow for a concentric reduction. In situations in which a traumatic hip dislocation or subluxation has occurred and the hip is concentrically reduced, the initial treatment

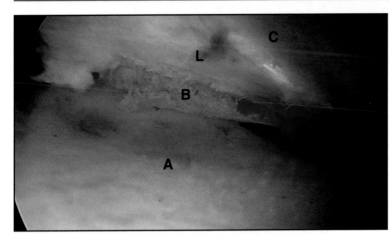

Figure 19-1. A posterior bony Bankart-type lesion of the right hip. The arthroscope is in the anterolateral portal and viewing posteriorly. A = posterior acetabular surface; B = fractured posterior acetabular rim (bony Bankart lesion); L = posterior acetabular labrum attached to the posterior rim fracture; C = posterior capsule, attached to the posterior bony Bankart.

is nonsurgical, with physical therapy to reestablish normal strength and range of motion of the affected hip. In posterior dislocations, posterior hip precautions with avoidance of flexion and adduction for 6 weeks is recommended. In anterior dislocations, extension and external rotation are avoided.[10] At 6 to 12 weeks postinjury, patients are reassessed for instability and mechanical symptoms, and magnetic resonance imaging (MRI) is obtained to assess for avascular necrosis.[1,10] In patients experiencing mechanical symptoms or a sense of instability, hip arthroscopy can be helpful in addressing intra-articular pathology that occurred as a result of their hip dislocation.

In a report of 14 professional athletes who sustained a hip dislocation and were unable to return to play at an average of 125 days after injury, Philippon et al[11] found that all 14 athletes had sustained labral tears and chondral injuries. They also noted that 12 athletes had injuries to the ligamentum teres and 9 had associated femoroacetabular impingement (FAI). After arthroscopic treatment of their hip pain, all 14 athletes were able to return to play at the professional level.

In another study, 17 patients experiencing mechanical hip symptoms at an average of 3 months after dislocation were treated with hip arthroscopy.[12] All 17 patients had femoral head chondral damage, 16 had acetabular chondral damage, 14 had anterior labral tears, 6 had posterior labral tears (Figure 19-1), and 14 had intra-articular loose bodies (Figure 19-2). At an average follow-up of 45 months, their Western Ontario and McMaster Universities Osteoarthritis Index scores had improved from 46 preoperatively to 87. Two patients had gone on to total hip arthroplasty, one for osteoarthritis and one for osteonecrosis.

FAI can be a risk factor for posterior hip dislocation and subluxation. Krych et al[13] reported a series of 22 athletes who had suffered a posterior instability episode that was confirmed by a posterior rim fracture. Eighteen of the 22 patients had FAI, and 16 of those had an injured hip as a result of a noncontact injury. They concluded that there is an association between posterior hip instability and FAI. They felt that preexisting FAI places the hip at a mechanical disadvantage and allows the femoral head to be levered posteriorly. Eleven of the 22 patients were treated nonoperatively. Of the 11 patients who required arthroscopic surgery, common findings included a posterior labral tear with rim fracture, anterior labral tear, loose bodies, chondral damage of the femoral head, and ligamentum teres avulsion. Twenty of the 22 patients were able to return to their sport.

In addition to true hip dislocations, traumatic subluxations can require arthroscopic surgery. Kashiwagi et al[8] reported a 10-year-old girl who presented with a persistently abducted hip and had increased medial joint space on plain x-rays following a fall that did not result in a true hip dislocation. At the time of surgery, interposition of the ligamentum teres with an attached osteochondral fragment of acetabular origin was blocking concentric reduction of the hip joint. Oh et al[14] reported 2 patients with persistent hip pain after hip subluxations who had osteochondral avulsions of the ligamentum teres, one from the femoral head and one from the acetabulum. Both were treated successfully with debridement of the osteochondral fragment and the ligamentum teres.

Figure 19-2. (A) Large loose bodies (LB) encountered in the posterior aspect of a left hip joint as a result of a posterior hip subluxation, viewed from the anterolateral portal. The femoral head (F), acetabulum (A), and posterior labrum (L) are seen. Note the synovitis in the posterior capsule (PC). (B) View of the left hip with the arthroscope in the anterolateral portal. Note the damage to the posterior aspect of the femoral head (F), which is the origin of the loose chondral bodies (LB). The pulvinar tissue (P) is inflamed. Also shown are the posterior labrum (L) and acetabulum (A). The cannula has been introduced through the posterolateral portal.

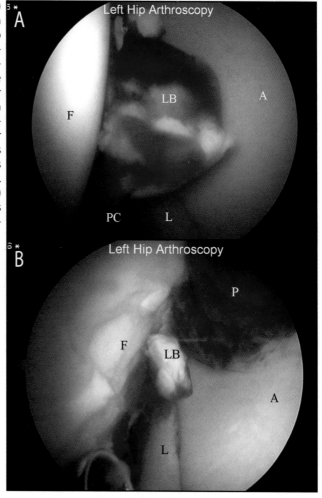

Arthroscopy also has a role in patients who have had traumatic hip injuries in addition to hip dislocations. In a series of 29 patients who sustained traumatic hip injuries, including pelvic ring fractures, acetabular fractures, proximal femur fractures, posterior hip dislocations, soft tissue injuries, and a gunshot wound, 59% had loose bodies, 93% had labral tears, and 48% had osteochondral injuries or chondral delamination.[15]

Occasionally, traumatic instability can lead to recurrent dislocations. In a case report,[16] a dancer who sustained an anterior hip dislocation as a result of an extension and external rotation maneuver went on to have 3 more anterior hip dislocations until she underwent arthroscopic surgery. At the time of surgery, she had a redundant anterior capsule, an anterior superior-to-posterior superior labral tear, an inflamed iliopsoas tendon, and a ligamentum teres tear. After arthroscopic labral repair, ligamentum teres debridement, partial iliopsoas tendon release, and anterior capsular plication, she was able to return to dance 6 months postoperatively.

Controversial Indications

Arthroscopy for All Hip Dislocations Acutely

Some surgeons offer arthroscopic surgery to all patients after hip dislocation in the acute phase. In one study, 36 patients underwent hip arthroscopy within a few days of dislocation, fracture dislocation, or wall fracture.[9] Thirty-three patients had bodies at the time of surgery; in 9 of those patients, the loose bodies were not detected on preoperative computed tomography (CT) scans. In the current authors' experience, many patients who sustain hip dislocations do not suffer long-term disability as a result of their injury, and routine arthroscopy of all hip dislocations is not necessary. There has been a case report of abdominal compartment syndrome causing cardiac arrest that occurred as a result of arthroscopy for loose body removal following open reduction and internal fixation of an acetabular fracture during which arthroscopic fluid extravasated along the fracture site.[17] In addition, the risk of fluid extravasation through the capsular defect would be increased in the acute setting.

PERTINENT PHYSICAL FINDINGS

1. The dynamic internal rotatory impingement test is positive for patients with posterior instability and those with anterior impingement.

2. The dynamic external rotatory impingement test is positive for patients with anterior/inferior instability and those with posterior impingement.

A true hip dislocation is fairly obvious on physical examination, whereas subtle instability or mechanical symptoms may be more challenging to detect. Posterior dislocations present with a flexed, adducted, and internally rotated leg, whereas anterior dislocations present with an externally rotated, slightly flexed, and abducted leg.[18] Subtle instability can be detected by the shuck test or piston test to the leg or by placing the hip in an apprehensive position. The dynamic internal rotatory impingement test looks for anterior impingement, but a sense of apprehension also indicates posterior instability. A positive dynamic external rotatory impingement test can indicate posterior/superior osseous impingement, but if there is apprehension, a positive test can indicate anterior or inferior instability. A positive posterior rim test indicates posterior impingement but also tests the anterior capsule, and a lateral rim impingement test indicates superior and posterior impingement and can indicate anterior and inferior instability (Table 19-2).[19] The presence of mechanical symptoms is usually best gathered from the history, but crepitus can occasionally be detected by the examiner placing his or her hand over the hip during manipulation of the joint.

PERTINENT IMAGING

1. Plain x-rays: anteroposterior (AP) pelvis and frog-leg lateral views of the affected hip (additional lateral views may be obtained if impingement is suspected)

2. Postreduction CT scan if the hip was truly dislocated to verify concentric reduction

3. MRI in the acute phase to document the extent of the soft tissue damage

4. MRI at 6 weeks postinjury to evaluate for avascular necrosis

At the time of injury, standard plain hip x-rays should be obtained. At the minimum, AP pelvis and frog-leg lateral views are required. Anterior hip dislocations can be missed if orthogonal views are not obtained (Figure 19-3). In addition, if hip subluxation is suspected, an obturator oblique view is likely to demonstrate a posterior rim fracture.[20] After closed reduction of a dislocated hip, AP pelvis and frog-leg lateral views are obtained to confirm reduction, and a CT scan of the hip is necessary to confirm a concentric reduction and assess for intra-articular loose bodies and rim or femoral head fractures that may be present. Once the hip has been reduced, MRI without contrast is helpful to determine the extent of the soft tissue injury and to have as a baseline to compare with future scans. A follow-up MRI is obtained 6 weeks after the hip dislocation to evaluate for avascular necrosis and to document soft tissue pathology. Moorman et al[20] documented a triad of

Table 19-2. Common Examinations for Instability and Impingement

Test	Tested Impingement	Tested Instability
DIRI	Anterior	Posterior
DEXRIT	Superior and posterior	Anterior and inferior
Posterior rim test	Posterior	Anterior
Lateral rim test	Superior and posterior	Anterior and inferior

DEXRIT = dynamic external rotatory impingement test; DIRI = dynamic internal rotatory impingement.

Reprinted with permission from Hal D. Martin, DO.

Figure 19-3. (A) AP pelvis x-ray of a woman who presented to the emergency department after sustaining a hyperextension injury to her left hip. When she was told there was nothing wrong with her hip, she refused to leave until further imaging was obtained. (B) CT scan of the left hip demonstrating an anterior hip dislocation.

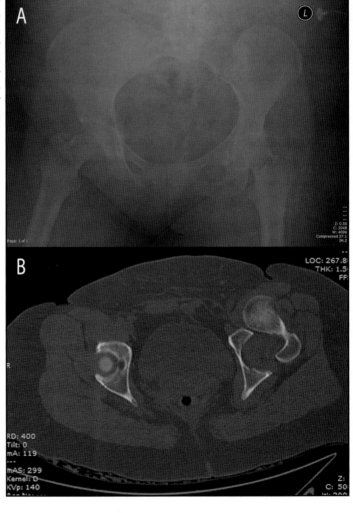

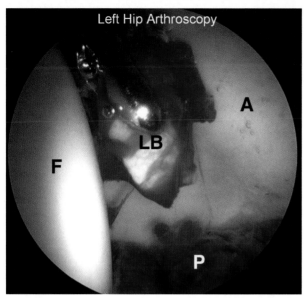
Left Hip Arthroscopy

Figure 19-4. A pituitary rongeur is used to remove intra-articular loose bodies (LB) through the anterior portal of this left hip. The arthroscope is in the anterolateral portal. Note the inflamed pulvinar tissue (P), femoral head (F), and acetabulum (A).

MRI findings following hip subluxation that include a posterior rim fracture, hemarthrosis, and rupture of the iliofemoral ligament. If surgical intervention is planned, documenting the presence of impingement is recommended to plan whether any bony resection is necessary.

EQUIPMENT

Standard hip arthroscopy equipment, including 70- and 30-degree arthroscopes, a traction table, and arthroscopy cannulas, are necessary to perform the operation. Additional equipment necessary for loose body removal includes straight and curved grasping devices; the authors prefer pituitary rongeurs (Figure 19-4) to morselize the loose bodies to allow for easy removal through closed or slotted cannulas. A large-bore (5.5-mm) suction-shaver device is useful for removing loose bodies and, if left open with the suction on, can aid in attracting loose bodies from difficult-to-reach places. Almost all hips that have dislocated have a labral tear; therefore, the surgeon needs to be prepared to repair the labrum if possible and debride it if it is an irreparable tear. For labral repair, hip-specific suture anchors are required and are available from most device companies. To pass sutures, a suture-penetrating device, such as a bird beak or suture shuttle, is acceptable. The current authors prefer to have both types of devices available to allow for greater flexibility in the repair technique. In addition, the surgeon should plan to close the capsulotomy; commercially available capsular closure devices are available, but the authors prefer to shuttle several sutures using a suture shuttle and a bird beak.

POSITIONING

The patient is positioned supine on the traction table. A standard fracture table may be used, or there are several traction attachments available from various companies that will attach to a standard operating table and allow traction to be applied to the hip joint. An oversized perineal post is used to protect the pudendal nerve, and the patient is positioned with the perineal post at the junction of the perineum and the medial thigh of the operative leg. Both feet are secured in traction boots, taking care to pad the superficial sensory nerves of the feet. Gentle traction is applied to the nonoperative leg at approximately 45 degrees to stabilize the pelvis against the perineal post. Traction is then applied to the operative leg in neutral abduction, with the hip in slight internal rotation. This can be accomplished by applying manual traction in 45 degrees of abduction followed by adducting the hip to neutral or by placing the hip in neutral abduction and cranking on traction per the technique of each individual table. When it is necessary to repair the posterior labrum, tilting the table 15 to 20 degrees away from the surgeon makes it easier to maneuver posteriorly.

STEP-BY-STEP DESCRIPTION OF THE PROCEDURE

The most common procedures performed to treat the sequelae of traumatic instability are loose body removal (Video 19-1), labral repair, chondral debridement, and capsulorrhaphy. Of these procedures, posterior labral repair and capsulorrhaphy are unique to traumatic instability cases (Video 19-2). Arthroscopic access is established in the typical fashion. For routine arthroscopy, many surgeons use a 2-portal technique, but when dealing with traumatic instability, it is imperative to establish the posterolateral portal as well. It is important to visualize the joint from the posterolateral portal to assess for loose bodies and damage to the posterior femoral head and the posteroinferior acetabulum. It is also important to have this portal in place because many labral tears occur posteriorly and inferiorly. Anchor placement and suture management is easiest through the posterolateral portal.

Posterior labral repair can be technically challenging because the rim of the acetabulum is thinner posteriorly than anteriorly. A small bony fragment is often associated with posterior labral tears. This piece is typically small enough to be excised or incorporated within the labral repair. The authors prefer to place the posterior anchors through the posterolateral portal while viewing from the anterolateral portal to avoid penetrating the articular cartilage with the drill bit or the anchor itself. Once the anchor has been placed, the labrum can be secured to the acetabulum by looping around the labrum or placing a stitch through the labrum (whichever is more appropriate for the tissue encountered). The posterior capsular tissue is usually not suitable for repair and is therefore left alone. Restoring the posterior labral seal typically imparts enough posterior stability. If cam and/or pincer impingement and anterior labral pathology are encountered, they should be addressed with the surgeon's preferred technique.

For patients with anterior instability or persistent anterior capsular tears at the time of surgery, an anterior capsular repair or capsulorrhaphy should be performed. The anterior capsule is repaired by passing sutures through the proximal limb of the capsule with a suture shuttle, penetrating the distal limb of the capsule with a suture retriever, and tying the sutures on the outside of the capsule. For patients with a redundant anterior capsule, an interportal capsulotomy is created, and a portion of the distal limb of the capsule is resected. Working in the peripheral compartment with the hip flexed to approximately 35 degrees, the capsule is then closed as previously described. This effectively advances the distal capsule proximally and eliminates the anterior capsular laxity.

POSTOPERATIVE PROTOCOL

Physical therapy is initiated within the first few days postoperatively, with the goal being to reestablish proper hip mechanics while protecting the repaired structures. In the case of a posterior labral repair, hip flexion is limited to 90 degrees for 6 weeks. A postoperative brace can be used if there is concern about patient compliance. For a patient who has had an anterior capsulorrhaphy, hyperextension is limited for 6 weeks, and a brace can be used if there is concern about patient compliance. The authors allow immediate weight bearing as tolerated with crutches until a normal gait pattern is established, and early activation of the gluteus medius is encouraged. Upright cardiovascular activity (eg, stair climbing, elliptical training, ultra G) is encouraged at 6 weeks postoperatively with a running progression commencing at 8 to 10 weeks. Ideally, at 3 months postoperatively, sport-specific activities and a functional progression are initiated. The goal is to return to full activity by 4 to 6 months postoperatively.

POTENTIAL COMPLICATIONS

Arthroscopic hip surgery is relatively safe, with the reported rate of major complications being less than 1%.[21] The most common complication is a transient neuropraxia of the pudendal and lateral femoral cutaneous nerves. Other complications include iatrogenic damage to the articular cartilage and labrum during access or as a result of manipulating the arthroscope. One specific risk when treating traumatic instability is penetration of the posterior acetabular articular surface during anchor placement or skiving off the posterior rim because the acetabulum is so thin posteriorly. Another consideration would be recurrent instability, particularly if the labrum is excised rather than repaired and/or the bony Bankart lesion is removed.

TOP TECHNICAL PEARLS FOR THE PROCEDURE

1. Establish a posterolateral portal as a part of the initial access.

2. Have a large-bore (5.5-mm) suction-shaver available for removal of loose bodies.

3. Use caution when placing posterior suture anchors because the posterior acetabulum is thin. Have small (1.5-mm) anchors available.

4. Be prepared to treat preexisting impingement.

5. When closing the capsule, consider not tying the second-to-last suture until the last suture has been passed to make it easier to pass and retrieve the final stitch.

REFERENCES

1. Shindle MK, Ranawat AS, Kelly BT. Diagnosis and management of traumatic and atraumatic hip instability in the athletic patient. *Clin Sports Med.* 2006;25(2):309-325.
2. Ferguson SJ, Bryant JT, Ganz R, Ito K. An in vitro investigation of the acetabular labral seal in hip mechanics. *J Biomech.* 2003;36(2):171-178.
3. Upadhyay SS, Moulton A. The long-term results of traumatic posterior dislocation of the hip. *J Bone Joint Surg Br.* 1981;63(4):548-551.
4. Mitchell JC, Giannoudis PV, Millner PA, Smith RM. A rare fracture-dislocation of the hip in a gymnast and review of the literature. *Br J Sports Med.* 1999;33(4):283-284.
5. Thompson VP, Epstein HC. Traumatic dislocation of the hip; a survey of two hundred and four cases covering a period of twenty-one years. *J Bone Joint Surg Am.* 1951;33(3):746-778.
6. Steward MJ, Millford LW. Fracture-dislocation of the hip; an end-result study. *J Bone Joint Surg Am.* 1954;36(2):315-342.
7. Svoboda SJ, Williams DM, Murphy KP. Hip arthroscopy for osteochondral loose body removal after a posterior hip dislocation. *Arthroscopy.* 2003;19(7):777-781.
8. Kashiwagi N, Suzuki S, Seto Y. Arthroscopic treatment for traumatic hip dislocation with avulsion fracture of the ligamentum teres. *Arthroscopy.* 2001;17(1):67-69.
9. Mullis BH, Dahners LE. Hip arthroscopy to remove loose bodies after traumatic dislocation. *J Orthop Trauma.* 2006;20(1):22-26.

10. Lynch TS, Terry MA, Bedi A, Kelly BT. Hip arthroscopic surgery: patient evaluation, current indications, and outcomes. *Am J Sports Med.* 2013;41(5):1174-1189.

11. Philippon MJ, Kuppersmith DA, Wolff AB, Briggs KK. Arthroscopic findings following traumatic hip dislocation in 14 professional athletes. *Arthroscopy.* 2009;25(2):169-174.

12. Ilizaliturri VM Jr, Gonzalez-Gutierrez B, Gonzalez-Ugalde H, Camach-Galindo J. Hip arthroscopy after traumatic hip dislocation. *Am J Sports Med.* 2011;39 suppl:50S-57S.

13. Krych AJ, Thompson M, Larson CM, Byrd JW, Kelly BT. Is posterior hip instability associated with cam and pincer deformity? *Clin Orthop Relat Res.* 2012;470(12):3390-3397.

14. Oh KJ, Pandher DS, Lee SH. Arthroscopic management of acute painful hip following occult subluxation: evidence-based case report. *Knee Surg Sports Traumatol Arthrosc.* 2007;15(11):1370-1374.

15. Khanna V, Harris A, Farrokhyar F, Choudur HN, Wong IH. Hip arthroscopy: prevalence of findings after traumatic injury of the hip. *Arthroscopy.* 2014;30(3):299-304.

16. Epstein DM, Rose DJ, Philippon MJ. Arthroscopic management of recurrent low-energy anterior hip dislocation in a dancer: a case report and review of literature. *Am J Sports Med.* 2010;38(6):1250-1254.

17. Bartlett CS, DiFelice GS, Buly RL, Quinn TJ, Green DS, Helfet DL. Cardiac arrest as a result of intraabdominal extravasation of fluid during arthroscopic removal of a loose body from the hip joint of a patient with an acetabular rim fracture. *J Orthop Trauma.* 1998;12(4):294-299.

18. Foulk DM, Mullis BH. Hip dislocation: evaluation and management. *J Am Acad Orthop Surg.* 2010;18(4):199-209.

19. Martin HD, Shears SA, Palmer IJ. Evaluation of the hip. *Sports Med Arthrosc.* 2010;18(2):63-75.

20. Moorman CT III, Warren RF, Hershman EB, et al. Traumatic posterior hip subluxation in American football. *J Bone Joint Surg Am.* 2003;85(7):1190-1196.

21. Harris JD, McCormick FM, Abrams GD, et al. Complications and reoperations during and after hip arthroscopy: a systematic review of 92 studies and more than 6,000 patients. *Arthroscopy.* 2013;29(3):589-595.

Please see videos on the accompanying website at

www.ArthroscopicTechniques.com

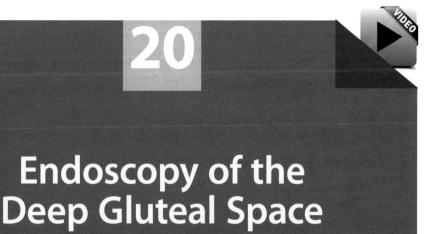

20

Endoscopy of the Deep Gluteal Space

Hal D. Martin, DO; Munif Ahmad Hatem, MD; and Ian J. Palmer, PhD

INTRODUCTION

Deep gluteal syndrome is characterized by nondiskogenic, extrapelvic sciatic nerve compression presenting with symptoms of pain and dysesthesias in the buttock area, hip, or posterior thigh and/or as radicular pain.[1] The nomenclature piriformis syndrome was widely used in the early years to characterize patients with deep gluteal pain because the piriformis muscle was considered the only structure to compress the sciatic nerve in the deep gluteal space.[2,3] However, the progress in diagnostic and surgical techniques has demonstrated several structures entrapping the sciatic nerve, including fibrous bands containing blood vessels,[4,5] gluteal muscles,[1] hamstring muscles,[6,7] the gemelli-obturator internus complex,[8,9] bone structures,[10] vascular abnormalities,[11,12] and space-occupying lesions.[13,14] Considering the variation of potential anatomical neural compromise, the term *deep gluteal syndrome* is preferred[1] to describe the entrapment of the sciatic nerve in the deep gluteal space. The sciatic nerve can also be affected in locations above and below the deep gluteal space, as in intrapelvic vascular and gynecologic abnormalities.[15] Furthermore, entrapments can occur in more than one place in the same nerve fiber or coexist with lumbosacral root compression. Because the sciatic nerve can be entrapped by structures around the hip, a comprehensive physical examination with a thorough understanding of anatomy and biomechanics is critical in cases of deep gluteal pain.

PERTINENT PHYSICAL FINDINGS

History and Physical Examination

A comprehensive physical examination, detailed history, and standardized radiographic interpretation are paramount in evaluating hip pain.[4,16,17] Lumbar spine, abdominal, and

Byrd JWT, Bedi A, Stubbs AJ, eds. *The Hip:*
AANA Advanced Arthroscopic Surgical Techniques (pp 241-249).
© 2016 AANA.

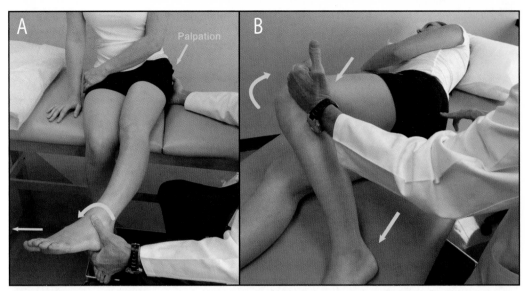

Figure 20-1. (A) Seated piriformis stretch test. The patient is in the seated position with the knee in extension. The examiner passively moves the flexed hip into adduction with internal rotation while palpating 1 cm lateral to the ischium (middle finger) and proximally at the sciatic notch (index finger). (B) Active piriformis test. With the patient in the lateral position, the examiner palpates the piriformis. The patient drives the heel into the examining table, thus initiating external hip rotation while actively abducting and externally rotating against resistance.

genitourinary problems are ruled out by history, physical examination, and ancillary testing. It is important to consider intrapelvic causes of sciatic nerve entrapment, particularly in patients with previous gynecologic surgical procedures and menses-related pain.[15,18]

Patients presenting with sciatic nerve entrapment often have a history of trauma and symptoms of sit-pain (inability to sit for > 30 minutes) lateral to the ischium and radicular pain of the affected leg.[4,19] Patients may present with neurological symptoms of abnormal reflexes or motor weakness.[20] Some symptoms may mimic a hamstring tear or intra-articular hip pathology, such as aching, burning sensation, or cramping in the buttock or posterior thigh. Symptoms of sit-pain should be differentiated from pudendal nerve entrapment, in which the pain is medial to the ischium.

The seated piriformis stretch test (Figure 20-1A) is a passive flexion, adduction, and internal rotation test performed as the examiner palpates the deep gluteal region.[16] The active piriformis test (Figure 20-1B) is an active abduction and external rotation test while the examiner monitors the piriformis. This active contraction may be held for 3 minutes to elicit symptoms (personal communication, Dr. Giancarlo Polesello, October 2013). The combination of the seated piriformis stretch test with the piriformis active test has shown a sensitivity of 91% and specificity of 80% for the endoscopic finding of sciatic nerve entrapment.[21]

Palpation of the gluteal structures is fundamental for the diagnosis of gluteal and sit-pain. The patient sits with the pelvis square to the examination table, and the ischial tuberosity (IT) serves as the reference point for palpation. Pain superolateral to the IT at the sciatic notch is characteristic of deep gluteal syndrome[4]; pain lateral to the IT is characteristic of ischial tunnel syndrome, or ischiofemoral impingement is considered; pain at the IT is possibly characteristic of hamstring tendinous pathologies; and for pain medial to the IT, pudendal nerve entrapment is considered.

Ischial tunnel syndrome, or hamstring syndrome, is described as pain in the lower buttock region that radiates down the posterior thigh to the popliteal fossa and is commonly associated with hamstring weakness.[6] This syndrome is related to sciatic nerve entrapment by scarring or a fibrotic band at the lateral insertion of the hamstring tendons to the IT.[6,7] Patients experience pain with sitting, stretching, and exercise, primarily running (sprinting and acceleration).[7,22] Palpable tenderness is located around the IT in the proximal hamstring region. An active knee flexion test against resistance, with 30 vs 90 degrees of knee flexion, evaluates the hamstring insertion on the lateral border of the semimembranosus.[7]

Ancillary Testing

Guided injections are useful to support the diagnosis of deep gluteal syndrome, mainly when the piriformis is involved. Computed tomography, fluoroscopy, ultrasonography, electroneuromyography, and magnetic resonance imaging (MRI) are useful to obtain more precise injections.[23] The association of physical examination and injection is also used to rule out intra-articular hip pathologies, nerve root compression at the lumbar spine, and pudendal nerve entrapment.

Electromyography and nerve conduction studies may assist with the diagnosis of deep gluteal syndrome. Piriformis entrapment of the sciatic nerve is often indicated by H-reflex disturbances of the tibial and/or fibular nerves.[24,25] It is important to compare side to side and perform a dynamic test with the knee in extension and hip in adduction with internal rotation. This position must be held for 3 minutes, which will tighten the piriformis muscle, compressing the sciatic nerve sufficiently to disturb nerve conduction distally. Patients presenting with symptoms of sciatic nerve entrapment may fail to exhibit paraspinal denervation even when radiculopathy coexists.[24]

The sciatic nerve anatomy and potential sources of compression can be assessed through high-resolution MRI. In addition to sciatic nerve compression assessment, MRI is important for ruling out spine issues, intra-articular hip pathology, and other differential diagnoses. Ultrasonography is a valuable method to guide nerve blocks and has been increasingly used for nerve assessment, with the advantages of dynamic evaluation and Doppler assessment of the vascular nerve supply.[11]

The diagnosis of sciatic nerve entrapment is established through the combination of physical examination, imaging studies, and piriformis injection testing.

ENDOSCOPIC ASSESSMENT AND DECOMPRESSION

Endoscopy is an effective approach for assessing for deep gluteal syndrome.[4] Advantages of endoscopy are that it is minimally invasive; it provides a magnified view of the sciatic nerve; and it allows evaluation of the entire deep gluteal space from the sciatic notch to the proximal thigh, including sciatic nerve biomechanics.

The supine technique without traction is used and modified by positioning the operating table in maximal contralateral patient tilt. The supine, as opposed to the prone, position allows for manual manipulation of the lower limb at the knee and hip joints for the full assessment of sciatic nerve kinematics. A relative contraindication for sciatic nerve decompression in this supine technique is knee recurvatum, considering the increased strain on the sciatic nerve. Nerve conduction and electroymyography are usually monitored intraoperatively and can demonstrate immediate improvement or change postrelease. Acute variations in nerve conduction intraoperatively may be observed due to fluid accumulation over time. For deep gluteal space visualization, a 70-degree, high-definition, long arthroscope with adjustable and lengthening cannulas is used.[4] The cannulas are opened to maintain the fluid flow when using the radiofrequency (RF) probe.[26] Fluid pressure is set to 60 mm Hg, with intermittent pressure increases up to 80 mm Hg. Three portals are used (Figure 20-2): anterolateral, posterolateral, and auxiliary posterolateral.[4,27] Frequent use of intraoperative fluoroscopy will confirm the proper location of the endoscopic view.

Endoscopy allows for a complete extrapelvic sciatic nerve visualization and safe nerve decompression in the deep gluteal space. The starting position[28] is established within the peritrochanteric space, and the arthroscope is rotated proximally. With the hip in a neutral position, inspect the peritrochanteric space through the anterolateral and posterolateral portals. Perform a greater

Figure 20-2. The anterolateral portal placement is 1 cm anterior and 1 cm superior to the greater trochanter outlined in blue. The posterolateral portal placement is 3 cm posterior to the greater trochanter and in line with the anterolateralportal. The auxiliary portal is positioned 3 cm posterior and 3 cm superior to the greater trochanter.

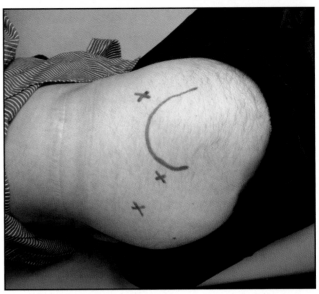

trochanteric bursectomy[29] with an arthroscopic shaver, releasing fibrous bands until the quadratus femoris is identified. A blunt probe can be used to release any fibrous bands at the level of the quadratus femoris. With the hip in internal rotation, evaluate the sciatic nerve color, epineural blood flow, epineural fat, and nerve motion (nerve motion requires internal and external rotation). Normal sciatic nerve appearance (Figure 20-3A) will have visible epineural blood flow and epineural fat. Normal nerve motion is discernible as a gliding along the border of the external rotator muscles with internal/external hip rotation. An abnormal sciatic nerve (Figure 20-3B) will appear white like a shoestring, will feel tight with probing, and will not glide with hip rotation. Check for greater trochanteric impingement by moving the hip into deep hip flexion and external rotation (Figure 20-3C). Normally, the sciatic nerve will glide posterolaterally to clear the greater trochanter. In cases of sciatic nerve entrapment by the greater trochanter or ischium, greater trochanteric osteoplasty or osteotomy may be a consideration.

After gross evaluation of the sciatic nerve, identify the vascular branches penetrating the nerve anteriorly just proximal to the quadratus femoris muscle. To protect the perineural sheath of the sciatic nerve, a blunt probe is used for dissection and probing. Fibrous bands may extend from the greater trochanteric bursa down to the sciatic nerve.[4] Fibrovascular scar bands are often present, which should be cauterized and released with arthroscopic scissors. In cases of thick and clustered fibrovascular bands resembling a bird's nest, alternating use of cauterization and release is necessary. Large-diameter fibrovascular bands may require ligature in addition to cauterization prior to release.[4]

Rotate the arthroscope distally and inspect the sciatic nerve at the ischial tunnel, hamstring origin, and sacrotuberous ligament. Identify and release any fibers from the sciatic nerve along this distal course. Rotate the arthroscope proximally and identify the obturator internus muscle and tendon. Release fibrous bands, probe, and check for the relation between the sciatic nerve and obturator internus tendon, which may penetrate the sciatic nerve. Next, move the long scope to the auxiliary or posterolateral portal when required (usually in obese patients). Identify the branch of the inferior gluteal artery, which crosses posterior to the sciatic nerve distal to the border of the piriformis muscle. This branch must be cauterized or ligated (when larger than 2 mm using 4/0 polydioxanone [Ethicon]) and released before the inspection of the piriformis muscle and tendon (Figure 20-4). A cadaveric study reported a mean distance of 8 mm (range, 4 to 14 mm) between the sciatic nerve and the crossing branch of the inferior gluteal vessel.[26] In addition, the temperature profile during activation of a monopolar RF device was safe at a distance of 3 to

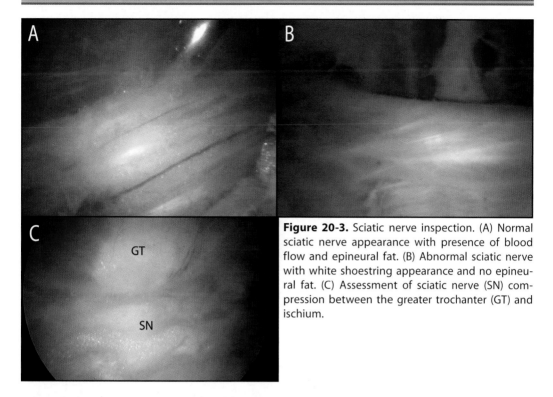

Figure 20-3. Sciatic nerve inspection. (A) Normal sciatic nerve appearance with presence of blood flow and epineural fat. (B) Abnormal sciatic nerve with white shoestring appearance and no epineural fat. (C) Assessment of sciatic nerve (SN) compression between the greater trochanter (GT) and ischium.

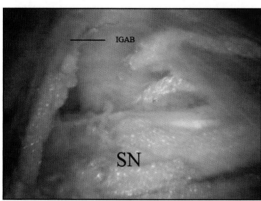

Figure 20-4. Proximal view with identification of a branch of the inferior gluteal artery (IGAB), which crosses the sciatic nerve (SN) posteriorly, which must be cauterized or ligated (when larger than 2 mm) prior to release.

10 mm to the sciatic nerve during activation times of 3, 5, and 10 seconds.[26] The standard approach to vessel cauterization is a 3-second interval of RF activation, maintaining continuous irrigation.

The piriformis muscle and tendon can now be identified. The piriformis tendon is often located proximal to the belly of the muscle, which will require probing. Shave the distal border of the piriformis to expose the tendon. Arthroscopic scissors are used for the release of the piriformis tendon. Pulling the scissors toward yourself during resection adds safety and ensures that only the tendon is released (Figure 20-5). Retraction of the sciatic nerve with a curved probe also adds safety any time the shaver or scissors are used near the sciatic nerve. Following piriformis tendon resection, shave the tendinous stump back 1 to 2 cm. Probe the sciatic nerve for tension and look for hidden muscle or tendon branches traversing the nerve. Perform the dynamic testing of sciatic nerve kinematics, probing the nerve during hip internal and external rotation with hip flexion and

Figure 20-5. Piriformis tendonotomy. PM = piriformis muscle and tendon; SN = sciatic nerve.

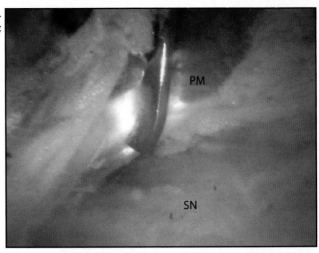

extension. Carefully note that the superior gluteal neurovascular structures exit the sciatic notch superior to the piriformis muscle.

A standardized technique and surgical experience for diagnosis and sciatic nerve decompression is mandatory to identify the sciatic nerve anatomy, avoid iatrogenic injury, and not overlook potential sources of sciatic nerve entrapment.

POSTOPERATIVE PROTOCOL

Physical therapy rehabilitation and patient compliance are critical to the outcomes of endoscopic sciatic nerve decompression. The goal of rehabilitation is to gain mobility and maintain movement of the hip joint. Patients feel much better after surgery and may want to take an aggressive approach regarding stretching and rehabilitation. However, stretch injury can cause neurapraxia and neuralgia. A 6% to 12% increase in nerve stretch can cause decreased nerve conduction.[30,31] To avoid overstretch injury, the Ilizarov osteogenesis principles of limb lengthening can be applied to rehabilitation by a slow progression of increased stretching. Kinematic motion of the sciatic nerve with knee flexion is different from that with knee extension. This factor is important for the understanding and application of physical therapy principles. The following is an outline for postoperative sciatic nerve decompression rehabilitation.

Full circumduction of the hip with knee flexion can begin on postoperative day 1. A knee brace is used to avoid knee extension and maintain a relaxed sciatic nerve when necessary. Use of the knee brace is dependent on the strain of the sciatic nerve, which is influenced by degree of femoral anteversion and the number of sites of entrapment. If increased tension is noticed postoperatively, the knee is locked at 45 degrees for 3 weeks, applying only nerve glides and circumduction. After week 4, knee extension can increase up to 10 degrees every 2 weeks as tolerated. Maintain circumduction, gentle nerve glides, and stretching maneuvers aimed at the external rotators (Figure 20-6). The piriformis stretch involves placing the hip in flexion, adduction, and internal rotation. Gradually progress the stretching by increasing the duration and intensity until a maximal stretch is obtained. The standard physical therapy protocol can begin as early as 4 weeks. Use caution in cases of previous abdominal surgery and femoral retroversion because strain parameters will be a dependent factor, and the nerve may be impinged in more than one location. The therapist should be diligent in recognizing these potential outcome factors. These physical therapy techniques are the same as those used in preoperative conservative treatment.

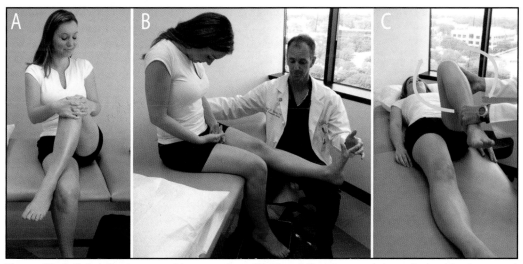

Figure 20-6. Rehabilitation stretching exercises. (A) The piriformis stretch is performed in the seated position. The patient brings the knee toward the opposite shoulder. (B) Sciatic nerve glides. The patient first performs cervical extension and plantarflexion of the ankle followed by cervical flexion with ankle dorsiflexion. (C) Hip circumduction is performed in the supine position with gentle passive circular movements, with the knee and ankle parallel to the body longitudinal axis (avoiding hip rotation).

The use of steroidal and nonsteroidal anti-inflammatory drugs has been useful after postoperative day 2. Additional physical therapy techniques may be helpful, including ultrasound and electrical stimulation. With a proper rehabilitation protocol, good to excellent outcomes can be achieved. The advancement in rehabilitation has proven beneficial in improving the outcomes of endoscopic sciatic nerve decompression.

RESULTS

Martin et al[4] reported a case series of 35 patients presenting with deep gluteal syndrome. Average duration of symptoms was 3.7 years, with an average preoperative visual analog score of 7, which decreased to 2.4 postoperatively. Preoperative modified Harris Hip Score was 54.4 and increased to 78 postoperatively. Twenty-one patients reported preoperative use of narcotics for pain, and 2 remained on narcotics postoperatively (unrelated to the initial complaint). Eighty-three percent of patients had no postoperative sciatic sit-pain.[4] Five patients experienced low modified Harris Hip Scores and modest pain relief postoperatively. This poor outcome group may be related to femoral retroversion and previous abdominal surgery.

POTENTIAL COMPLICATIONS

Among 200 national and international cases, complications continue to be low.[32] It is important to assess acetabular and femoral version, which has an effect on sciatic nerve biomechanics. To help avoid postsurgical stretch injury, it is recommended that intra-articular work be performed separately from extra-articular work. Due to the length of time from diagnosis to treatment and recovery, the psychological toll of the pain cycle can be frustrating. Preoperative psychiatric and cognitive behavior evaluation is helpful for any condition lasting longer than 6 months with social disruption. Participation in a pain club is not recommended and may be a negative outcome predictor. Complications have involved hematoma brought on by early postoperative use of nonsteroidal anti-inflammatory drugs with excessive postoperative activity. Concomitant pudendal and sciatic nerve complaints are often resolved; however, in 2 cases, the pudendal complaints worsened, most likely due to intrapelvic involvement.

CONCLUSION

Endoscopy of the deep gluteal space provides a standardized approach to sciatic nerve assessment and decompression. This endoscopic approach appears useful in detecting sciatic nerve pathology in addition to assessment and treatment of the ischiofemoral space and the proximal hamstring/ischial tunnel. By understanding the anatomy and biomechanics and applying clinical tests and diagnostic strategies, adequate treatment of all 4 layers can be obtained as a part of a comprehensive treatment plan and rehabilitation program.

TOP TECHNICAL PEARLS FOR THE PROCEDURE

1. Careful patient selection should include a preoperative psychological evaluation.
2. Proper portal placement is used to ensure adequate visualization.
3. The surgeon must have a thorough understanding of the deep gluteal space anatomy.
4. Carefully dissect around the sciatic nerve with a blunt probe and retract the nerve with a curved retractor.
5. Positive outcomes require a proper physical therapy protocol and patient compliance to physical therapy.

REFERENCES

1. McCrory P, Bell S. Nerve entrapment syndromes as a cause of pain in the hip, groin and buttock. *Sports Med.* 1999;27(4):261-274.
2. Robinson DR. Pyriformis syndrome in relation to sciatic pain. *Am J Surg.* 1947;73(3):355-358.
3. Yeoman W. The relation of arthritis of the sacro-iliac joint to sciatica, with an analysis of 100 cases. *Lancet.* 1928;2:1119-1122.
4. Martin HD, Shears SA, Johnson JC, Smathers AM, Palmer IJ. The endoscopic treatment of sciatic nerve entrapment/deep gluteal syndrome. *Arthroscopy.* 2011;27(2):172-181.
5. Vandertop WP, Bosma NJ. The piriformis syndrome: a case report. *J Bone Joint Surg Am.* 1991;73(7):1095-1097.
6. Puranen J, Orava S. The hamstring syndrome. A new diagnosis of gluteal sciatic pain. *Am J Sports Med.* 1988;16(5):517-521.
7. Young IJ, van Riet RP, Bell SN. Surgical release for proximal hamstring syndrome. *Am J Sports Med.* 2008;36(12):2372-2378.
8. Cox JM, Bakkum BW. Possible generators of retrotrochanteric gluteal and thigh pain: the gemelli-obturator internus complex. *J Manipulative Physiol Ther.* 2005;28(7):534-538.
9. Meknas K, Kartus J, Letto JI, Christensen A, Johansen O. Surgical release of the internal obturator tendon for the treatment of retro-trochanteric pain syndrome: a prospective randomized study, with long-term follow-up. *Knee Surg Sports Traumatol Arthrosc.* 2009;17(10):1249-1256.

10. Miller A, Stedman GH, Beisaw NE, Gross PT. Sciatica caused by an avulsion fracture of the ischial tuberosity. A case report. *J Bone Joint Surg Am.* 1987;69(1):143-145.

11. Labropoulos N, Tassiopoulos AK, Gasparis AP, Phillips B, Pappas PJ. Veins along the course of the sciatic nerve. *J Vasc Surg.* 2009;49(3):690-696.

12. Papadopoulos SM, McGillicuddy JE, Albers JW. Unusual cause of 'piriformis muscle syndrome.' *Arch Neurol.* 1990;47(10):1144-1146.

13. Beauchesne RP, Schutzer SF. Myositis ossificans of the piriformis muscle: an unusual cause of piriformis syndrome. A case report. *J Bone Joint Surg Am.* 1997;79(6):906-910.

14. Chen WS. Sciatica due to piriformis pyomyositis: report of a case. *J Bone Joint Surg Am.* 1992;74(10):1546-1548.

15. Possover M. Laparoscopic management of endopelvic etiologies of pudendal pain in 134 consecutive patients. *J Urol.* 2009;181(4):1732-1736.

16. Martin H. Clinical examination and imaging of the hip. In: Byrd J, Guanche C, eds. *AANA Advanced Arthroscopy: The Hip.* Philadelphia, PA: Saunders; 2010:3-30.

17. Martin HD, Kelly BT, Leunig M, et al. The pattern and technique in the clinical evaluation of the adult hip: the common physical examination tests of hip specialists. *Arthroscopy.* 2010;26(2):161-172.

18. Possover M, Schneider T, Henle KP. Laparoscopic therapy for endometriosis and vascular entrapment of sacral plexus. *Fertil Steril.* 2011;95(2):756-758.

19. Benson ER, Schutzer SF. Posttraumatic piriformis syndrome: diagnosis and results of operative treatment. *J Bone Joint Surg Am.* 1999;81(7):941-949.

20. Papadopoulos EC, Khan SN. Piriformis syndrome and low back pain: a new classification and review of the literature. *Orthop Clin North Am.* 2004;35(1):65-71.

21. Martin HD, Kivlan BR, Palmer IJ, Martin RL. Diagnostic accuracy of clinical tests for sciatic nerve entrapment in the gluteal region. *Knee Surg Sports Traumatol Arthrosc.* 2014;22(4):882-888.

22. Migliorini S, Merlo M. The hamstring syndrome in endurance athletes. *Br J Sports Med.* 2011;45(4):363.

23. Filler AG, Haynes J, Jordan SE, et al. Sciatica of nondisc origin and piriformis syndrome: diagnosis by magnetic resonance neurography and interventional magnetic resonance imaging with outcome study of resulting treatment. *J Neurosurg Spine.* 2005;2(2):99-115.

24. Fishman LM, Wilkins AN. Piriformis syndrome: electrophysiology vs. anatomical assumption. In: Fishman LM, Wilkins AN, eds. *Functional Electromyography.* New York, NY: Springer US; 2011:77-93.

25. Jawish RM, Assoum HA, Khamis CF. Anatomical, clinical and electrical observations in piriformis syndrome. *J Orthop Surg Res.* 2010;5(1):3.

26. Martin HD, Palmer IJ, Hatem M. Monopolar radiofrequency use in deep gluteal space endoscopy: sciatic nerve safety and fluid temperature. *Arthroscopy.* 2014;30(1):60-64.

27. Martin HD, Hatem MA, Champlin K, et al. The endoscopic treatment of sciatic nerve entrapment/deep gluteal syndrome. *Tech Orthop.* 2012;27(3):172-183.

28. Martin H. Diagnostic arthroscopy. In: Kelly BT, Philippon MJ, eds. *Arthroscopic Techniques of the Hip: A Visual Guide.* Thorofare, NJ: SLACK Incorporated; 2009:29-48.

29. Voos JE, Rudzki JR, Shindle MK, Martin H, Kelly BT. Arthroscopic anatomy and surgical techniques for peritrochanteric space disorders in the hip. *Arthroscopy.* 2007;23(11):1246.e1-1246.e5.

30. Coppieters MW, Alshami AM, Babri AS, Souvlis T, Kippers V, Hodges PW. Strain and excursion of the sciatic, tibial, and plantar nerves during a modified straight leg raising test. *J Orthop Res.* 2006;24(9):1883-1889.

31. Wall EJ, Massie JB, Kwan MK, Rydevik BL, Myers RR, Garfin SR. Experimental stretch neuropathy: changes in nerve conduction under tension. *J Bone Joint Surg Br.* 1992;74(1):126-129.

32. Proceedings from the International Society of Hip Arthroscopy Annual Meeting; October 10-12, 2013; Munich, Germany.

Please see videos on the accompanying website at

www.ArthroscopicTechniques.com

21

Endoscopy of Proximal Hamstring Injuries

Carlos A. Guanche, MD

INTRODUCTION

Hamstring injuries are common in athletic populations and can affect all levels of athletes, with several studies showing the rate of muscle strains to be as high as 22.2%.[1-10] Although some studies suggest that contact activities are the cause of proximal hamstring injuries, most have shown that more than 90% occur without contact, with the classic injury being a water skier who gets pulled up by the boat.[5-11]

There is a continuum of hamstring injuries that can range from musculotendinous strains to avulsion injuries.[1,2] In one study, 12.3% of 170 hamstring injuries were tendon tears; the majority (90.5%) were muscle belly injuries.[12] Most hamstring strains do not require surgical intervention and resolve with various modalities and rest. The hamstring complex consists of the biceps femoris, semitendinosus, and semimembranosus. These muscles work together to extend the hip, flex the knee, and externally rotate the hip and knee.[11] The complex has a strong bony attachment on the ischial tuberosity (IT), with the footprint on the ischium comprising the semitendinosus and the long head of biceps femoris, beginning as a common proximal tendon and footprint and a distinct semimembranosus footprint (Figure 21-1).[13] This footprint is medial and anterior to the crescent-shaped footprint of the common insertion of the semitendinosus and long head of the biceps femoris (see Figure 21-1). This chapter details the endoscopic access to the hamstring origin and the management of injuries to this complex.

INDICATIONS

▶ Acute tear of the hamstring origin
▶ Partial, chronic tear of the hamstring origin

Byrd JWT, Bedi A, Stubbs AJ, eds. *The Hip: AANA Advanced Arthroscopic Surgical Techniques* (pp 251-261).
© 2016 AANA.

Figure 21-1. Normal anatomy of the hamstring origin. (A) Left hip viewed from posteriorly. The origin of the biceps and semitendinosus (B/ST) muscles, which have been incised, are shown (arrows). (B) The hamstring origin has been everted to show the footprint on the ischium.

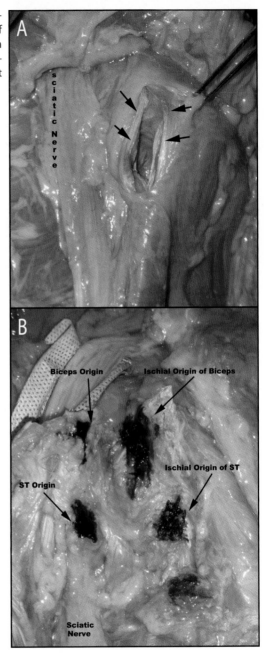

- ▶ Chronic ischial bursitis that is refractory to nonsurgical care
- ▶ Patients receiving conservative treatment, including at least 6 weeks of physical therapy and 2 ultrasound-guided ischial injections[14]

Relative Indications

- ▶ Large, retracted tear that has chronic atrophy noted on magnetic resonance imaging (MRI). In these cases, the procedure will likely require extensive mobilization and use of a graft for reconstruction of the avulsed segment. This may be attempted in an endoscopic fashion but may ultimately require an open approach.

The indications for endoscopic surgery in this area are evolving, and specific surgeons' surgical abilities must be taken into consideration. The other critical tenet is that even with the best of skills, it is possible that the procedure may need to be aborted, and a traditional open approach may ultimately be necessary to successfully address the pathology, particularly in cases of significant distal retraction.

The advantages of the endoscopic technique are that it is a more direct approach; it avoids elevation of the gluteus maximus; and, with the use of endoscopic magnification to better visualize the sciatic nerve, it should improve the management of these injuries and reduce the morbidities associated with the open approach.

PERTINENT PHYSICAL FINDINGS

Proximal hamstring injuries can be categorized as complete tendinous avulsions, partial tendinous avulsions, apophyseal avulsions, and degenerative (tendinosis).[15] Degenerative tears of the hamstring origin are more insidious in onset and are commonly seen as an overuse injury in middle- and long-distance runners. The mechanism of injury in these patients is presumably repetitive irritation of the medial aspect of the hamstring tendon along the lateral aspect of the tuberosity where the bursa resides. This rubbing ultimately causes an attritional tear of the tendon. The clinical examination in these patients is somewhat different. Physical examination is typically performed with the patient in the prone position.

- ▶ With acute avulsions, a popping or tearing sensation is described, along with associated pain and bruising over the posterior hip.[16,17] Acute symptoms include weakness with active knee flexion, a sensation of instability, or difficulty controlling the leg.
- ▶ Inspection and palpation of the posterior thigh may reveal muscle spasm. Ecchymosis may only be observed if the fascial covering is also disrupted. Palpation of the entire posterior thigh is important to localize the injury. In acute injuries, there is typically focal tenderness and swelling.
- ▶ Acute or chronic tears may cause a pins-and-needles sensation in the sciatic nerve distribution, much like sciatica.[17,18] This may be due to acute compression by a hematoma in the proximity of the sciatic nerve or chronic scarring and tethering of the tendon to the nerve.
- ▶ In chronic ischial bursitis, symptoms include buttock or hip pain and localized tenderness overlying the IT.
- ▶ Clinically, those most affected tend to sit with the painful buttock elevated off their seat.
- ▶ One examination technique positions the patients prone, and they are asked to actively tension their hamstring tendon. This is then compared with the passive tendon tension while sitting. Decreased tension as compared with the normal side suggests a proximal tendon rupture.[16]

PERTINENT IMAGING

If there is a high level of suspicion for a proximal hamstring injury, routine and advanced imaging is performed.

- ▶ Plain x-rays of the pelvis and a lateral view of the affected hip help rule out apophyseal avulsions, particularly in adolescent athletes.
- ▶ MRI is used to assess the proximal hamstring origin. A complete rupture of all 3 tendons is common and is most easily identified on MRI with accurate measurement of the amount of

Figure 21-2. Coronal T2-weighted MRI of complete 3-tendon rupture of the proximal hamstring on the right. The left side is shown for comparison. IT = ischial tuberosity; SM = intact semimembranosus origin; ST/B = semitendinosus/biceps avulsion.

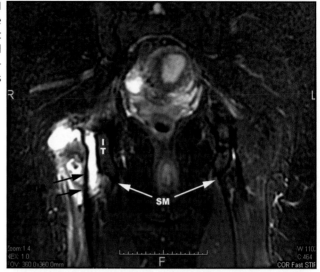

Figure 21-3. Coronal T2-weighted MRI of a right hip showing the sickle sign (red arrow) indicating fluid within the ischial bursa. The white arrow indicates a normal attachment. IT = ischial tuberosity.

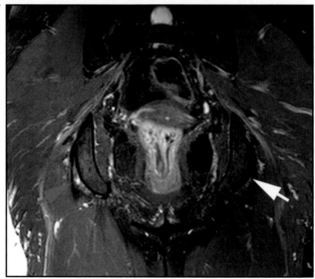

retraction possible (Figure 21-2).[19] All 3 MRI planes (coronal, sagittal, and axial) should be used to define the tear pattern.

▶ Partial hamstring origin tears are more difficult to diagnose. Partial insertional tears with no significant retraction can be seen on MRI as a sickle sign (Figure 21-3). These are typically partial avulsions of the common biceps and semitendinosus origin.

▶ Ultrasound is highly accurate in evaluating partial tears and insertional tendinosis.[20] Its potential for bedside use, as a dynamic test, may detect more subtle injuries, particularly in the athletic population (Figure 21-4).[13]

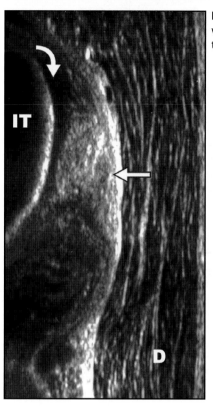

Figure 21-4. Ultrasound image of the hamstring origin (arrow) with the ischial bursa (curved arrow). D=distal; IT=ischial tuberosity.

EQUIPMENT

- ► Standard arthroscopic equipment
- ► Standard-length instruments
  - ▷ 30-degree arthroscope
  - ▷ Extended-length arthroscopic cannulas
- ► Suture anchors with multiple suture strands (double or triple)
- ► Suture-passing instrumentation typically used in rotator cuff repairs
  - ▷ Wire passers
  - ▷ Penetrators
  - ▷ Needle-passing devices
- ► Fluid inflow pump
- ► Hinged knee brace fixed at 90 degrees of flexion for postoperative immobilization

STEP-BY-STEP DESCRIPTION OF THE PROCEDURE

The patient is positioned prone following the induction of anesthesia, with all prominences and neurovascular structures protected. The table is flat (as opposed to the open repair, where the table is slightly flexed) to help maintain the space between the gluteal musculature and the ischium. The posterior aspect of the hip is then sterilized, assuring that the leg and thigh are free and allowing repositioning intraoperatively (Figure 21-5).

Figure 21-5. Positioning of the patient in the prone position with the leg draped free. View is of a right hip setup. The table is flat with no flexion. The surgeon and assistant are positioned ipsilateral. The arthroscopic equipment is positioned on the contralateral side.

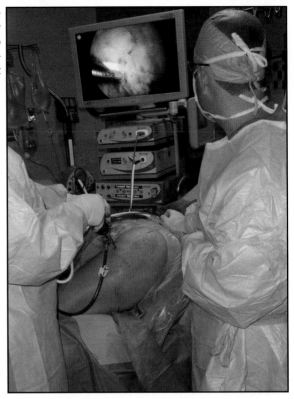

Figure 21-6. Portals for the endoscopic approach. The medial (MP) and lateral (LP) portals are routinely established. The other 2 (distal and proximal portals) are established later, if necessary, to anchor insertion and suture management. DP = distal portal; PP = proximal portal; SN = sciatic nerve.

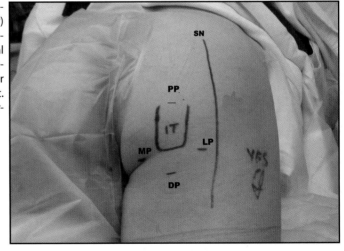

Two portals are then created slightly distal to the palpable IT, one 2 cm medial and one 2 cm lateral (Figure 21-6). The lateral portal is established first. This is done using blunt dissection with a switching stick because the gluteus maximus muscle is penetrated and the submuscular plane is created. The switching stick serves to palpate the prominence of the tuberosity and identify the medial and lateral borders of the ischium. The medial portal is then established, taking care to palpate the medial aspect of the ischium. A 30-degree arthroscope is inserted in the lateral portal, and an electrocautery device is placed in the medial portal. In some cases, a 70-degree arthroscope may be useful (eg, when one of the tendons is distally retracted and visualizing the tendon with the 30-degree scope is difficult). The space between the ischium and the gluteus muscle is then

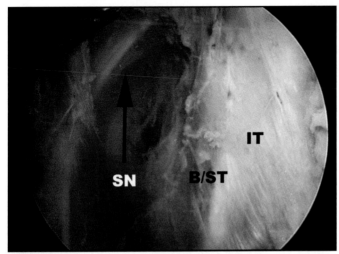

Figure 21-7. Normal endoscopic exposure in a left hip viewed from the lateral portal showing the sciatic nerve (SN), common biceps/semitendinosus (B/ST) lateral ischium. Note the tool entering from the medial portal. IT = ischial tuberosity.

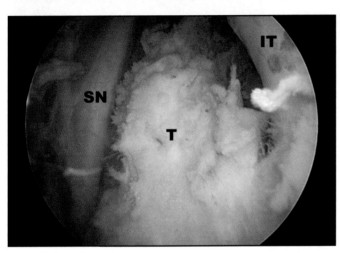

Figure 21-8. Sciatic nerve (SN) and its proximity to an avulsion of the hamstring from the ischium (IT). T = avulsed tendon.

developed, taking care to stay along the central and medial portions of the ischium to avoid damage to the sciatic nerve. The lateral aspect is then exposed with the use of a switching stick as a soft tissue dissector. With the lateral aspect identified, the dissection continues anteriorly and laterally toward the known area of the sciatic nerve (Figure 21-7). A methodical release of any soft tissue bands is then undertaken in a proximal-to-distal direction to mobilize the nerve and protect it throughout the repair of the hamstring. In acute disruptions that have some scarring, significant bands are often encountered.

Once the nerve is identified and protected, attention is then directed to the area of the tendon origin. The tip of the ischium is identified through palpation with the instruments. The tendinous origin is then inspected to identify obvious tearing (Figure 21-8). In acute tears, the area is frequently obvious, and the tendon is often retracted distally. Occasionally, however, the tendon sheath is intact, and the area of avulsion is only obvious by palpation and feeling for the tendon defect deep to the sheath along the distal and lateral ischium. In acute cases, a large hematoma may need to be evacuated. It is important to protect the sciatic nerve during this portion of the procedure because it is sometimes obscured by the hematoma.

In incomplete tears, an endoscopic knife can be used to longitudinally split the tendon along its fibers. The hamstring is then undermined, and the partial tearing is debrided with an oscillating shaver. The lateral wall of the ischium is cleared of devitalized tissue, and a bleeding bed

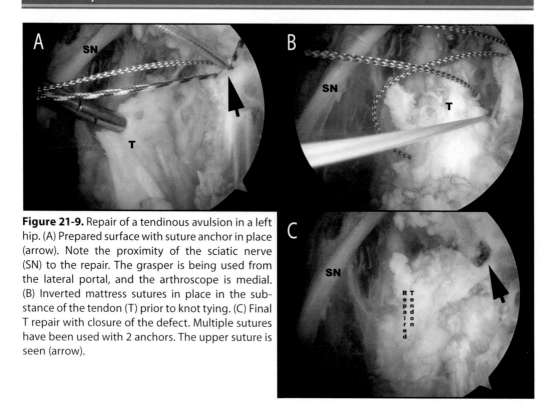

Figure 21-9. Repair of a tendinous avulsion in a left hip. (A) Prepared surface with suture anchor in place (arrow). Note the proximity of the sciatic nerve (SN) to the repair. The grasper is being used from the lateral portal, and the arthroscope is medial. (B) Inverted mattress sutures in place in the substance of the tendon (T) prior to knot tying. (C) Final T repair with closure of the defect. Multiple sutures have been used with 2 anchors. The upper suture is seen (arrow).

is established in preparation for the tendon repair. The lateral and distal ischium and the ischial bursa can also be debrided and cleared of inflamed tissues as the lateral ischial tissue is mobilized. By retracting the anterior tissues, the bursa can be entered and debrided.

Depending on the type of tear and the angle of approach for suture anchors, 2 additional portals may be established. One is approximately 4 to 6 cm distal to the tip of the ischium and equidistant from the medial and lateral portals. This portal is used for grabbing a retracted tendon insertion of suture anchors and for suture management. The second portal is proximal to the ischium about 4 to 6 cm above the tip. This can be used for holding the tendon in place while suturing and for anchor placement in some cases.

Various suture-passing devices can then be used for the repair. The principles are essentially the same as those used in arthroscopic rotator cuff repair. Once all of the sutures are passed through the tissue of the avulsed hamstring, the sutures are tied and a solid repair of the tendon is completed. In general, one suture anchor is used per centimeter of detachment (Figure 21-9). The tendon should be placed on the lateral aspect of the IT and lie down flat to allow optimal bony healing and prevent prominence. It is important to remember to flex the knee at least 30 degrees while mobilization and tying are taking place because this allows for a more secure and anatomical repair.

POSTOPERATIVE PROTOCOL

Postoperatively, the patient is fitted with a hinged knee brace that is fixed at 90 degrees of flexion for 4 weeks to limit weight bearing, restrict excursion of the hamstring tendons, and protect the repair. At 4 weeks, the knee is gradually extended by about 15 degrees per week to allow full weight bearing by 8 weeks, while maintaining the use of crutches. Physical therapy is instituted at 4 weeks postoperatively. Isotonic (6 weeks) and isokinetic (8 weeks) strengthening and aqua therapy are initiated with progression of core pelvic and closed-chain exercises. Dry land and sport-specific training are initiated at 12 weeks, with return to full sports participation between 5 and 8 months. This is predicated on full passive motion and no pain in the hamstring origin.

POTENTIAL COMPLICATIONS

The endoscopic approach has been developed over the past 2 years, and the procedure has been used in a group of 25 of the author's patients. All patients underwent the surgery as described, with 2 patients requiring abandonment of the procedure as a result of a failure of visualization of any of the pertinent structures and fear of fluid extravasation. All patients underwent suture anchor fixation, with no anchor complications to date. Two patients initially complained of numbness over the posterior thigh but had resolution of their symptoms by 6 weeks postoperatively. No wound complications or sciatic nerve dysfunction occurred. One patient (with preoperative refractory ischial bursitis) had a subsequent guided injection as a result of recurrent ischial pain. One patient had deep venous thrombosis of the surgical extremity 8 weeks following the procedure.

More generally, the 3 main nervous structures at risk to iatrogenic injury are the posterior femoral cutaneous, inferior gluteal, and sciatic nerves.[21,22] The sciatic nerve is in close proximity to the IT as it runs along the lateral aspect. With the endoscopic technique, the need for retraction is essentially nonexistent because the nerve is identified and visualized during the repair, but no retraction is necessary.

A concern unique to the endoscopic approach is fluid extravasation into the pelvis as a result of the fluid used in the distension of the potential space around the hamstring origin. Every effort should be made to regularly check the abdomen for evidence of abdominal distension. Likewise, unusual blood pressure decreases that may be due to fluid compression from retroperitoneal extravasation need to be kept in mind. In general, an attempt should be made to maintain the fluid inflow pressures as low as is feasible for good visualization, and an attempt should be made to keep track of fluid ingress and egress volumes to assure that extravasation is avoided.

DISCUSSION

The surgical approach for hamstring repair may be slightly intimidating for surgeons because it is not a common area for surgical treatment that is encountered throughout orthopedic training. It is recommended that a first-time repair be performed in the acute setting in a fairly slender patient to allow for an easier approach to the IT. Recognition of proximal hamstring ruptures allows possible treatment with this minimally invasive repair. Using the delineated guidelines and appropriate judgment for the repair of these injuries should give good functional results in a less traumatic fashion. In addition, further refinement of the endoscopic technique is in its earliest phases; the extent that this technique can be used in all tears remains to be seen. It allows for a more thorough assessment of the entire constellation of findings, including sciatic nerve involvement. Further studies are necessary to document the outcomes of the technique and compare it with traditional open procedures.

TOP TECHNICAL PEARLS FOR THE PROCEDURE

1. Position the patient prone in the neutral position with no hip flexion to allow the sub-gluteal space to be larger.

2. The initial portals need to be more distal than is thought. It is important to approach the tendon avulsion site from below rather than directly over the area of injury.

3. The sciatic nerve should be identified and protected throughout the case. Even in cases of an acute injury, it important to know where the nerve is at all times so that suture repair is safely completed with no nerve injury.

4. Avoid prolonged postoperative immobilization with secure fixation because there is the potential for a knee flexion contracture.

5. Be ready to connect the 2 initial portals and complete the procedure in an open fashion, particularly in early phases of the learning curve.

REFERENCES

1. Brown T. Thigh. In: DeLee JC, Miller MD, eds. *Orthopaedic Sports Medicine: Principles and Practice.* Vol 2. Philadelphia, PA: Saunders; 2003:1481-1523.

2. Clanton TL. Invited editorial/introduction to nitric oxide and the respiratory musculature: a short history of nitric oxide in skeletal muscle function. Comparative biochemistry and physiology. *Comp Biochem Physiol A Mol Integr Physiol.* 1998;119(1):165-166.

3. Speer KP, Lohnes J, Garrett WE Jr. Radiographic imaging of muscle strain injury. *Am J Sports Med.* 1993;21(1):89-95.

4. Garrett WE Jr, Rich FR, Nikolaou PK, Vogler JB III. Computed tomography of hamstring muscle strains. *Med Sci Sports Exerc.* 1989;21(5):506-514.

5. Elliott MC, Zarins B, Powell JW, Kenyon CD. Hamstring muscle strains in professional football players: a 10-year review. *Am J Sports Med.* 2011;39(4):843-850.

6. Culpepper MI, Niemann KM. High school football injuries in Birmingham, Alabama. *South Med J.* 1983;76(7):873-875.

7. Dick R, Ferrara MS, Agel J, et al. Descriptive epidemiology of collegiate men's football injuries: National Collegiate Athletic Association Injury Surveillance System, 1988-1989 through 2003-2004. *J Athl Train.* 2007;42(2):221-233.

8. Moretz A III, Rashkin A, Grana WA. Oklahoma high school football injury study: a preliminary report. *J Okla State Med Assoc.* 1978;71(3):85-88.

9. Powell JW, Barber-Foss KD. Injury patterns in selected high school sports: a review of the 1995-1997 seasons. *J Athlet Train.* 1999;34(3):277-284.

10. Shankar PR, Fields SK, Collins CL, Dick RW, Comstock RD. Epidemiology of high school and collegiate football injuries in the United States, 2005-2006. *Am J Sports Med.* 2007;35(8):1295-1303.

11. Mueller FO, Blyth CS. North Carolina high school football injury study: equipment and prevention. *J Sports Med.* 1974;2(1):1-10.

12. Koulouris G, Connell D. Evaluation of the hamstring muscle complex following acute injury. *Skeletal Radiol.* 2003;32(10):582-589.

13. Miller SL, Gill J, Webb GR. The proximal origin of the hamstrings and surrounding anatomy encountered during repair: a cadaveric study. *J Bone Joint Surg Am.* 2007;89(1):44-48.

14. Zissen MH, Wallace G, Stevens KJ, Fredericson M, Beaulieu CF. High hamstring tendinopathy: MRI and ultrasound imaging and therapeutic efficacy of percutaneous corticosteroid injection. *AJR Am J Roentgenol.* 2010;195(4):993-998.

15. Klingele KE, Sallay PI. Surgical repair of complete proximal hamstring tendon rupture. *Am J Sports Med.* 2002;30(5):742-747.

16. Sallay PI, Ballar G, Hamersly S, Schrader M. Subjective and functional outcomes following surgical repair of complete ruptures of the proximal hamstring complex. *Orthopedics.* 2008;31(11):1092.

17. Sarimo J, Lempainen L, Mattila K, Orava S. Complete proximal hamstring avulsions: a series of 41 patients with operative treatment. *Am J Sports Med.* 2008;36(6):1110-1115.

18. Mica L, Schwaller A, Stoupis C, Penka I, Vomela J, Vollenweider A. Avulsion of the hamstring muscle group: a follow-up of 6 adult non-athletes with early operative treatment: a brief report. *World J Surg.* 2009;33(8):1605-1610.

19. Brucker PU, Imhoff AB. Functional assessment after acute and chronic complete ruptures of the proximal hamstring tendons. *Knee Surg Sports Traumatol Arthrosc.* 2005;13(5):411-418.

20. Zissen MH, Wallace G, Steven KJ, Fredericson M, Beaulieu CF. High hamstring tendinopathy: MRI and ultrasound imaging and therapeutic efficacy of percutaneous corticosteroid injection. *AJR Am J Roentgenol.* 2010;195(4):993-998.

21. Lempainen L, Sarimo J, Mattila K, Vaittinen S, Orava S. Proximal hamstring tendinopathy: results of surgical management and histopathologic findings. *Am J Sports Med.* 2009;37(4):727-734.

22. Lempainen L, Sarimo J, Heikkilä J, Mattila K, Orava S. Surgical treatment of partial tears of the proximal origin of the hamstring muscles. *Br J Sports Med.* 2006;40(8):688-691.

Please see videos on the accompanying website at

www.ArthroscopicTechniques.com

22

Common Complications of Hip Arthroscopy and Their Management

Fotios Paul Tjoumakaris, MD and John P. Salvo, MD

INTRODUCTION

Hip arthroscopy has advanced considerably over the past 2 decades. This advancement has come in 2 forms: technique and usage. A recent study demonstrated that the use of hip arthroscopy by Part II examinees of the American Board of Orthopaedic Surgery increased by 600% from 2006 to 2010.[1] With this increase in the number of procedures has come the ability to address a wide array of pathology, from labral tears to osseous impingement in the form of cam and pincer deformity.[2] The majority of the increase in usage has come in the form of treatment of femoroacetabular impingement (FAI). Whereas previously this pathology was treated in an open fashion with surgical dislocation, the majority of patients today can be treated by an arthroscopic approach.[3]

Hip arthroscopy, although less invasive, presents significant challenges to the arthroscopist and has a complication rate that ranges from 0.41% to 7.5%.[1,4,5] Although the majority of these complications are minor in nature, in rare instances they can be catastrophic for the patient and require repeat surgery or result in life-threatening illness. The learning curve for acquiring the skills for hip arthroscopy is fairly steep, and it is increasingly believed that advanced training in hip arthroscopy may be required to present this option to patients.[6] For this reason, a thorough understanding of the potential risks of surgery and the most common complications is paramount in managing patient expectations and minimizing morbidity from the procedure. This chapter introduces the most common complications encountered during hip arthroscopy, outlines the most optimal methods of detection, and provides helpful guidance to minimize the incidence of these events.

Byrd JWT, Bedi A, Stubbs AJ, eds. *The Hip:*
AANA Advanced Arthroscopic Surgical Techniques (pp 263-272).
© 2016 AANA.

Figure 22-1. Femoral head gouge seen at revision hip arthroscopy. View from the anterolateral portal and gouge from the modified anterior portal.

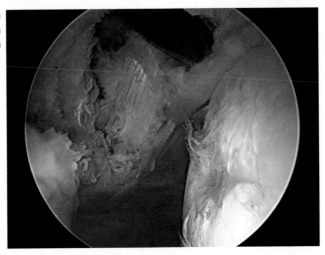

COMPLICATION 1: IATROGENIC ARTICULAR CARTILAGE/SOFT TISSUE INJURY (LABRUM)

Injuries to the articular cartilage during initial joint access or labral penetration during spinal needle, trocar, or cannula placement are among the most common complications to occur during hip arthroscopy. The hip is a constrained joint that requires traction for access. Inadequate traction or portal placement can equally be causative of this complication. Patients with difficult distraction, osteoarthritis, and profunda or protrusio deformity have been shown to be at higher risk of iatrogenic cartilage injury during hip arthroscopy.[7] Damage to the femoral head (Figure 22-1) or acetabular articular cartilage may hasten the development of osteoarthritis and may necessitate the need for hip replacement in severe instances; however, the majority of cases involve minor scuffing of the articular cartilage of the femoral head. Iatrogenic labral penetration may occur during initial portal placement and can occur in up to 20% of patients.[8] Damage to the labrum may compromise the ability to perform a repair, impair the stabilizing effect of the labrum, and result in the loss of the suction-seal phenomenon about the hip joint. During labral repair, medialization of the labrum can occur as a result of improper anchor placement and can also impair the ability of the labrum to dissipate force. Finally, anchor penetration of the articular cartilage can occur during anchor insertion and result in damage to the acetabular cartilage. This can result in a compromised joint with inadequate repair of the acetabular labrum.

Remedies

Articular Cartilage Scuffing/Labral Injury

- ▶ Use fluoroscopy to visualize adequate joint distraction and during establishment of the initial anterolateral portal because this is the one portal that is created blindly.
- ▶ After venting the joint with the spinal needle, reposition the needle and confirm smooth entrance into the joint to minimize the risk of labral penetration.
- ▶ Point the bevel of the spinal needle toward the femoral head during venting of the joint and portal placement.
- ▶ Consider placing the initial needle anterior to the superior femoral head to avoid labral penetration.[9]

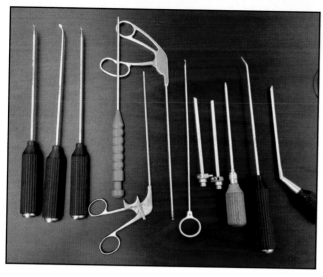

Figure 22-2. Basic instrumentation for hip arthroscopy. Cannulated smooth-edge trocars, appropriate length of arthroscopic instruments, and curved or flexible instrumentation increases the chances of a successful procedure.

▶ All other portals are established with arthroscopic visualization of the guide pin and trocar.

▶ Use of instruments specifically designed for hip arthroscopy (longer length, curved, or flexible) is recommended (Figure 22-2).

▶ Use appropriate and full-thickness capsulotomies to allow free movement of instruments in the joint.

▶ Avoid advancing the trocar too far in the joint.

▶ Perform meticulous technique during anchor drilling to ensure appropriate position of the labral repair and avoid iatrogenic cartilage injury.

  ▷ Use a distal portal for percutaneous anchor placement to allow an appropriate angle on the acetabular rim to minimize risk of iatrogenic joint penetration (Figure 22-3A).

▶ When tying arthroscopic knots, drill and place all anchors prior to tying sutures (Figure 22-3B). The mobility of the labrum after preparation for repair provides improved visualization of the acetabular rim and anchor placement as close to the rim edge as possible. When using knotless anchors, drilling all anchors prior to passing sutures may facilitate the repair.

▶ Use small-diameter suture retrievers for suture passage to avoid labral damage (Figure 22-4).

▶ When possible, use vertical mattress stitches in the labrum to allow a better reduction to the acetabulum without blunting and everting the labrum (Video).

▶ Anchors should be cautiously placed at the 3-o'clock position, and consider using curved anchors here to avoid medial penetration and irritation of the iliopsoas tendon.

▶ Observe the acetabular cartilage during anchor drilling (Video).

COMPLICATION 2: INADEQUATE TREATMENT OF FEMOROACETABULAR IMPINGEMENT (UNDERCORRECTION/OVERRESECTION)

One of the most common reasons for the necessity of revision hip arthroscopy is due to inadequate resection of bony impingement during the index procedure. In a recent investigation of 37 patients undergoing revision hip arthroscopy, the authors found that 95% of patients had

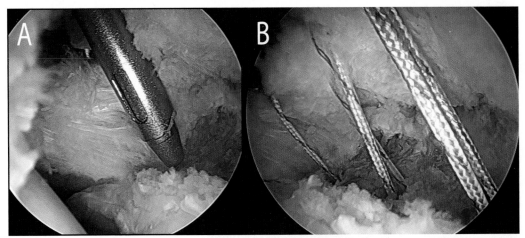

Figure 22-3. (A) Viewing from the anterolateral portal, the drill guide is in the mid-anterior portal, allowing appropriate angle for drilling in the acetabulum. (B) Three anchors in the acetabular rim at the edge without penetration of the acetabulum allow for anatomic reduction.

Figure 22-4. Small-diameter suture passers minimize iatrogenic labral damage during suture passing.

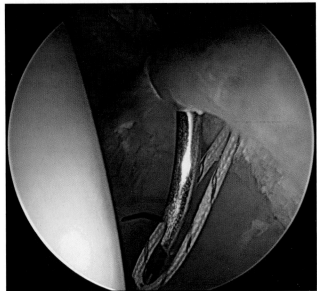

residual FAI, and 97% had radiographic evidence of persistent impingement.[10] As the pathophysiology of FAI becomes more understood, there is increased awareness among surgeons and radiologists about the recognition of lesions that can commonly impinge. Patients with residual impingement may report pain in the anterior hip and groin and with sitting or rotation of the joint and often present with positive signs of impingement (pain with flexion, adduction, and internal rotation). Although underresection of a cam or pincer lesion can often be remedied by revision surgery, overresection of a cam lesion can result in femoral neck fracture and require internal fixation or hip replacement. In a cadaveric study, it was shown that 30% of the anterolateral quadrant of the femoral head-neck junction could be safely resected without affecting the load-bearing capacity of the proximal femur.[11] Amounts greater than this led to a significant decrease in energy required to produce a femoral neck fracture. Patients with a femoral neck fracture may report increased and sudden pain, inability to ambulate, and rotational deformity of the lower limb. In addition to an excessive resection, notching the head-neck junction may also place increased stress at this

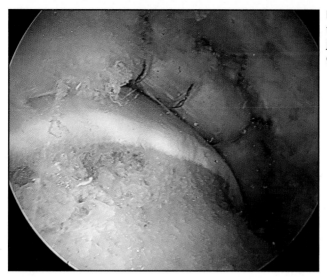

Figure 22-5. Post labral repair and femoroplasty. Contour of the head-neck junction has been restored, and bony conflict has resolved.

site and be responsible for fracture with excessive weight-bearing activities.[12] Overresection of the acetabulum may lead to iatrogenic instability, which can be a devastating complication.

Remedies

► Carefully plan for the resection of any cam or pincer lesion by obtaining preoperative x-rays (anteroposterior, lateral, and Dunn views) in addition to 3-dimensional imaging (computed tomography and magnetic resonance imaging).

► Evaluate the head-neck junction with fluoroscopy after patient positioning on multiple views and during the procedure with dynamic arthroscopic analysis to confirm adequate resection.

► Perform appropriate capsulotomies for exposure. Lack of visualization is a common cause of underresection of FAI, especially cam. Consider traction sutures in the capsule or T capsulotomies for complete exposure of the cam lesion.

   ▷ If the surgeon performs a T capsulotomy, it should be repaired at the end of the procedure if possible to restore integrity to the iliofemoral ligament.

► Avoid cortical notching greater than 4- or 6-mm depths, and contour the femoral head-neck junction appropriately to address the bony conflict (Figure 22-5).

► Avoid resection of more than 30% of the femoral head-neck junction.

► Obtain routine x-rays for all patients postoperatively to assess for correction of FAI.

COMPLICATION 3: NEUROLOGIC COMPLICATIONS/ VASCULAR INJURY AND AVASCULAR NECROSI

Neurologic complications during hip arthroscopy may be due to various factors: portal placement close to at-risk structures, compression, prolonged hip traction time or excessive amount of traction, and iatrogenic injury from the procedure itself. With portal placement, the lateral femoral cutaneous nerve (LFCN) is the most likely structure to be injured and may result in painful numbness or burning on the anterolateral aspect of the thigh. Demographic differences exist (eg, male vs female, thin vs obese, White vs Hispanic) in where these structures (ie, femoral, sciatic, and LFCN) lie in relation to various anatomic landmarks, such as the anterior superior iliac spine and greater trochanter.[13] The risk of traction or compression on the pudendal nerve has been well documented and may result in perineal numbness or sexual dysfunction. This complication may be as high as 2%, and patients should be counseled about this risk preoperatively.[14] Traction may also compromise the sciatic nerve and may be more due to the amount of traction weight applied rather than the total traction time.[15] Injury to the common peroneal nerve and femoral nerve may also occur from traction, and in the case of the femoral nerve, iatrogenic injury can occur from excessive medial portal placement or during repair of a torn labrum and/or pincer resection. The risk of permanent nerve injury is low after hip arthroscopy and may be limited to 1% of cases.[5] All patients should be examined postoperatively to document a thorough neurovascular examination and confirm that no neuropraxia exists. When there is a reported deficit, the majority of patients will improve by 1 year postoperatively.[16] Supportive care is often administered to treat these conditions, such as nerve-stabilizing medications, desensitization therapy, or tendon transfers where permanent dysfunction exists.

Although vascular injury can occur after hip arthroscopy, it is rare. Injury to the inferior gluteal artery from laceration or pseudoaneurysm and occlusion at the ankle from a traction boot have been reported in the literature.[5] Injury to the lateral epiphyseal branch of the medial femoral circumflex artery can occur with femoral osteoplasty and may result in avascular necrosis (AVN) of the femoral head, requiring hip replacement. Other known risk factors for AVN are excessive traction, increased intra-articular hip pressure, and partial capsulectomy.[4]

Remedies

▶ Traction time should be documented and limited whenever possible.

▶ The least amount of traction necessary to adequately distract the joint should be applied.

▶ Newer perineal posts have abundant padding and should be used against the perineum during traction (Figure 22-6).

▶ Avoid entrapment of the scrotum and labia during traction.[4]

▶ Placing the anterolateral portal and mid-anterior portals in the safe zone (lateral to the anterior superior iliac spine and inferior to the trochanteric line) can help minimize injury to the LFCN and femoral nerve.

▶ Dissection proximal to the acetabulum should be performed with caution.

▶ Surgery in the peritrochanteric space should involve identification of how close in proximity the sciatic nerve is to any planned release or incision.

▶ Avoid femoral osteoplasty beyond the lateral synovial fold without directly visualizing and protecting the superior retinacular vessels.

▶ Avoid high intra-articular pump pressures during arthroscopy.

  ▷ A 50–mm Hg pump pressure is typically adequate for visualization.

COMPLICATION 4:
POSTOPERATIVE HIP INSTABILITY

Cases of postoperative hip instability have been reported in the literature after hip arthroscopy.[17] The reasons for postoperative hip instability can be multifactorial. Excessive rim trimming (essentially creating a dysplastic hip), capsulotomy, or capsular resection; overzealous labral resection; inadequate labral repair; and partial resection of the ligamentum teres have been posited as potential reasons.[18] Excessive hip traction and performing hip arthroscopy on patients with

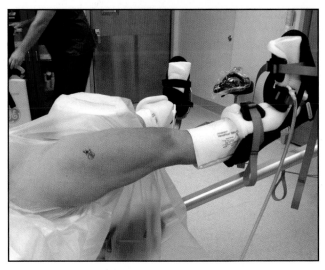

Figure 22-6. Hip distractor with thick padding on the perineal post and on the operative and nonoperative legs to minimize the risk of compression damage.

hip dysplasia with center-edge angles less than 20 degrees can also be significant risk factors. A recent investigation demonstrated that the results of hip arthroscopy in patients with borderline hip dysplasia can be favorable; however, capsular plication was performed concomitantly, with labral preservation likely contributing to the improved outcomes.[19] Patients with postoperative hip instability require emergent closed reduction and many may ultimately require revision surgery to repair the capsule and/or labrum. If instability persists, patients are at risk for AVN, progressive joint deterioration, and future total hip replacement.

Remedies

► Avoid excessive traction during surgery.

► Limit the extent of the capsulotomy or capsular resection.

► When possible, perform labral preservation surgery instead of resection.
  ▷ Consider capsular repair or plication (Figure 22-7).

► Critically evaluate patients with hip dysplasia and be cautious when recommending arthroscopic intervention.
  ▷ Management of the capsule and ability to repair the labrum anatomically is critical to a good outcome for hip arthroscopy in hip dysplasia (see Figure 22-7).

► Limit the amount of pincer or acetabular resection.

► Minimize capsulotomies in borderline dysplasia, and perform capsular repair and/or plication.

► Consider routine x-rays in all patients postoperatively.

COMPLICATIONS 5: MISCELLANEOUS

Patients undergoing routine hip arthroscopy are at risk for additional musculoskeletal and medical complications. These may include heterotopic ossification (HO), superficial and deep venous thrombosis (DVT), pulmonary embolism, septic arthritis, wound infection, abdominal compartment syndrome, reflex sympathetic dystrophy (or complex regional pain syndrome), hypothermia, and death.

Figure 22-7. Capsular repair/closure at the end of the procedure allows for appropriate tension for capsular healing. In borderline dysplasia, capsular closure is important, and capsular plication is considered on an individual basis.

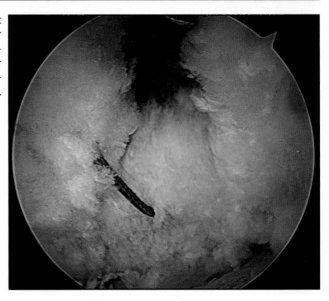

The risk of HO after hip arthroscopy is more common in patients who undergo surgery to resect cam or pincer lesions and in those who do not receive nonsteroidal anti-inflammatory drugs as prophylaxis postoperatively.[20] The majority of patients who are diagnosed with HO by postoperative x-rays have limited clinical manifestations or functional impairment, despite the high incidence rate of 44% reported in a recent study.[21]

There is limited information on the risk of DVT after hip arthroscopy. Although this is a known complication in many open and arthroscopic orthopedic procedures, the exact incidence is currently unknown. There is a case report in the literature of contralateral leg DVT after hip arthroscopy; however, recommending routine prophylaxis is currently not settled science.[22] Postoperatively, patients should be examined for excessive calf or leg swelling, pain in the leg or calf, or shortness of breath indicating embolic disease. When there is doubt, an ultrasound should be obtained, and further medical therapy with anticoagulants is often palliative/curative.

Fluid extravasation into the abdominal compartment during hip arthroscopy has been reported. Abdominal compartment syndrome, death, and cardiac arrest can occur secondary to this phenomenon. This can occur more commonly with psoas tendon release, arthroscopy after acute pelvic trauma, and excessive operative time with high fluid pressures.[4,23] Cardinal signs of this complication are a tight abdominal compartment on palpation and intraoperative hypotension.

Septic arthritis and superficial wound infections may occur after hip arthroscopy. Although the risk of this complication is low, the majority of patients are prophylactically administered antibiotics preoperatively and monitored throughout their postoperative course for signs and symptoms. Irrigation and debridement of the joint may be required for patients with postoperative septic arthritis, while oral antibiotics may adequately treat the majority of superficial wound infections. A sudden increase in pain with limitation in motion and guarding, erythema at the incisions, and a systemic response to sepsis may be present, indicating an underlying infection.

Remedies

▶ Consider nonsteroidal anti-inflammatory drug prophylaxis postoperatively to limit the risk of HO.

▶ Consider thromboprophylaxis with aspirin, fractionated heparin, or other anticoagulants for patients at risk for DVT/pulmonary embolism.

▶ Avoid hip arthroscopy acutely after pelvic or acetabular trauma/fracture.

- ► Monitor abdominal compartment softness during the procedure.
- ► Avoid high arthroscopy pump pressures.
- ► Perform iliopsoas release toward the end of the procedure.[4]
- ► Monitor the patient for intraoperative hypotension.
- ► Routine antibiotic prophylaxis for all patients may reduce the risk of infection.

CONCLUSION

Hip arthroscopy has grown considerably over the past 15 years, with many patients benefiting greatly from the advances offered by a modern arthroscopic technique. As with any procedure, expanding indications are often accompanied by a risk of new and unforeseen complications. There is no substitute for routine postoperative follow-up so that prompt recognition and treatment can be offered to patients to optimize their outcome. Surgeons who are educated about minimizing complications intra- and postoperatively can help avoid many of the most common complications and are better equipped to discuss these issues with their patients during the informed decision-making process. Although complications may never be eliminated, reducing the risk introduced by the surgical team is paramount to achieving the best outcome for patients.

TOP TECHNICAL PEARLS FOR THE PROCEDURE

1. The surgeon must be meticulous in creating the arthroscopic portals and capsulotomies to avoid iatrogenic damage to the articular cartilage and labrum.
2. Minimize traction time and traction force to avoid traction/compression injuries.
3. While drilling for the anchors, view the acetabular articular cartilage to ensure there is no penetration or undermining from the drill and hence the anchors, which are typically larger than the drill hole.
4. Do a thorough dynamic exam arthroscopically after cam decompression accompanied by appropriate fluoroscopic views to ensure resolution of the bony conflict.
5. Consider capsular repair on an individual basis and strongly consider repair or capsulorrhaphy in patients with dysplasia or instability.

REFERENCES

1. Bozic KJ, Chan V, Valone FH III, Feeley BT, Vail TP. Trends in hip arthroscopy utilization in the United States. *J Arthroplasty.* 2013;28(8 suppl):140-143.
2. Guanche CA, Bare AA. Arthroscopic treatment of femoroacetabular impingement. *Arthroscopy.* 2006;22(1):95-106.
3. Ganz R, Gill TJ, Gautier E, Ganz K, Krügel N, Berlemann U. Surgical dislocation of the adult hip a technique with full access to the femoral head and acetabulum without the risk of avascular necrosis. *J Bone Joint Surg Br.* 2001;83(8):1119-1124.

4. Gupta A, Redmond JM, Hammarstedt JE, Schwindel L, Domb BG. Safety measures in hip arthroscopy and their efficacy in minimizing complications: a systematic review of the evidence. *Arthroscopy.* 2014;30(10):1342-1348.

5. Harris JD, McCormick FM, Abrams GD, et al. Complications and reoperations during and after hip arthroscopy: a systematic review of 92 studies and more than 6,000 patients. *Arthroscopy.* 2013;29(3):589-595.

6. Hoppe DJ, de Sa D, Simunovic N, et al. The learning curve for hip arthroscopy: a systematic review. *Arthroscopy.* 2014;30(3):389-397.

7. McCarthy JC, Lee JA. Hip arthroscopy: indications, outcomes, and complications. *Inst Course Lect.* 2006;55:301-308.

8. Badylak JS, Keene JS. Do iatrogenic punctures of the labrum affect the clinical results of hip arthroscopy? *Arthroscopy.* 2011;27(6):761-767.

9. Aoki SK, Beckmann JT, Wylie JD. Hip arthroscopy and the anterolateral portal: avoiding labral penetration and femoral articular injuries. *Arthrosc Tech.* 2012;1(2):e155-e160.

10. Philippon MJ, Schenker ML, Briggs KK, Kuppersmith DA, Maxwell RB, Stubbs AJ. Revision hip arthroscopy. *Am J Sports Med.* 2007;35(11):1918-1921.

11. Mardones RM, Gonzalez C, Chen Q, Zobitz M, Kaufman KR, Trousdale RT. Surgical treatment of femoroacetabular impingement: evaluation of the effect of the size of the resection. *J Bone Joint Surg Am.* 2005;87(2):273-279.

12. Wijdicks CA, Balldin BC, Jansson KS, Stull JD, LaPrade RF, Philippon MJ. Cam lesion femoral osteoplasty: in vitro biomechanical evaluation of iatrogenic femoral cortical notching and risk of neck fracture. *Arthroscopy.* 2013;29(10):1608-1614.

13. Watson JN, Bohnekamp F, El-Bitar Y, Moretti V, Domb BG. Variability in locations of hip neurovascular structures and their proximity to arthroscopic portals. *Arthroscopy.* 2014;30(4):462-467.

14. Pailhé R, Chiron P, Reina N, Cavaignac E, Lafontan V, Lafosse JM. Pudendal nerve neuralgia after hip arthroscopy: retrospective study and literature review. *Orthop Traumatol Surg Res.* 2013;99(7):785-790.

15. Telleria J, Safran MR, Harris AH, Gardi JN, Glick JM. Risk of sciatic nerve traction injury during hip arthroscopy–is it the amount or duration? An intraoperative nerve monitoring study. *J Bone Joint Surg Am.* 2005;87(12):273-279.

16. Dippmann C, Thorborg K, Kraemer O, Winge S, Hölmich P. Symptoms of nerve dysfunction after hip arthroscopy: an under-reported complication? *Arthroscopy.* 2014;30(2):202-207.

17. Austin DC, Horneff JG III, Kelly JD IV. Anterior hip dislocation 5 months after hip arthroscopy. *Arthroscopy.* 2014;30(10):1380-1382.

18. Mei-Dan O, McConkey MO, Brick M. Catastrophic failure of hip arthroscopy due to iatrogenic instability: can partial division of the ligamentum teres and iliofemoral ligament cause subluxation? *Arthroscopy.* 2012;28(3):440-445.

19. Domb BG, Stake CE, Lindner D, El-Bitar Y, Jackson TJ. Arthroscopic capsular plication and labral preservation in borderline hip dysplasia: two-year clinical outcomes of a surgical approach to a challenging problem. *Am J Sports Med.* 2013;41(11):2591-2598.

20. Beckmann JT, Wylie JD, Kapron AL, Hanson JA, Maak TG, Aoki SK. The effect of NSAID prophylaxis and operative variables on heterotopic ossification after hip arthroscopy. *Am J Sports Med.* 2014;42(6):1359-1364.

21. Rath E, Sherman H, Sampson TG, Ben Tov T, Maman E, Amar E. The incidence of heterotopic ossification in hip arthroscopy. *Arthroscopy.* 2013;29(3):427-433.

22. Greene JW, Deshmukh AJ, Cushner FD. Thromobembolic complications in arthroscopic surgery. *Sports Med Arthrosc.* 2013;21(2):69-74.

23. Ladner B, Nester K, Cascio B. Abdominal fluid extravasation during hip arthroscopy. *Arthroscopy.* 2010;26(1):131-135.

Please see videos on the accompanying website at

www.ArthroscopicTechniques.com

SECTION V

Controversies and Future Considerations

23

Is There a Role for Arthroscopy in Hip Instability and Dysplasia?

Indications and Technique

Benjamin G. Domb, MD and Chris Stake, DHA

INTRODUCTION

The role of hip arthroscopy in the treatment of femoroacetabular impingement (FAI) has been well delineated.[1-4] However, there are patients with intra-articular hip pain and labral tears on x-ray who do not demonstrate FAI. In the patient population without FAI, hip instability should be considered as a cause of hip pain and cartilage injury. In contrast to shoulder instability, in which frank dislocation or subluxation occurs due to the lack of inherent stability provided by the bony articulation, it is postulated that hip instability is subtle and occurs as micromotion.

Generally, there are 2 primary etiologies of hip instability: bony instability and ligamentous laxity. Patients with atraumatic bony instability are those with borderline dysplasia as defined as a lateral center-edge angle of Wiberg[5] from 18 to 25 degrees. This instability type is caused by acetabular undercoverage in the setting of mild dysplasia, and definitive treatment remains controversial. Other patients with instability have normal acetabular coverage and greater ligamentous laxity. These patients are often female and have signs of hyperlaxity on general ligament laxity testing using the Beighton-Horan scale.[6] Surgeons should consider this clinical diagnosis in the setting of nondysplastic x-rays, findings of ligamentous laxity, and hip pain. Often, bony dysplasia and collagen disorders occur simultaneously and represent a difficult challenge for hip arthroscopists.

Hip preservation in overtly dysplastic skeletally mature patients is best managed surgically with periacetabular osteotomy. In patients with severe dysplasia (lateral center-edge [LCE] angles < 15 degrees), one can achieve good clinical results with periacetabular osteotomy.[7,8] Conversely, treatment of patients with borderline dysplasia remains controversial. Arthroscopists have been wary of patients with acetabular undercoverage because of the mixed results of arthroscopy in dysplasia.[9-13] For patients with borderline dysplasia and/or ligamentous instability, a surgical approach that uses capsular plication with an inferior capsular shift and preservation of labral function with labral repair has been used and has shown good results.[13]

Byrd JWT, Bedi A, Stubbs AJ, eds. *The Hip:*
AANA Advanced Arthroscopic Surgical Techniques (pp 275-281).
© 2016 AANA.

Figure 23-1. AP x-ray of the right hip. The LCE angle is measured from the middle of the femoral head to the edge of the lateral sourcil against a vertical line. Measurements from 18 to 25 degrees are considered borderline dysplasia.

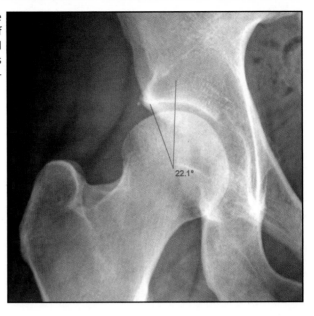

22.1°

INDICATIONS

▶ Unresponsive to conservative treatments and intra-articular hip pain

▶ Shows signs of instability

▶ Ligamentous laxity (Beighton score > 6)

▶ Radiographic signs of borderline dysplasia (LCE < 25 degrees; Figure 23-1): anteroposterior (AP) hip x-ray with LCE angle

Controversial Indications

▶ Moderate to severe dysplasia with an LCE of 15 to 20 degrees

PERTINENT PHYSICAL FINDINGS

▶ Physical examination of the hip with range of motion (ROM) and strength testing

▶ Anterior impingement test to assess hip pain and possibly support the presence of a labral tear (Figure 23-2A)

▶ The Dial test is used to detect anterior capsule laxity with the patient supine and the hip in neutral extension. The leg is internally rotated, released, and allowed to externally rotate. External rotation of the affected hip greater than the contralateral limb or greater than 45 degrees is considered a positive test.[14]

▶ The preferred method to detect instability is with an anterior apprehension test with the patient in the prone or lateral position. The affected hip is abducted and maximally externally rotated with posterior pressure applied to the greater trochanter to translate the femoral head anteriorly. Pain recreated in this position indicates a positive test (Figure 23-2B).

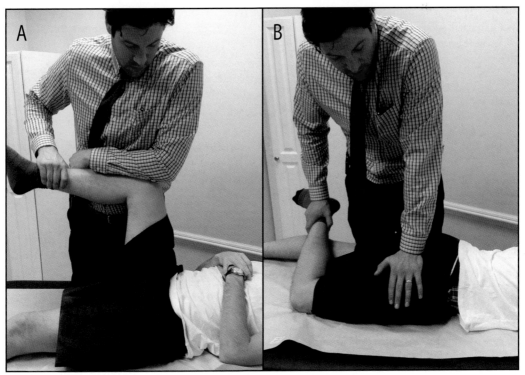

Figure 23-2. (A) Demonstration of the anterior impingement test. The hip is flexed, adducted, and internally rotated. Reproduction of symptomatic pain is a positive test. (B) Demonstration of the prone anterior apprehension test. With the patient in the prone position, the hip is in extension while the examiner externally rotates the hip and applies an anteriorly directed force by applying pressure posteriorly over the greater trochanter. Reproduction of pain is a positive test.

Pertinent Imaging

▸ Standing and supine AP pelvis views are obtained to analyze the dynamic nature of pelvic tilt. Often, a crossover sign seen on supine films will be absent on standing films, indicating a mobile pelvis.[15,16] In the standing position (the more functional position), pincer impingement findings are fewer and indicate instability as opposed to pincer impingement.

▸ False-profile view: Acetabular coverage is assessed (LCE angle and acetabular inclination on the AP pelvis view and anterior CE angle on the false-profile view).

▸ 45-degree Dunn view

▸ Cross-table lateral views

▸ Preoperative magnetic resonance arthrogram is obtained for assessment of labral and chondral damage. A large-volume arthrogram can give signs of capsule laxity when there is a large (> 5-mm) separation of the capsule from the femoral neck.[17]

Equipment

Two cannulas are used to aid in suture management. Hip-length cannulas, measuring 11 cm in length, are preferred so the soft tissue is not caught at the cannula opening. An acute-angle, wire-passing device (Suture Lasso; Arthrex, Inc) is used for the suture-shuttle technique. This wire is then retrieved with a sharp Penetrator Suture Retriever (Arthrex), a 15-degree upcurved device that can easily penetrate the thick iliofemoral ligament. Long, large-diameter, absorbable sutures are used. The authors prefer 60-cm-long, dyed, #2 Vicryl suture (Ethicon, Inc) that can withstand arthroscopic knot-tying techniques.

POSITIONING

The preferred position is supine and out of traction. At the completion of the hip arthroscopy procedure, the hip is flexed to 45 degrees in neutral rotation. An assistant is necessary to control the internal and external rotation because these changes significantly affect visualization during the procedure.

STEP-BY-STEP DESCRIPTION OF THE PROCEDURE

The patient is positioned in a modified supine position on a traction table with a well-padded perineal post. Access to the hip is performed under fluoroscopy, and the capsulotomy is performed in line with the labrum using a sharp Beaver blade (Smith & Nephew) to preserve capsule tissue for later repair. A T-cut along the axis of the femoral neck is generally not performed, except in cases of distal and/or posterior cam morphology. A patient with instability generally has a capsule that is easily mobilized with instruments so that a T-cut is not necessary. At the completion of the central compartment procedures, the hip is released from traction, and the hip is flexed approximately 45 degrees to access the peripheral compartment.

At the completion of peripheral compartment procedures and femoroplasty, attention is turned to the capsule plication. During the central and peripheral compartment procedures, capsule tissue must be preserved to allow for later repair. With the arthroscope in the anterolateral portal and a shaver in the anterior portal, the muscle overlying the capsule edges is removed. A hip-length cannula is placed through the anterior portal and the distal lateral accessory portal. The cannulas are positioned to have the distal lateral accessory portal positioned more medial than the anterior cannula. This cannula position is important for suture management and to achieve the oblique passage of sutures (Figure 23-3). A suture-shuttle technique is used, with a 90-degree Suture Lasso passed through the proximal limb of the capsule and shuttled into the medial synovial fold. The Penetrator Suture Retriever is used to penetrate the distal limb of the capsule slightly more medial to the point where the wire is passed through the proximal limb.

Once the retriever has penetrated the capsule, it is aimed into the medial synovial fold to retrieve the wire. This wire is then brought out of the cannula and exchanged for a #1 or #2 dyed absorbable suture. This suture passage creates an oblique orientation of the suture across the capsule edges (Figure 23-4). This is repeated to allow for 4 to 6 sutures to be placed. Sutures are left untied until the passage of all sutures is completed to prevent closure of the working space. Suture management outside of the cannulas is critical to prevent tangling during knot tying. A clamp is placed on each pair of sutures and oriented such that the surgeon knows which are medial-to-lateral sutures. After completion of the capsule closure, the arthroscope is left in the peripheral compartment, and the leg is brought into neutral extension to assure there is no separation of the capsule.

POSTOPERATIVE PROTOCOL

A brace is used for 2 weeks postoperatively to protect against extension greater than 0 degrees, which can place tension on the capsule and labral repair. Patients are restricted to 2 weeks of

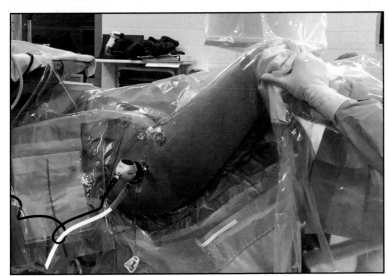

Figure 23-3. Cannula arrangement for the capsule plication. The proximal cannula is directed more laterally, and the distal cannula is directed more medial in the peripheral space. The arthroscope is in the anterolateral portal.

20-lb foot-flat weight bearing with crutches. Physical therapy is begun as early as postoperative day 1 to begin passive ROM with continuous passive motion or a stationary bicycle. Postoperative ROM restrictions include limited extension greater than 0 degrees, external rotation greater than 30 degrees, and flexion greater than 90 degrees for 6 weeks.

POTENTIAL COMPLICATIONS

The capsule plication procedure is one of the more technically demanding procedures performed in hip arthroscopy and can lead to longer operative times. Complications from longer operative times include anesthesia complications, hypothermia, and fluid extravasation. Because this is performed without traction, traction-related complications are not relevant. The most critical complication is from fluid extravasation. Working in the peripheral compartment creates more fluid extravasation. If an iliopsoas release has been performed, the conduit that has been created increases the risk of retroperitoneal compartment syndrome. Frequent palpation of the abdomen should be performed to assure no abdominal fluid extravasation is occurring. The authors recommend checking with the anesthesiologist for changes in perfusion pressures if the procedure becomes prolonged. As with the shoulder, with capsule plications comes the risk of overtightening the joint. To prevent overtightening, avoid capsule resection during the initial capsulotomy. The authors prefer to use a sharp Beaver blade to cut the capsule with avoidance of capsule removal during labral repair and femoroplasty. Failure of the suture repair is a potential complication that can be avoided by using large-diameter sutures, taking large bites of capsule tissue with suture passage, and using multiple sutures. Before removing the scope, extend the leg to neutral from the flexed position while viewing the repair to assure no separation has occurred.

CONCLUSION

Arthroscopic capsule plication with a capsule shift can benefit patients with hip instability. Advanced hip arthroscopy skills are required to successfully accomplish this important last step in hip arthroscopy.

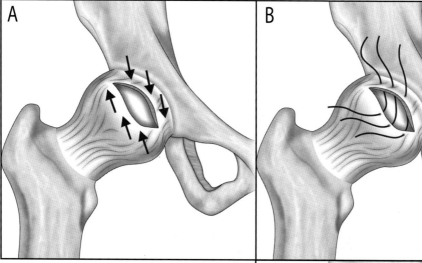

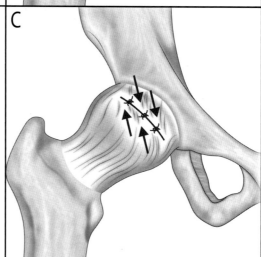

Figure 23-4. (A) The aim of capsule closure is to shift the distal edge of the capsule in a superolateral direction. (B) Sutures are passed through the proximal edge and retrieved through the distal edge, beginning with the medial end of the capsulotomy. (C) After all sutures are passed, they are tied sequentially from medial to lateral to achieve the shift of capsule.

Top Technical Pearls for the Procedure

1. Intra-articular work is performed with preservation of the capsule to allow for later repair. Obliteration of the capsule during labral repair will leave inadequate tissue for repair.

2. Removal of the soft tissue and muscle that lies just anterior to the capsule will aid in suture passing and retrieval.

3. Because the goal is to plicate the iliofemoral ligament, it is vital to work from medial to lateral so the inferior limb of the capsule can be penetrated medially.

4. Because it is a small space, sutures can become tangled during passing and tying. Outside of the cannula, align paired sutures together so that sequential tying can be done from medial to lateral.

5. Tie sutures after they are all passed. Tying sutures as you go closes down the space and makes passing of lateral sutures difficult.

REFERENCES

1. Byrd JW, Jones KS. Arthroscopic management of femoroacetabular impingement: minimum 2-year follow-up. *Arthroscopy.* 2011;27(10):1379-1388.
2. Larson CM, Giveans MR. Arthroscopic management of femoroacetabular impingement: early outcomes measures. *Arthroscopy.* 2008;24(5):540-546.
3. Nho SJ, Magennis EM, Singh CK, Kelly BT. Outcomes after the arthroscopic treatment of femoroacetabular impingement in a mixed group of high-level athletes. *Am J Sports Med.* 2011;39 suppl:14S-19S.
4. Philippon MJ, Briggs KK, Yen YM, Kuppersmith DA. Outcomes following hip arthroscopy for femoroacetabular impingement with associated chondrolabral dysfunction: minimum two-year follow-up. *J Bone Joint Surg Br.* 2009;91(1):16-23.
5. Wiberg G. Studies on dysplastic acetabular and congenital subluxation of the hip joint with special reference to the complication of osteoarthritis. *Acta Chir Scand.* 1939;83(suppl 58):28-38.
6. Beighton P, Horan F. Orthopaedic aspects of the Ehlers-Danlos syndrome. *J Bone Joint Surg Br.* 1969;51(3):444-453.
7. Matheney T, Kim YJ, Zurakowski D, Matero C, Millis M. Intermediate to long-term results following the bernese periacetabular osteotomy and predictors of clinical outcome: surgical technique. *J Bone Joint Surg Am.* 2010;92 suppl 1 pt 2:115-129.
8. Steppacher SD, Tannast M, Ganz R, Siebenrock KA. Mean 20-year followup of Bernese periacetabular osteotomy. *Clin Orthop Relat Res.* 2008;466(7):1633-1644.
9. Byrd JW, Jones KS. Hip arthroscopy in the presence of dysplasia. *Arthroscopy.* 2003;19(10):1055-1060.
10. Matsuda DK. Acute iatrogenic dislocation following hip impingement arthroscopic surgery. *Arthroscopy.* 2009;25(4):400-404.
11. Mei-Dan O, McConkey MO, Brick M. Catastrophic failure of hip arthroscopy due to iatrogenic instability: can partial division of the ligamentum teres and iliofemoral ligament cause subluxation? *Arthroscopy.* 2012;28(3):440-445.
12. Parvizi J, Bican O, Bender B, et al. Arthroscopy for labral tears in patients with developmental dysplasia of the hip: a cautionary note. *J Arthroplasty.* 2009;24(6 suppl):110-113.
13. Domb BG, Stake CE, Lindner D, El-Bitar Y, Jackson TJ. Arthroscopic capsular plication and labral preservation in borderline hip dysplasia: two-year clinical outcomes of a surgical approach to a challenging problem. *Am J Sports Med.* 2013;41(11):2591-2598.
14. Boykin RE, Anz AW, Bushnell BD, Kocher MS, Stubbs AJ, Philippon MJ. Hip instability. *J Am Acad Orthop Surg.* 2011;19(6):340-349.
15. Henebry A, Gaskill T. The effect of pelvic tilt on radiographic markers of acetabular coverage. *Am J Sports Med.* 2013;41(11):2599-2603.
16. Pullen WM, Henebry A, Gaskill T. Variability of acetabular coverage between supine and weightbearing pelvic radiographs. *Am J Sports Med.* 2014;42(11):2643-2648.
17. Magerkurth O, Jacobson JA, Morag Y, Caoili E, Fessell D, Sekiya JK. Capsular laxity of the hip: findings at magnetic resonance arthrography. *Arthroscopy.* 2013;29(10):1615-1622.

Please see videos on the accompanying website at

www.ArthroscopicTechniques.com

The Role of Arthroscopy in Pediatric Hip Disorders

Slipped Capital Femoral Epiphysis and Legg-Calvé-Perthes Disease

Patrick Vavken, MD, MSc and Yi-Meng Yen, MD, PhD

INTRODUCTION

Intra-articular pathology of the hip resulting in hip and groin pain is becoming increasingly recognized as a significant cause of morbidity in children and adolescents. Pediatric hip disorders, particularly slipped capital femoral epiphysis (SCFE) and Legg-Calvé-Perthes disease (LCPD) and their late sequela, have also been identified as important risk factors of early-onset osteo-arthritis.[1] Healed SCFE and LCPD often result in complex femoral and acetabular deformities leading to femoroacetabular impingement. Gross[2] was among the first to publish on the use of hip arthroscopy in children with hip dysplasia, LCPD, and SCFE. With improved instrumentation and techniques, hip arthroscopy is becoming a major tool in the treatment of pediatric hip disorders. The obvious advantages of hip arthroscopy include its being minimally invasive, having lower morbidity, and reducing recovery time. In cases in which open surgery, such as a periacetabular pelvic osteotomy, must be performed, hip arthroscopy can be used as an adjunctive procedure to perform intra-articular work.[3] This chapter focuses on hip arthroscopy for SCFE and LCPD.

ARTHROSCOPIC TREATMENT OF SLIPPED CAPITAL FEMORAL EPIPHYSIS

SCFE is the most common pediatric hip disorder, affecting approximately 11 in every 100,000 skeletally immature children. In a typical SCFE, the structural integrity of the proximal femoral physis is compromised, leading to the epiphysis remaining reduced in the acetabulum while the proximal femoral metaphysis displaces anteriorly. This results in the loss of sphericity of the femoral head-neck junction and creates a cam deformity. In addition, there is frequently a

Byrd JWT, Bedi A, Stubbs AJ, eds. *The Hip: AANA Advanced Arthroscopic Surgical Techniques* (pp 283-294). © 2016 AANA.

Figure 24-1. The Southwick slip angle is measured by the head-shaft angle of the affected SCFE side subtracted from the head-shaft angle of the normal side as measured on the frog-leg lateral x-ray.

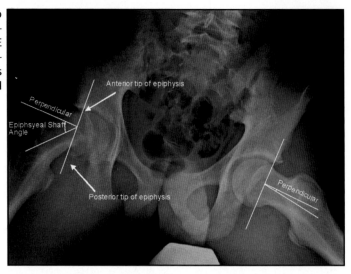

resultant retrotorsion of the femur. SCFE severity is generally described by the degree of slippage or the slip angle. Described by Southwick,[4] mild is defined as 0 to 30 degrees, moderate as 30 to 60 degrees, and severe as greater than 60 degrees (Figure 24-1). Rab[5] performed computer modeling of SCFE cases and demonstrated that even mild slips lead to inclusion of the proximal femur against the acetabulum and moderate-to-severe slips lead to impaction of the proximal femur against the acetabular rim. There has been some evidence that the physis can remodel, but studies by Lee et al[6] and Leunig et al[7] have shown that even mild slips with less than 3 months of symptoms had labral and chondral damage intraoperatively. These more recent studies corroborate the pioneering work of Futami et al[8] in 1985 that used hip arthroscopy prior to in situ pinning; this demonstrated the anterolateral acetabular cartilage damage and posterolateral labral damage in conjunction with hematoma and synovitis.

In situ pinning with screw fixation is considered the treatment of choice for mild-to-moderate SCFE. Severe slips can be treated with open methods, including a modified Dunn or other intertrochanteric osteotomy.[4] Recent evidence has shown that even patients with less than 30 degrees of slip angle have a 30% chance of hip pain and decreased Tegner and Lysholm scoring 6 to 14 years postoperatively.[9] Fifteen percent of former SCFE patients show radiographic changes consistent with arthritis at age 45 years[10] compared with 1.7% in the normal population of the same age.[11] Using delayed gadolinium-enhanced magnetic resonance imaging (MRI) of cartilage, a cartilage-specific MRI technique, rather than crude plain films, Zilkens et al[12] showed that 85% of patients with SCFE with an alpha angle greater than 60 degrees had objective proof of cartilage degeneration despite Tönnis grade 0 x-rays and high Harris Hip Scores (HHS) 11 years after in-situ fixation. These studies started a shift in the paradigm for the treatment of SCFE by facilitating the use of hip arthroscopy in the earlier treatment and analysis of SCFE.

INDICATIONS

▶ Symptomatic femoroacetabular impingement (FAI) and decreased hip range of motion (ROM) from mild SCFE
▶ Pain and difficulty with activities of daily living from mild SCFE
▶ Evidence of intra-articular derangement with mechanical symptoms

Controversial Indications

▶ For concomitant hip dysplasia with SCFE, consider hip arthroscopy as an adjunctive procedure to periacetabular osteotomy.

▶ Symptomatic FAI and decreased hip ROM from moderate SCFE: In these cases, careful examination of the deformity is necessary to determine whether restoration of "normal" can be achieved with arthroscopy alone. Impingement due to retroversion of the femur of less than 0 degrees or coxa vara may not be adequately corrected by arthroscopy alone.

Contraindications

▶ Significant loss of joint space due to chondrolysis or arthrosis

▶ Severe SCFE: Hip arthroscopy can be used to address intra-articular pathology, but the bony deformity should be addressed with intertrochanteric or derotational osteotomies or modified Dunn osteotomy.

PERTINENT PHYSICAL FINDINGS

▶ Physical findings consistent with typical FAI

▶ In cases of moderate-to-severe SCFE, hip flexion will be accompanied by obligate external rotation, referred to as the Drehmann sign.

▶ With a more lateral extension of the cam deformity, there can be pain with abduction and external rotation.

PERTINENT IMAGING

▶ Plain x-rays, including well-centered anteroposterior pelvis, bilateral Dunn, or frog-leg lateral and bilateral false-profile views are usually sufficient for preoperative planning in mild SCFE.

▶ In moderate SCFE, low-dose computed tomography (CT) may be helpful to delineate the extent of the cam deformity and can aid in the determination of the femoral version. The exact location of the screw can be ascertained and may contribute to screw impingement.

▶ MRI can be helpful to examine intra-articular pathology, particularly labral and chondral disease. However, most SCFE hips have been pinned in situ with metallic hardware, and even if composed of titanium, the metallic artifact on an MRI may make the images uninterpretable.

EQUIPMENT

Standard hip arthroscopic equipment is used, including a fracture table or hip scope extension, a C-arm, a 70-degree arthroscope, and hip arthroscopy instruments. The typical body mass index for SCFE patients tend to be high, and extra-long instrumentation may be necessary. In addition, if hardware is present from a previous in situ pinning, the necessary brand of instrumentation should be on hand for screw removal.

Figure 24-2. Intraoperative fluoroscopy of a patient with mild SCFE after screw removal.

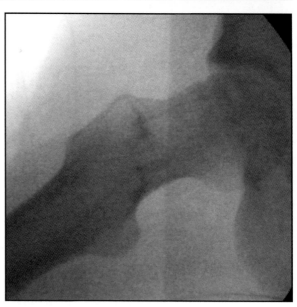

POSITIONING

Hip arthroscopy for SCFE can be performed in the supine or lateral position. The authors' preferred method is the supine position on a fracture table that allows for independent traction on both lower extremities. The authors perform hip arthroscopy under general anesthesia with neuromuscular blockade and a fascia iliac block.

STEP-BY-STEP DESCRIPTION OF THE PROCEDURE

The technique for hip arthroscopy for SCFE is the same as has been described in Sections II and III of this book. Special considerations for SCFE involve screw management and careful resection of the metaphyseal cam lesion.

When hip arthroscopy is used as an adjunct to a primary SCFE, in situ pinning of the SCFE should be performed first without traction on the fracture table or hip extension table. Fluoroscopy should be able to fully visualize the hip. In situ pinning is performed by ensuring that the pin is placed through the metaphysis and in the center-center position of the epiphysis. A 7.0-mm, fully threaded cannulated screw is most commonly used. Traction of the affected leg should be instituted slowly and under fluoroscopy to ensure that the epiphysis does not displace.

In residual SCFE, the hardware can be removed prior to the hip arthroscopy, and the surgeon should inform the patient of potential hardware breakage and that this step of the operation could be time consuming (Figure 24-2). The advantage of removing the hardware first is to potentially remove obstructions to visualization once the camera is moved into the peripheral compartment. Most often, the screw is placed in the anterior metaphysis, and this can cause tethering or scarring of the capsule around the screw entry. Alternatively, the screw can be removed after central compartment arthroscopy and potentially under direct visualization.

Once the hardware has been addressed, a diagnostic arthroscopy can be conducted in the central compartment. Standard arthroscopic portals are established after traction of the affected limb. SCFE patients often have a high body mass index, and multiple portals or extra-long instrumentation may be needed. A generous capsulotomy should be performed, especially when the cam deformity

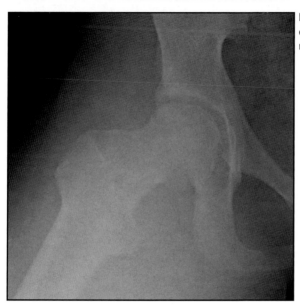

Figure 24-3. The same SCFE patient after osteochondroplasty of the femoral head-neck junction.

extends posterolaterally. In some cases, it may be difficult to distract the joint due to abundant scar tissue formation from insertion of the in situ screw; in these cases, arthroscopy can be started in the peripheral compartment with the hip in flexion, and the central compartment can be entered after the capsulotomy is completed. The acetabular and femoral cartilage, synovium, labrum, and ligamentum teres should be assessed. Chondral damage should be addressed by chondroplasty with or without microfracture. Labral pathology should be repaired if possible; otherwise, a debridement can be done.

Attention can then be turned to the peripheral compartment after the central compartment issues are completely addressed. The location and extent of the cam lesion due to the metaphysis of the proximal femur in a SCFE is different from idiopathic FAI, and careful preoperative planning is necessary. Accessory portals, such as one that Dienst et al[13] described in the soft spot one-third of the way between the anterior superior iliac spine and the trochanter, can be useful. Flexion and extension of the hip will help in visualization of the anterior and posterior neck, respectively. Hyperextension of the hip may be necessary to reach all pertinent parts of the metaphysis. Care should be taken to identify the synovial folds because these contain the retinacular vessels, which can be in close proximity to the cam lesion. The osteoplasty should include resection of part of the physis itself, even in young patients (Figure 24-3). Fluoroscopy and a dynamic examination should be used to confirm adequate resection.

The capsule and the portals can then be closed by standard techniques.

Postoperative Protocol

Most patients are able to be discharged on the day of surgery, although a minority stay over-night for pain control. All patients who have a proximal femoral osteochondroplasty are made touchdown weight bearing with crutches with a foot-flat gait. Patients are kept on crutches for 4 to 6 weeks. Continuous passive motion is generally used for 6 to 8 hours a day for 2 weeks, unless microfracture was performed, in which case the duration may be increased to 8 weeks. Although there have been no reported cases of deep venous thrombosis or pulmonary embolism in pediatric patients undergoing hip arthroscopy, patients who are 13 years old or older or patients on oral contraception can be prescribed 81 mg of aspirin daily. Physical therapy is initiated early in the postoperative period. Patients undergo 4 phases of rehabilitation, first focusing on ROM exercises, then muscle endurance, strengthening, and eventual sport-specific exercises. Impact sports are limited for at least 4 months postoperatively.

POTENTIAL COMPLICATIONS

Potential complications associated with hip arthroscopy for SCFE are largely the same as in adult hip arthroscopy, including, but not limited to, traction injuries, nerve palsies, infection, iatrogenic damage, and underresection. A dedicated analysis of complications after pediatric hip arthroscopy done at the authors' institution showed a complication rate of 1.8%, including transient pudendal nerve palsy, instrument breakage, and suture abscesses. Osteonecrosis and growth disturbances have luckily only been a theoretical risk in the authors' experience. If hardware removal is performed concurrent with the hip arthroscopy, complications of this procedure, such as hardware breakage or retained hardware, should be discussed.

TOP TECHNICAL PEARLS FOR THE PROCEDURE

1. In post-SCFE patients whose physes have fused, screw removal is recommended prior to hip arthroscopy in the peripheral compartment because the screw can tether the capsule.

2. The cam morphology from a SCFE consists of the prominence of the metaphysis and may be more extensive than idiopathic FAI. Care should be taken to adequately understand the location of the cam morphology with multiple views on plain x-rays or advanced imaging. Cases of significantly increased epiphyseal tilt or translation should be addressed with more definitive procedures, including surgical dislocation and/or osteotomy.

3. Considerations for body habitus should be taken into account, including longer equipment and the use of multiple arthroscopic portals.

4. Generous capsulotomy should be performed to allow access to the cam morphology. Consider closing the capsule after a generous capsulotomy.

5. Extension and traction is sometimes necessary to resect the posterior cam morphology that can be common in moderate SCFE.

ARTHROSCOPIC TREATMENT OF LEGG-CALVÉ-PERTHES DISEASE

LCPD is an idiopathic avascular necrosis of the proximal femoral epiphysis with considerable variety in presentation and course of disease. The pathogenesis of the disease passes through multiple stages: initial avascular necrosis, fragmentation of the epiphysis, resorption, collapse, and reossification or healing. Although some healed cases show little or no changes in femoral head shape, most are of moderate severity and will result in lasting changes in hip morphology.[14] These changes can affect the femoral head and acetabulum, which can result in complex deformities resulting in FAI, instability, or both. The diagnosis of active LCPD is made with plain x-rays, although CT may be useful in complex cases. Initial severity of LCPD is graded by the Catterall

Table 24-1. Stulberg Classification

CLASS	X-RAY FINDINGS	PROGNOSIS	AMENABLE TO ARTHROSCOPIC TREATMENT
I	Near-normal hip	Excellent	Yes
II	Enlarged head that deviates no more than 2 mm from concentric circles on anteroposterior and frog-leg lateral views, as well as a short neck and steep acetabulum	Excellent	Yes
III	Nonspherical, ovoid femoral heads	Prearthritic	Yes
IV	Femoral head flattening of at least 1 cm of the weight-bearing area on one or both views	Future arthritis very likely	Questionable
V	Flattened femoral head with a central collapse and an incongruent acetabulum	Future arthritis very likely	Questionable

Adapted from Stulberg SD, Cooperman DR, Wallensten R. The natural history of Legg-Calvé-Perthes disease. *J Bone Joint Surg Am.* 1981;63(7):1095-1108 and Herring JA, Kim HT, Browne R. Legg-Calve-Perthes disease. Part I: Classification of radiographs with use of the modified lateral pillar and Stulberg classifications. *J Bone Joint Surg Am.* 2004;86(10):2103-2120.

or Herring classification systems, whereas a post-LCPD hip is graded most commonly by the Stulberg classification, which provides a predictor for symptoms and function with time and serves as guideline for treatment options (Table 24-1).[15,16]

At these different stages of the disease, different reasons for pain have been suggested. In active LCPD, Catterall class IV and V, hinge abduction, and limb-length discrepancy are considered major causes of discomfort and immobility.[17] Grossbard[18] hypothesized that intra-articular pathology, such as osteochondritis dissecans and labral tears, were responsible for pain and mechanical symptoms. In the post-LCPD hip, extra-articular impingement, pathologic femoral torsion, and unbalanced acetabular retroversion has been described.[19] Snow et al[20] described FAI in LCPD as a reason for painful limitation of ROM in remodeled hips without radiographic changes.

The first formal longitudinal study on hip arthroscopy in LCPD was published by Suzuki et al[21] in 1994. They found substantial hypertrophic synovitis and hypervascularity inside the hip joint, which they linked to femoral head hypertrophy and subluxation due to a mass effect, which led to improved ROM after hip arthroscopy. These data were corroborated later by Majewski et al,[22] who used arthroscopic hydraulic mobilization for patients with LCPD, which improved ROM and pain. In 2001, O'Leary et al[23] published a series of 86 consecutive hip arthroscopies in 83 patients, 9 of whom had LCPD. Mean age was 21 years, and all reported primarily mechanical symptoms. Symptomatic relief was achieved in 8 of 9 patients, and one underwent total hip arthroplasty. In 2005, Kocher et al[24] published a case series of 54 consecutive cases in patients aged 18 years and younger. In 8 patients with LCPD, a significant improvement of the modified HHS from 49.5 to 80.1 points was seen over the 17-month follow-up. Most recently, Freeman et al[25] followed 22 patients (23 hips) with a median age of 27 years over 2 years after hip arthroscopy for LCPD and reported an improvement in the modified HHS from 56.5 to 85 points.

INDICATIONS

- FAI secondary to LCPD can be addressed by arthroscopy to improve impingement-free ROM and restore joint congruency and stability. Stulberg I to III hips are amenable to arthroscopic treatment.
- Mechanical symptoms such as clicking, catching, or locking that may be due to a torn labrum, chondral flaps, chondral loose bodies, or a combination of these from LCPD are suitable for arthroscopic intervention.

Controversial Indications

- Stulberg IV and V hips can sometimes be treated by arthroscopy alone but may require additional open procedures.

Contraindications

- Significant arthrosis of the joint
- Significant versional or gross deformity of the proximal femur
- For incongruity of the joint once a patient has developed secondary instability or a complex mismatch between the enlarged femoral head and misshapen acetabulum, arthroscopic treatment is unlikely to be of benefit. Depending on the shape and degree of coxa magna of the femoral head, a periacetabular osteotomy, Chiara osteotomy, shelf procedure, or other acetabular procedure should be considered. Hip arthroscopy can be used as an adjunct in these procedures.
- For extra-articular impingement due to coxa breva, patients with LCPD may develop a relatively high-riding greater trochanter as a consequence of the proximal femoral physis arrest and collapse. This extra-articular impingement can be a cause of limited ROM and dysfunction. Arthroscopy has little role in this instance and should be treated by a trochanteric advancement with relative neck lengthening.

PERTINENT PHYSICAL FINDINGS

- Examination for patients with LCPD is similar to FAI. The impingement test is usually positive.
- Extra-articular impingement of the greater trochanter onto the ilium should be tested with the patient in abduction.
- Attention to the amount of leg-length discrepancy can give the examiner an idea of the amount of coxa breva of the hip.

PERTINENT IMAGING

- Plain x-rays, including well-centered anteroposterior pelvis, bilateral Dunn lateral, and bilateral false-profile views, should be obtained.
  - ▷ Plain x-rays classify the post-LCPD deformity based on the Stulberg classification. Treatment can be generally based on this classification system.
    - ▷ A Stulberg I or II LCPD hip with FAI findings is a good candidate for arthroscopic intervention because treatment with femoral head-neck osteoplasty is similar to patients with primary FAI.

- ▷ Patients with Stulberg III are more difficult to treat but have the potential to do well with arthroscopic hip surgery.
- ▷ In general, patients with Stulberg IV or V are not as amenable to arthroscopic treatment because of the severity of the femoral head deformity and the presence of coexisting acetabular retroversion or dysplasia with resultant instability (Figure 24-4).
- ▶ A CT scan can be helpful with severe acetabular and femoral head deformities.
- ▶ MRI is often useful for ascertaining labral and chondral damage and assessing for loose bodies in the joint.

EQUIPMENT

Standard arthroscopic equipment is used, including a fracture table, C-arm, 70-degree arthroscope, and hip instruments. Because loose bodies are to be expected, a range of graspers or suction tips can be helpful.

POSITIONING

Hip arthroscopy for LCPD can be performed in the supine or lateral position. The authors' preferred method is the supine position on a fracture table that allows for independent traction on both lower extremities. The authors perform hip arthroscopy under general anesthesia with muscular relaxation and a nerve (fascia iliac) block.

STEP-BY-STEP DESCRIPTION OF THE PROCEDURE

The technique for hip arthroscopy for LCPD is the same as has been described in Sections II and III of this book.

Standard portals may need to be modified in patients with LCPD secondary to trochanteric overgrowth, coxa magna and/or breva, and prior surgical reconstruction of the acetabulum. The anterolateral portal may be more proximal than normal, and the use of accessory portals may be needed. The liberal use of fluoroscopy is recommended to avoid iatrogenic damage to the hip joint. If access to the central compartment cannot be established, an outside-in technique moving from the peripheral to the central compartment is an alternative.[13]

After access to the central compartment, inspection of the joint can be conducted. Commonly, loose bodies may be encountered, most times originating from the femoral head. A thorough inspection of the central and peripheral compartments should be conducted for loose bodies. Alternating suction and fluid flow is useful to find loose bodies. They should be removed with arthroscopic graspers, shavers, or suction (Figure 24-5). Chondral surfaces can be inspected, and chondroplasty or microfracture can be performed on the acetabulum, femoral head, or both. Labral pathology is also commonly found and may be addressed by labral debridement or repair of the labrum with suture anchors.

Once work is completed in the central compartment, the peripheral compartment can be addressed. A generous capsulotomy is helpful with the increased femoral head-neck size. Recontouring of the femoral head-neck junction will depend on the Stulberg classification, with Stulberg I/II hips more amenable to a suitable osteochondroplasty (see Figure 24-5); however, even Stulberg III/V hips can be attempted. With the LCPD hip, the amount of recontouring that can be conducted will depend on preoperative templating and how ovoid the femoral head-neck junction is. The use of liberal

Figure 24-4. Residual LCPD in a Stulberg III/IV hip.

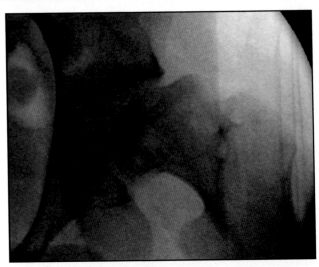

Figure 24-5. Loose chondral body and degeneration of the ligamentum teres.

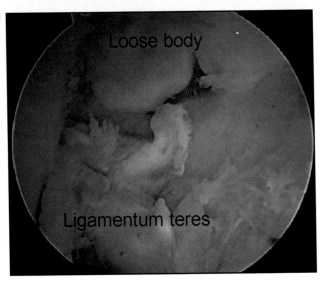

fluoroscopy and dynamic examination will guide the osteochondroplasty. It is rare that an LCPD head can be actually made truly spherical, particularly a Stulberg III/V femoral head (Figure 24-6).

Capsule closure can be performed, particularly in patients who are ligamentously lax or complain of instability.

POSTOPERATIVE PROTOCOL

The postoperative management is similar to that of arthroscopic treatment of SCFE.

POTENTIAL COMPLICATIONS

Potential complications associated with hip arthroscopy for LCPD are largely the same as in hip arthroscopy for SCFE.

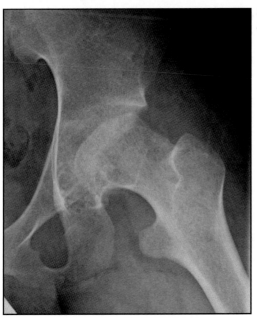

Figure 24-6. The same Stulberg IV hip after osteo-chondroplasty of the femoral head-neck junction.

TOP TECHNICAL PEARLS FOR THE PROCEDURE

1. Proper preoperative planning is necessary for success. Plain x-rays allow identification of the Stulberg class and assessment of whether open or arthroscopic methods are more reasonable.
2. Remove all loose bodies in the peripheral and central compartments.
3. Beware of a high greater trochanter and the possibility of trochanteric-ilium impingement. A trochanteric transfer or effective head-neck lengthening may need to be performed using an open procedure.
4. Use fluoroscopy liberally to assess for areas of femoral head-neck resection.
5. Repair the labrum if possible, avoiding acetabular resection if it will compromise congruity of the joint.

REFERENCES

1. Thomas GE, Palmer AJ, Batra RN, et al. Subclinical deformities of the hip are significant predictors of radiographic osteoarthritis and joint replacement in women: a 20 year longitudinal cohort study. *Osteoarthritis Cartilage.* 2014;22(10):1504-1510.
2. Gross R. Arthroscopy in hip disorders in children. *Orthop Rev.* 1977;6:43-49.
3. Leunig M, Ganz R. The evolution and concepts of joint-preserving surgery of the hip. *Bone Joint J.* 2014;96(1):5-18.
4. Southwick WO. Compression fixation after biplane intertrochanteric osteotomy for slipped capital femoral epiphysis. A technical improvement. *J Bone Joint Surg Am.* 1973;55(6):1218-1224.
5. Rab GT. The geometry of slipped capital femoral epiphysis: implications for movement, impingement, and corrective osteotomy. *J Pediatr Orthop.* 1999;19(4):419-424.

6. Lee CB, Matheney T, Yen YM. Case reports: acetabular damage after mild slipped capital femoral epiphysis. *Clin Orthop Relat Res.* 2013;471(7):2163-2172.

7. Leunig M, Horowitz K, Manner H, Ganz R. In situ pinning with arthroscopic osteoplasty for mild SCFE: a preliminary technical report. *Clin Orthop Relat Res.* 2010;468(12):3160-3167.

8. Futami T, Kasahara Y, Suzuki S, Seto Y, Ushikubo S. Arthroscopy for slipped capital femoral epiphysis. *J Pediatr Orthop.* 1992;12(5):592-597.

9. Fraitzl CR, Kafer W, Nelitz M, Reichel H. Radiological evidence of femoroacetabular impingement in mild slipped capital femoral epiphysis: a mean follow-up of 14.4 years after pinning in situ. *J Bone Joint Surg Br.* 2007;89(12):1592-1596.

10. Boyer DW, Mickelson MR, Ponseti IV. Slipped capital femoral epiphysis. Long-term follow-up study of one hundred and twenty-one patients. *J Bone Joint Surg Am.* 1981;63(1):85-95.

11. Dagenais S, Garbedian S, Wai EK. Systematic review of the prevalence of radiographic primary hip osteoarthritis. *Clin Orthop Relat Res.* 2009;467(3):623-637.

12. Zilkens C, Miese F, Bittersohl B, et al. Delayed gadolinium-enhanced magnetic resonance imaging of cartilage (dGEMRIC), after slipped capital femoral epiphysis. *Eur J Radiol.* 2011;79(3):400-406.

13. Dienst M, Seil R, Kohn DM. Safe arthroscopic access to the central compartment of the hip. *Arthroscopy.* 2005;21(12):1510-1514.

14. Stalzer S, Wahoff M, Scanlan M. Rehabilitation following hip arthroscopy. *Clin Sports Med.* 2006;25(2):337-357.

15. Stulberg SD, Cooperman DR, Wallensten R. The natural history of Legg-Calvé-Perthes disease. *J Bone Joint Surg Am.* 1981;63(7):1095-1108.

16. Herring JA, Kim HT, Browne R. Legg-Calve-Perthes disease. Part I: Classification of radiographs with use of the modified lateral pillar and Stulberg classifications. *J Bone Joint Surg Am.* 2004;86(10):2103-2120.

17. Catterall A. The natural history of Perthes' disease. *J Bone Joint Surg Br.* 1971;53(1):37-53.

18. Grossbard GD. Hip pain during adolescence after Perthes' disease. *J Bone Joint Surg Br.* 1981;63(4):572-574.

19. Ganz R, Slongo T, Turchetto L, Massè A, Whitehead D, Leunig M. The lesser trochanter as a cause of hip impingement: pathophysiology and treatment options. *Hip Int.* 2013;23 suppl 9:S35-S41.

20. Snow SW, Keret D, Scarangella S, Bowen JR. Anterior impingement of the femoral head: a late phenomenon of Legg-Calvé-Perthes disease. *J Pediatr Orthop.* 1993;13(3):286-289.

21. Suzuki S, Kasahara Y, Seto Y, Futami T, Furukawa K, Nishino Y. Arthroscopy in 19 children with Perthes' disease. Pathologic changes of the synovium and the joint surface. *Acta Orthop Scand.* 1994;65(6):581-584.

22. Majewski M, Hasler CC, Kohler G. Arthroscopic mobilization of the hip joint in children with aseptic necrosis of the femur head. *J Pediatr Orthop B.* 2010;19(2):135-139.

23. O'Leary JA, Berend K, Vail TP. The relationship between diagnosis and outcome in arthroscopy of the hip. *Arthroscopy.* 2001;17(2):181-188.

24. Kocher MS, Kim YJ, Millis MB, et al. Hip arthroscopy in children and adolescents. *J Pediatr Orthop.* 2005;25(5):680-686.

25. Freeman CR, Jones K, Byrd JW. Hip arthroscopy for Legg-Calvè-Perthes disease: minimum 2-year follow-up. *Arthroscopy.* 2013;29(4):666-674.

25

The Role of Computer Modeling and Navigation in Arthroscopic Hip Surgery

Andrew W. Kuhn, BA; Eric P. Tannenbaum, MD;
James R. Ross, MD; and Asheesh Bedi, MD

INTRODUCTION

Femoroacetabular impingement (FAI) is broadly defined to encompass the morphological abnormalities of the femoral head-neck junction and/or acetabular rim, which can present as hip pain and limited range of motion (ROM) and lead to early-onset osteoarthritis. Conservative management, open dislocation, and arthroscopic surgery have all been used to treat patients with this condition. Systematic reviews of high-level evidence have demonstrated similar clinical outcomes when open and arthroscopic treatments of FAI are compared.[1,2] An arthroscopic approach, however, may disrupt less of the surrounding tissue envelope and neurovascular structures, reducing possible intra- and postoperative complications, as well as shortening rehabilitation time.[3] For these reasons, the number of hip arthroscopies for treating FAI has steadily increased worldwide.[4] Yet, arthroscopy of the hip joint is often considered more complex and technically challenging for even a skilled arthroscopist.

The difficulty in visualization and spatial awareness of central and peripheral compartments of the hip are due to their depth and surrounding anatomy, including neurovascular structures. Poor visualization and/or poor spatial awareness of the joint may result in over- or underresection of the bony abnormality, increasing the risk of femoral neck fracture, hip dislocation, failed hip preservation surgery, or the need for revision surgery.

Preoperatively, surgeons primarily rely on 2-dimensional (2D) imaging modalities in assessing the hip for signs of FAI. Pelvic x-rays in the anteroposterior plane, as well as dedicated hip x-rays in the form of a frog-leg lateral, extended-neck lateral (Dunn), and false-profile views, are used in identifying the various forms of cam and/or pincer pathomorphology. The femoral head-neck junction is commonly assessed by means of the alpha angle. The alpha angle is a quantifiable measure of the asphericity of the femoral head and is calculated by measuring the angle formed between a line connecting the center of the femoral head to the center of the femoral neck and a line connecting the center of the femoral head to the point where the distance from the outer cortex to the center of the head exceeds the radius.[5] The head-neck offset ratio is another form of measurement that is

Byrd JWT, Bedi A, Stubbs AJ, eds. *The Hip:*
AANA Advanced Arthroscopic Surgical Techniques (pp 295-302).
© 2016 AANA.

useful in detecting cam pathomorphology. It is calculated by drawing a line bisecting the lateral axis of the femoral neck and 2 parallel lines, 1 tangent to the anterior femoral neck and 1 tangent to the anterior femoral head; the perpendicular distance between the 2 parallel lines is then measured as the offset distance. The offset distance relative to the diameter of the femoral head is known as the head-neck offset ratio.[6] Magnetic resonance imaging (MRI) and magnetic resonance arthrography demonstrate applicability in identifying chondral lesions of the femoral head and acetabular labrum. Although MRI may be used to grade chondral pathology, advanced MRI modalities, such as delayed gadolinium-enhanced MRI of cartilage techniques, have reported sensitivity ranges of 63% to 88% and specificity ranges of 37% to 63% for the detection of chondral lesions.[7,8] Two-dimensional computed tomography (CT) images are also valuable in computing the alpha angle, as well as femoral and acetabular version. Yet, inherent difficulties exist in defining, locating, and correlating these 2D structural images to a patient's actual anatomy. The advent of 3-dimensional (3D) modeling of the hip joint from 2D CT images may prove useful in identifying and comprehensively treating the osseous pathomorphology, potentially lowering the risk of under- or overresection.

PERTINENT IMAGING

High-resolution CT scans of the patient in the supine position are used to reconstruct 3D models of the hip. Often, the patient's feet are taped toward each other to limit the amount of movement during the scan. The 2D CT digital imaging and communications in medicine data are automatically segmented to isolate and separate the acetabulum and femoral head from other surrounding tissue.[9] The data are then imported into software programs, such as Mimics (Materialise), HipMotion (University of Bern, Switzerland), Visualization Toolkit (Kitware, Inc), and Dyonics Plan (Smith & Nephew), to create 3D models of the hip.

Patient-specific, preoperative 3D models may be useful in locating and defining bony abnormalities of femoral head-neck junction contributing to FAI. When retrospectively read, 3D CT images were compared with intraoperative findings of cam lesion deformity, and a moderate kappa agreement of 0.48 was observed.[10] Applying analytic software to these 3D models may increase the accuracy of alpha-angle calculation. Milone et al[11] compared differences in the mean alpha angle and cam location as determined by a novel CT-based software program (A2 Surgical), plain x-rays, and CT imaging (Figure 25-1). They concluded that the software-based 3D imaging measured larger alpha angles in a more anterosuperior location compared with plain x-rays and CT imaging.[11] Software is currently being developed to automatically illustrate abnormalities on the surface of the femoral head and head-neck junction preoperatively.[12] The software is able to report lesion location, extent, and height in 3D.

Preoperative computer modeling of the hip could potentially assist surgeons in quantitatively and qualitatively assessing abnormal pathoanatomy of the hip when standard x-rays are limited in utility.

PREOPERATIVE MANIPULATION OF COMPUTER MODELS AND PREDICTION SOFTWARE

Current technology allows patient-specific 2D CT digital imaging and communications in medicine data to be uploaded into 3D software programs that are capable of dynamically manipulating the joint and, in particular, measuring preoperative virtual ROM until osseous contact occurs (Figures 25-2 and 25-3). The first installation of software, HipMotion, used specifically for hip preservation surgery, compared the virtual and actual ROMs of plastic and asymptomatic cadaveric hips and found an intraclass coefficient value of almost 1.00.[13] The second part of the study used the software to compare patients with asymptomatic hips with hips with FAI and found that the latter had significantly decreased flexion, internal rotation at 90 degrees of

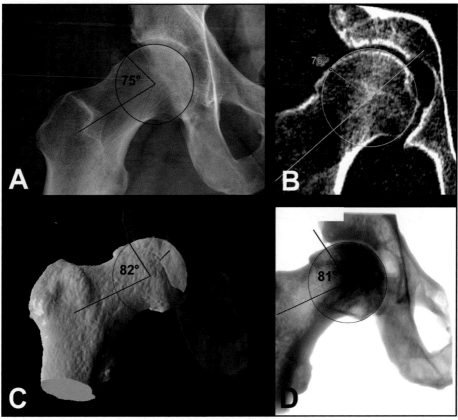

Figure 25-1. Methods of alpha-angle calculation demonstrated on the same patient. (A) Dunn x-ray with the leg in 45 degrees of flexion, 20 degrees of abduction, and neutral rotation. (B) Reformatted CT scan along the axis of the femoral neck to correspond with the Dunn x-ray. (C) Three-dimensional model with the leg positioned for maximum alpha-angle measurement at the 2-o'clock position. (D) Corresponding virtual fluoroscopic x-ray to profile the maximum alpha-angle measurement.

flexion, and abduction. In addition to virtually determining preoperative ROM, a similar study reported on using virtual resection (Figure 25-4) to predict the postoperative ROM in patients with FAI.[14] Virtual resection parameters were defined based on current surgical corrections and were programmed into the software. In a recent study, when pre- and postoperative virtual ROMs were compared with actual ROMs before and after arthroscopic treatment for FAI, an excellent correlation was observed, with no significant differences noted between them as determined by one-tailed paired *t* tests.[15] These studies indicate that virtual ROM software may be valuable in patient-specific preoperative planning and prediction of postoperative ROM in patients with FAI.

Intraoperative Computer Navigation

The described advances in preoperative 3D modeling of the hip may also assist the surgeon intraoperatively with surgical correction of the osseous pathomorphology. The first proposed computer-aided navigation system for arthroscopic hip surgery used encoder linkages for position tracking of arthroscopic instruments.[16] A base pin was inserted into the patient's ipsilateral hip, and the linkage system was connected. A preoperatively generated patient-specific 3D model of the hip was displayed on a screen, and the instruments were shown relative to the patient's anatomy

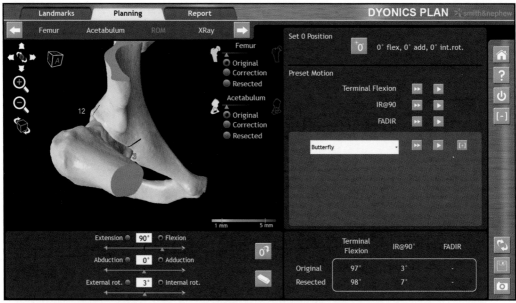

Figure 25-2. Simulated ROM can be performed on patient-specific 3D models. In the Dyonics Plan software, the pelvis is fixed and the femur is free to move about the proscribed rotational axis against the acetabulum. The femur can be moved until osseous contact occurs. In this example, internal rotation at 90 degrees of flexion is performed, and collision occurs at 3 degrees of internal rotation. (Reprinted with permission from Tannenbaum EP, Ross JR, Bedi A. Pros, cons and future possibilities for use of computer navigation in hip arthroscopy. *Sports Med Arthrosc.* 2014;22[4]:e33-e41. © 2014 Wolters Kluwer Health.)

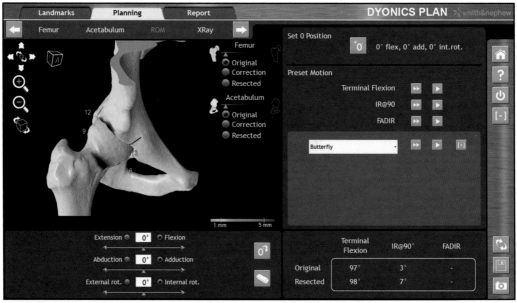

Figure 25-3. After simulation of internal rotation at 90 degrees of flexion, the femur can be placed in a neutral position to visualize the areas of osseous collision (blue) on the acetabular rim and the femoral head-neck junction. (Reprinted with permission from Tannenbaum EP, Ross JR, Bedi A. Pros, cons and future possibilities for use of computer navigation in hip arthroscopy. *Sports Med Arthrosc.* 2014;22[4]:e33-e41. © 2014 Wolters Kluwer Health.)

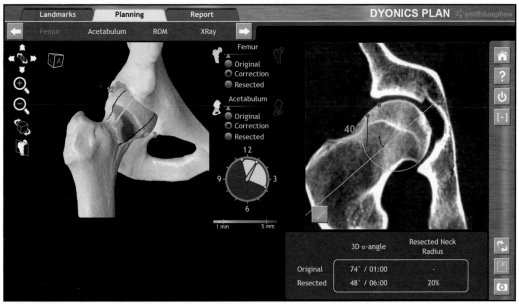

Figure 25-4. Dyonics Plan software allows the ability to perform surgical planning via virtual resection in ways similar to the software described by Kubiak-Langer et al.[14] Virtual resection is demonstrated by the green shading on the proximal femur and acetabular rim. The axial-reformatted slice at 1 o'clock is used as a template to perform femoroplasty to correct the alpha angle to 40 degrees. (Reprinted with permission from Tannenbaum EP, Ross JR, Bedi A. Pros, cons and future possibilities for use of computer navigation in hip arthroscopy. *Sports Med Arthrosc.* 2014;22[4]:e33-e41. © 2014 Wolters Kluwer Health.)

(Figure 25-5). The authors tested the system on hip joint models and asked subjects to complete a specified simulated arthroscopic task.[17] Nonnavigated subjects took significantly longer and had greater tool path length. In another study, a modified computer navigation system used for total hip replacement, BrainLAB Hip CT (Brainlab, Inc), was tested for its utility in hip arthroscopy.[18] Navigated outcomes were compared with nonnavigated outcomes of patients treated arthroscopically for FAI. Intraoperative fluoroscopic navigation, cross-matched with patient-specific 3D CT scans, did not increase the rate of operative success, and operative time was significantly longer. However, this study leads credence to the importance of preoperative planning because this prototype did not allow for it and, furthermore, did not highlight the zone(s) of impingement or amount of resected bone. In another study that used computer navigation and dynamic 2D CT sagittal and axial images, surgeons of varying levels of arthroscopic experience all successfully resected the bony lesion contributing to FAI in patients. These results demonstrate the potential for intraoperative computer navigation systems to increase the surgeon's visualization and spatial awareness. In effect, the steep learning curve associated with mastering hip arthroscopy, the probability of under- or overresection, and the risk for revision surgery may all be lessened.

COMPUTER MODELING AND NAVIGATION: A FULL APPROACH

Computer-assisted planning and navigation systems are currently being developed to assist surgeons from the preoperative planning stages to actual surgical treatment. A relatively new application[19] based on the MARVIN application framework uses preoperative ROM analysis on patient-specific 3D models, where virtual resection can be performed. When this dynamic model is used

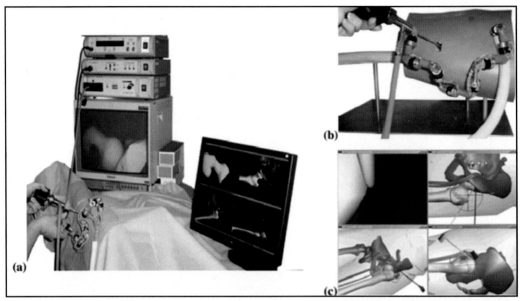

Figure 25-5. Computer-aided arthroscopic hip surgery system. (a) System setup. (b) Encoder linkage tracks an arthroscopic camera applied to a hip joint model. (c) Snapshot of a computer display shows the surgical tools and patient anatomy from multiple angles. (Reprinted with permission from Monahan E, Shimada K. Verifying the effectiveness of a computer-aided navigation system for arthroscopic hip surgery. *Stud Health Technol Inform.* 2008;132:302-307.)

intraoperatively, the planned resection area is shown as a highlighted color-coded distance map aiding the surgeon in resection depth awareness. When the resection of the bony lesion starts, the application changes the color-coded map in real time to prevent excessive or inadequate resection (Figure 25-6).

Similarly, another newly developed software program, Dyonics Plan System, allows surgeons to preoperatively view a 3D CT model of the femur and pelvis and perform dynamic ROM simulation. It also allows for intraoperative guidance instead of using an imageless guided system with encoder linkages; however, this software uses intraoperative fluoroscopic images, which have been found to correlate well with the 3D CT-generated images.[20] Surgeons are able to view the various virtual fluoroscopic views and compare these with intraoperative fluoroscopy to assist comprehensive correction of the cam- and pincer-type pathomorphologies.

FUTURE IMPLICATIONS AND LIMITATIONS

Computer modeling and navigation could play a major role in improving outcomes and reducing intra- and postoperative complications for patients undergoing arthroscopic treatment for FAI. The recent developments, however, are still in their infancy. No study has empirically shown improved clinical results. Food and Drug Administration approval has yet to be granted for these systems, and comparative trials need to be conducted. Most of these modeling systems use preoperative CT images to reconstruct the skeletal components and bony impingement of the hip yet lack insight into acetabular pathoanatomy. Acetabular coverage, from a volumetric standpoint, has yet to be defined and is a current area of investigation. Furthermore, the ROM simulation software is programmed on the basis of bony anatomy and does not account for surrounding soft tissue structures, such as the labrum, cartilage, and capsule. Future models that incorporate soft tissue and bony anatomy may provide greater benefit, understanding, and clinical utility. Lastly, these models have been shown to work only for concentric hip joints. The dynamic center of rotation

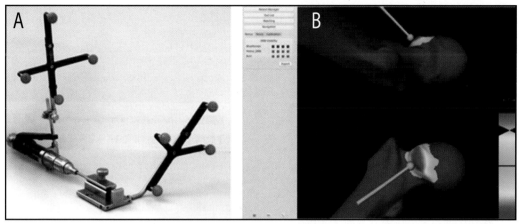

Figure 25-6. (A) Electric Pen Drive (Synthes GmbH) with a mounted ring clamp and attached dynamic reference base fitted into the custom-made calibration block for the calibration of the tool axis and burr tip. (B) Screenshot of the navigation application. The reaming area of interest is presented as a color-coded distance map according to the planned situation. The color-coded burr guides the surgeon in regard to the reaming distance. (Reprinted with permission frrom Ecker TM, Puls M, Steppacher SD, et al. Computer-assisted femoral head-neck osteochondroplasty using a surgical milling device an in vitro accuracy study. *J Arthroplasty.* 2012;27[2]:310-316.)

seen in dysplastic hips makes it more difficult to dynamize the 3D CT models to accurately define areas of impingement; however, this topic is currently under investigation. Segmentation of 2D CT data with a severely deformed proximal femur, such as Perthes' disease or residual slipped capital femoral epiphysis, may also result in difficulty with modeling and dynamization.

Although challenges still exist, advances have been made in computer modeling and navigation specific for arthroscopy of the hip. Three-dimensional, patient-specific CT models can be used preoperatively to assess abnormal bony pathoanatomy. Dynamic ROM simulations can be applied to these models in an attempt to predict pre- and postoperative ROM. In addition, these models have the potential to be integrated intraoperatively to assist surgeons with real-time bony resection. These advances could potentially improve outcomes in those affected by FAI and other related hip disorders that require an arthroscopic approach to treatment.

TOP TECHNICAL PEARLS FOR THE PROCEDURE

1. Use 3-dimensional computer modeling to visualize the hip joint preoperatively and improve spatial awareness.

2. Simulate preoperative hip range of motion based on patient-specific computer-generated models to help identify potential zones of impingement.

3. Predict postoperative hip range of motion after virtually resecting patient-specific computer-generated models preoperatively.

4. Use computer modeling and navigation intraoperatively to help reduce operative time and tool path length, thus improving patient outcomes.

5. Potentially reduce under- or overresection of bony lesions intraoperatively by using a patient-specific, preoperatively generated model or plan.

REFERENCES

1. Bedi A, Chen N, Robertson W, Kelly BT. The management of labral tears and femoroacetabular impingement of the hip in the young, active patient. *Arthroscopy*. 2008;24(10):1135-1145.
2. Ng VY, Arora N, Best TM, Pan X, Ellis TJ. Efficacy of surgery for femoroacetabular impingement: a systematic review. *Am J Sports Med*. 2010;38(11):2337-2345.
3. Botser IB, Smith TW Jr, Nasser R, Domb BG. Open surgical dislocation versus arthroscopy for femoroacetabular impingement: a comparison of clinical outcomes. *Arthroscopy*. 2011;27(2):270-278.
4. Imam S, Khanduja V. Current concepts in the diagnosis and management of femoroacetabular impingement. *Int Orthop*. 2011;35(10):1427-1435.
5. Nötzli HP, Wyss TF, Stoecklin CH, Schmid MR, Treiber K, Hodler J. The contour of the femoral head-neck junction as a predictor for the risk of anterior impingement. *J Bone Joint Surg Br*. 2002;84(4):556-560.
6. Eijer H, Leunig M, Mahomed M, Ganz R. Cross-table lateral radiograph for screening of anterior femoral head-neck offset in patients with femoro-acetabular impingement. *Hip Int*. 2001;11:37-41.
7. Lattanzi R, Petchprapa C, Glaser C, et al. A new method to analyze dGEMRIC measurements in femoroacetabular impingement: preliminary validation against arthroscopic findings. *Osteoarthritis Cartilage*. 2012;20(10):1127-1133.
8. Bittersohl B, Hosalkar HS, Apprich S, Werlen SA, Siebenrock KA, Mamisch TC. Comparison of preoperative dGEMRIC imaging with intra-operative findings in femoroacetabular impingement: preliminary findings. *Skeletal Radiol*. 2011;40(5):553-561.
9. Zoroofi RA, Sato Y, Sasama T, et al. Automated segmentation of acetabulum and femoral head from 3-D CT images. *IEEE Trans Inf Technol Biomed*. 2003;7(4):329-343.
10. Heyworth BE, Dolan MM, Nguyen JT, Chen NC, Kelly BT. Preoperative three-dimensional CT predicts intraoperative findings in hip arthroscopy. *Clin Orthop Relat Res*. 2012;470(7):1950-1957.
11. Milone MT, Bedi A, Poultsides L, et al. Novel CT-based three-dimensional software improves the characterization of cam morphology. *Clin Orthop Relat Res*. 2013;471(8):2484-2491.
12. Kang RW, Yanke AB, Espinoza Orias AA, Inoue N, Nho SJ. Emerging ideas: novel 3-D quantification and classification of cam lesions in patients with femoroacetabular impingement. *Clin Orthop Relat Res*. 2013;471(2):358-362.
13. Tannast M, Kubiak-Langer M, Langlotz F, Puls M, Murphy SB, Siebenrock KA. Noninvasive three-dimensional assessment of femoroacetabular impingement. *J Orthop Res*. 2007;25(1):122-131.
14. Kubiak-Langer M, Tannast M, Murphy SB, Siebenrock KA, Langlotz F. Range of motion in anterior femoroacetabular impingement. *Clin Orthop Relat Res*. 2007;458:117-124.
15. Bedi A, Dolan M, Hetsroni I, et al. Surgical treatment of femoroacetabular impingement improves hip kinematics: a computer-assisted model. *Am J Sports Med*. 2011;39 suppl:43S-49S.
16. Monahan E, Shimada K. Computer-aided navigation for arthroscopic hip surgery using encoder linkages for position tracking. *Stud Health Technol Inform*. 2006;119:393-398.
17. Monahan E, Shimada K. Verifying the effectiveness of a computer-aided navigation system for arthroscopic hip surgery. *Stud Health Technol Inform*. 2008;132:302-307.
18. Brunner A, Horisberger M, Herzog RF. Evaluation of a computed tomography-based navigation system prototype for hip arthroscopy in the treatment of femoroacetabular cam impingement. *Arthroscopy*. 2009;25(4):382-391.
19. Ecker TM, Puls M, Steppacher SD, et al. Computer-assisted femoral head-neck osteochondroplasty using a surgical milling device an in vitro accuracy study. *J Arthroplasty*. 2012;27(2):310-316.
20. Ross JR, Bedi A, Stone RM, et al. Intraoperative fluoroscopic imaging to treat cam deformities: correlation with 3-dimensional computed tomography. *Am J Sports Med*. 2014;42(6):1370-1376.

Please see videos on the accompanying website at

www.ArthroscopicTechniques.com

26

Special Considerations for Revision Hip Arthroscopy

Eilish O'Sullivan, PT, DPT, OCS, SCS and Bryan T. Kelly, MD

INTRODUCTION

As the volume of hip arthroscopy procedures completed has increased, there has been a parallel increase in the number of revision hip arthroscopies. Hip arthroscopy is a nascent field that is rapidly evolving, with a significant learning curve associated with the procedure. The body of literature concerning revision hip arthroscopy is slowly expanding, with a dearth of evidence on outcomes. Hip arthroscopy has evolved rapidly over the past 10 years, from the isolated labral debridements in the early stages to the bony corrections and capsular closures of today. In some cases, these isolated debridements may not eradicate the root cause of the patient's pain, and as much of the literature has demonstrated, inadequate decompression or failure to address underlying structural issues is the most frequent cause for revision surgery.

One of the first series on revision hip arthroscopy was published by Philippon et al[1] in 2007. In their series of 37 revision surgeries (68% female), 87% of the procedures were for labral injuries, 59% for lysis of adhesions, 32% for instability, and 32% for residual bony impingement. The second procedure was performed at a mean of 20.5 months from the primary procedure. Two patients converted to total hip replacements at 7 and 9 months postoperatively, respectively. Three patients required repeat revision surgery, one for instability and 2 for new injuries. Thirty-six of 37 patients had radiographic evidence of impingement that was not addressed at the primary surgery or not addressed fully. Similarly, Heyworth et al[2] found that 79% of patients undergoing revision arthroscopy demonstrated bony impingement on x-rays. Of those with impingement, 9 out of the 19 patients had bony decompression performed in the primary procedure.

Outcomes of revision arthroscopy have been published recently.[3-5] Mean follow-up ranged from 23 to 36 months. Conversion to total hip replacement or surface replacement ranged from 0% to 8.5% in these series. Contrary to many authors, Aprato et al[3] found that only 31% of their cohort required surgery for femoroacetabular impingement (FAI). The revision surgery success

Byrd JWT, Bedi A, Stubbs AJ, eds. *The Hip:*
AANA Advanced Arthroscopic Surgical Techniques (pp 303-313).
© 2016 AANA.

in the series by Aprato et al[3] was found to decline from 1 to 3 years but was improved from the preoperative scores. Larson et al[5] found that patients undergoing revision hip arthroscopy for the correction of residual impingement made significant gains as evidenced by increases in functional outcome scores, but they were not as great as the increases made in a matched cohort of patients undergoing primary surgery for the correction of FAI. Domb et al[4] found moderate improvements in patient-reported outcomes following revision surgery and indicated predictors for successful revision, including labral defects, residual or unaddressed FAI, or heterotopic ossification (HO). Risk factors associated with revision hip preservation surgery have been examined, highlighting that patients undergoing revision were more likely to be young and female and have greater impairment as demonstrated by preoperative outcome scores as compared with a primary surgery cohort.[6] The greatest risk factor for a failed hip arthroscopy is the presence of advanced cartilage wear.[7]

In the revision setting, patients have often been in pain for a prolonged period and may have developed compensatory pathologies over time, which may further contribute to their pain and dysfunction. One should approach these patients systematically and identify all of the contributing factors to the patient's pain from deep to superficial. This begins with assessment of the bony morphology. The completeness of a prior decompression (if it was performed), the presence of other previously unidentified mechanical problems, and the status of the cartilage should also be evaluated. Femoral version is another key component because increased femoral anteversion may be protective to a certain extent in the setting of cam morphology, and femoral retroversion may magnify the effects of subtle impingement. One must be sure that the joint is amenable to an arthroscopic procedure, especially in the setting of revision surgery, and must be aware of the limitations of the arthroscope. These limitations include extreme femoral version (whether ante- or retroverted), pronounced coxa vara or valga, or anterior or lateral acetabular undercoverage. These factors may be more suitably addressed through an open procedure.

The capsule, ligaments, and labrum are assessed next through a combination of radiographic imaging and physical examination. Persistent capsular laxity may occur following hip arthroscopy if the capsule is not closed, or capsular injury may occur following the procedure. In a series examining capsular integrity in patients undergoing revision hip arthroscopy for reasons other than residual FAI, no patients with capsular closure at the time of primary surgery displayed capsular defects on magnetic resonance arthrography.[8] Periarticular musculature is evaluated subsequently because there may often be issues, such as abductor dysfunction, that may increase joint-reactive forces. Other secondary compensatory muscular dysfunction includes adductor and rectus abdominis tendinopathies (core muscle dysfunction) and proximal hamstring tendinopathies, which should be assessed for. The capsuloligamentous structures are assessed with a combination of physical examination (strength and muscle-length testing) and MRI findings. Infrequently, a fractional lengthening of the psoas may be indicated in the setting of psoas impingement and/or symptomatic internal coxa saltans. One must be mindful of the patient's femoral version when assessing the appropriateness of the psoas release because increased femoral anteversion has been demonstrated to be associated with inferior outcomes.[9] Finally, one must look for neurologic contributions to the patient's pain, which may span from local structures, such as the lateral femoral cutaneous, genitofemoral, iliohypopogastric, ilioinguinal, and pudendal nerves to the lumbosacral nerve roots.

INDICATIONS

▶ Persistent pain and decreased functional mobility following primary arthroscopy
▶ Most frequently, unaddressed or incompletely addressed impingement

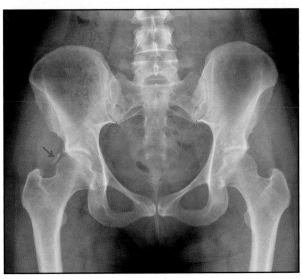

Figure 26-1. Capsular HO following right hip arthroscopy as indicated by arrow.

- ▷ Most commonly, the superoposterior and lateral portions of the cam lesion (difficult to access) and the subspine region
- ▶ Recurrent labral tear (often occurring in the setting of residual impingement)
- ▶ Lysis of adhesions (most frequently capsulolabral) in the setting of persistent stiffness and pain
- ▶ Excision of symptomatic heterotopic bone formation causing pain and/or limited range of motion (ROM) is another indication for revision arthroscopy (Figure 26-1).
- ▶ Persistent capsular laxity may occur following hip arthroscopy if the capsule is not closed, or capsular injury may occur following the procedure.
- ▶ Psoas impingement and/or symptomatic internal coxa saltans

Controversial Indications

- ▶ In the setting of significant labral deficiency, labral augmentation may be warranted. Autograft (usually a local portion of the indirect head of the rectus femoris or iliotibial band) or allograft (usually tibialis anterior or semitendinosus) may be used.
- ▶ Some patients with limited areas of cartilage wear and obvious impingement may be considered for revision surgery.

PERTINENT PHYSICAL FINDINGS

- ▶ Impingement testing
  - ▷ Subspine impingement may be assessed for with passive straight hip flexion; the patient will report pain and/or pinching at end range and will likely have decreased ROM.
  - ▷ Restriction in internal rotation at 90 degrees of hip flexion may indicate residual superolateral cam abutting the anterior acetabulum.
- ▶ Capsular laxity/anterior apprehension assessment may be completed with the patient supine in a Thomas test position, with the affected leg off the edge of the table. The examiner

Figure 26-2. Traumatic capsular disruption (arrows indicate edges of capsule) following an anterior dislocation 6 months after primary right hip arthroscopy.

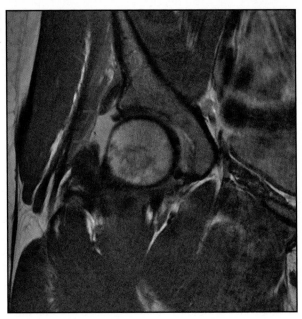

brings the affected leg into extension and external rotation while observing for signs of pain or apprehension.

▸ A diagnostic intra-articular injection is especially helpful in the setting of potential revision surgery because there are many pain generators about the hip joint, and it may aid in determining whether the pain is intra-articular.

PERTINENT IMAGING

▸ Plain x-rays, including well-positioned anteroposterior, elongated femoral neck, and false-profile views, as required to initially assess for joint spacing and adequacy of correction

▸ MRI is used to determine capsular integrity (Figure 26-2), highlight possible cartilage injury, and assess for labral injury and compensatory musculotendinous injuries.

   ▷ T2 mapping and T1 rho and delayed gadolinium-enhanced MRI of cartilage imaging allow for greater appreciation of the cartilage integrity.

   ▷ Magnetic resonance arthrography may be useful in the setting of capsular insufficiency.

▸ Computed tomography (CT) scanning with 3-dimensional reconstruction is critical for determining the areas of residual impingement and the dynamic morphological profile of the joint (Figure 26-3).

   ▷ Allows for calculation of the alpha angle and the location of the maximum alpha angle; the acetabular version at 1, 2, and 3 o'clock; femoral version; and the morphology of the subspine.

   ▷ Areas of HO may also be better delineated with CT scanning (Figure 26-4).

▸ The role of computer navigation, computer-assisted dynamic evaluation and planning, and dynamic ultrasound may be useful but are currently incompletely defined.

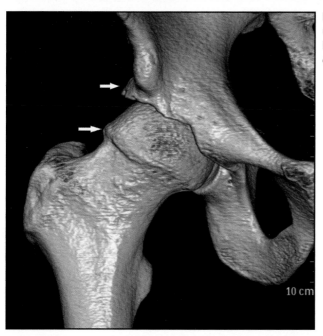

Figure 26-3. Right hip with residual/unaddressed impingement in primary hip arthroscopy, with sub-spine/rim and cam morphology present.

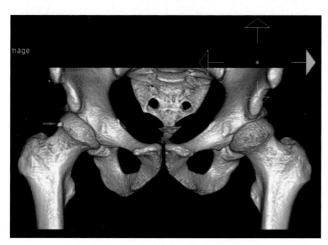

Figure 26-4. CT scan with 3D reconstruction of the pelvis. Small area of anterior HO in the capsule of the right hip is indicated by the arrow.

EQUIPMENT

- ▶ Fracture table
- ▶ C-arm fluoroscope
- ▶ Dedicated hip arthroscopy set, including extra-long cannulas with coupled obturators to place over flexible guidewires, flexible and slotted cannulas, a 70-degree arthroscope with use of a 30-degree arthroscope as needed, flexible guidewires, and spinal needles
- ▶ Extended straight and curved shaver blades and burrs
- ▶ Flexible radiofrequency probes
- ▶ Anchor system (including drill and drill guide)
- ▶ Fluid management system

POSITIONING

The patient is positioned supine on the fracture table as originally described by Byrd.[10] A large perineal post is used and should be well padded to minimize the likelihood of the patient developing pudendal neuropraxia. The feet are secured in boots, which should be well padded to protect against superficial peroneal nerve irritation.

To stabilize the patient's pelvis, minimal countertraction may be applied. Twenty-five to 50 lb of traction is applied to the operative leg while in approximately 30 degrees of abduction, and then it is brought to neutral adduction. The ease with which the suction-seal of the hip is broken may indicate a less stable hip. Fluoroscopic imaging is used to confirm adequate distraction of approximately 10 mm across the femoroacetabular joint. The goal is consistent positioning with safe setup for the patient that allows appropriate access to the joint.

STEP-BY-STEP DESCRIPTION OF THE PROCEDURE

The procedure is done in a stepwise process to systematically address the pathology within the joint. A consistent approach minimizes errors. Three portals are generally used—the anterolateral, mid-anterior, and distal anterolateral accessory portals—and have been determined to be within the safe zone.[11] The anterolateral portal is established first at the anterior border of the superior aspect of the greater trochanter. It is established 1 to 2 cm superior and 1 to 2 cm anterior to the greater trochanter. The portal is established just posterior to the iliotibial band, and once established, a spinal needle is advanced through it into the hip joint in close proximity to the femoral head. The portals should be spaced at least 6 cm apart to allow adequate maneuverability of instruments.

The second portal established is the mid-anterior portal, which is established under arthroscopic guidance. This is approximately 2 cm lateral and distal the intersection of a horizontal line from the anterior superior iliac spine and a vertical line from the tip of the greater trochanter. The mid-anterior portal poses less potential harm to the lateral femoral cutaneous nerve than the traditional anterior portal. Following this, the distal anterolateral accessory portal is established, which is helpful for anchor placement when labral refixation is required. This portal is in line with the anterolateral portal and approximately 6 cm distal to it. One must proceed with care into the joint because previous surgery may have left capsular scarring and adhesions, making access slightly more difficult.

Once the portals have been established, the interportal capsulotomy is created between the mid-anterior and lateral portals. This increases the ease of visualization of rim and labrum pathology and should be completed several millimeters away from its attachment to allow for repair at the completion of the procedure.

Upon entry to the joint, a systematic evaluation of the intra-articular structures should commence with the articular cartilage on the femoral and acetabular sides of the joint. The presence and location of synovitis should be noted. The integrity of the ligamentum teres should be examined, as well as possible foveal inflammation. The joint capsule is examined for attenuation or frank injury (Figure 26-5). The labrum is assessed for injury.

Following the capsulotomy, adhesions between the capsule and labrum or femoral neck are identified and, if present, must by lysed to reestablish the normal capsulolabral recess (Figure 26-6). Electrocautery may be used to remove the adhesions, but one must proceed with caution to avoid injuring the labrum.

Exposure of the acetabulum is achieved through dissection subperiosteally, which allows for rim decompression if necessary. If a rim decompression is performed, one must be mindful of the extent of the decompression because iatrogenic instability has occurred in the setting of overresection of the rim. The subspine is also exposed with this approach and may be decompressed at this point. Care must be taken to protect the direct head of the rectus femoris during the resection.

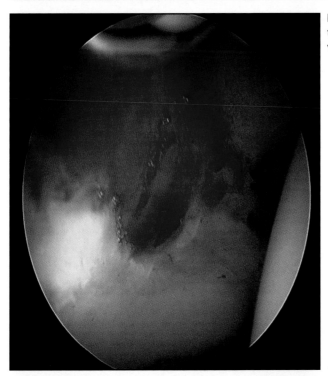

Figure 26-5. Frank capsular disruption following right hip arthroscopy as viewed from the anterolateral portal.

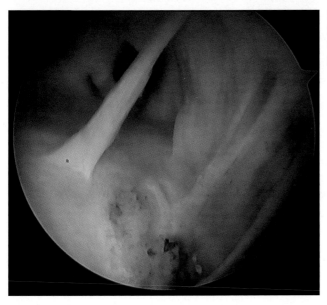

Figure 26-6. Capsulolabral adhesions found during revision right hip arthroscopy as viewed from the mid-anterior portal.

A failed labral repair may be addressed with labral refixation if possible; if that is not possible, debridement of the frayed tissue should occur. If the labrum is amenable to refixation, the acetabular rim must be prepared down to a bed of bleeding bone. Distal portal usage for the suture anchors allows for a trajectory that is parallel to the joint surface and avoids joint penetration. Evaluation for poor anchor placement should be carefully performed to assess for joint perforation or medial penetration through the base of the anterior inferior iliac spine with potential injury to the psoas. Misplaced anchors may need to be removed.

Figure 26-7. Decompression of a residual cam lesion in a right hip. Black arrow indicates labral refixation, and blue arrow indicates cam decompression as viewed from the mid-anterior portal.

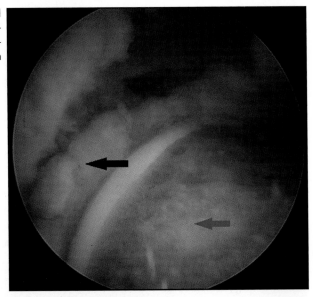

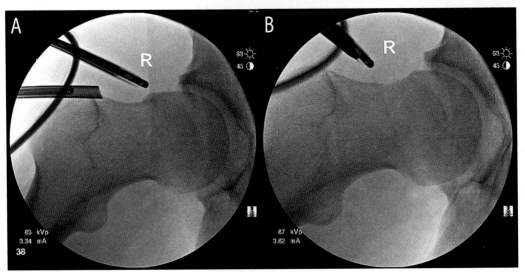

Figure 26-8. Intraoperative fluoroscopic images of the cam decompression during right revision hip arthroscopy (A) prior to decompression and (B) following decompression.

Once the rim and labrum have been addressed, traction is released, and attention is shifted to the peripheral compartment. In the setting of incomplete or unaddressed femoral-sided impingement, complete exposure of the bony deformity is imperative. The T capsulotomy allows for the most comprehensive visualization, including the femoral neck. The interval separating the medial and lateral limbs of the iliofemoral ligament is identified with a switching stick, and then a blade is used to cut the capsule along the femoral neck toward the intertrochanteric groove. Dynamic fluoroscopy assists the direct visualization to perform the femoroplasty. The cam deformity should be sequentially addressed from superior, superolateral, anterior, anterolateral, and inferior portions (Figure 26-7). The retinacular vessels should be visualized. Restoration of adequate head-neck offset is confirmed with fluoroscopy (Figure 26-8).

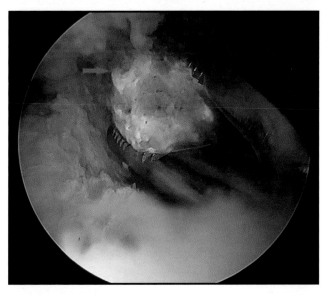

Figure 26-9. Excision of anterior capsular HO (arrow) in a right hip as viewed from the anterolateral portal.

If psoas impingement is suspected and there is erythema and labral injury at anteromedial aspect (2:30 to 3 o'clock), a fractional lengthening of the psoas may be considered in the absence of excessive femoral anteversion. This is accomplished through a small capsular window at the level of the acetabulum. This should be completed as one of the last portions of the procedure and without traction applied to avoid potential retroperitoneal fluid extravasation.

For arthroscopic HO removal, the central compartment is surveyed first under traction to assess for any concomitant intra-articular processes. For very large fragments, a mini-open approach may be required. To excise the HO, fluoroscopy is used to determine the location of the fragment. Spinal needles may be used to localize the HO. A cannula is then inserted over the spinal needle (Figure 26-9).

In the setting of instability, a capsular imbrication may be considered, with closure of the T capsulotomy, as well as proximal-to-distal closure. The T portion of the capsulotomy is closed first with side-to-side simple sutures with a penetrating suture passer and retriever through the limbs of the capsulotomy. If necessary, capsular tissue may be advanced to the indirect head of the rectus femoris to ensure stability (Figure 26-10).

After all central and peripheral compartment pathology has been addressed, a dynamic arthroscopy should be completed to assess for any residual impingement.

POSTOPERATIVE PROTOCOL

The postoperative protocol will be dictated by the exact procedures performed, with the most restrictive guidelines prevailing in dictating the patient's progression postoperatively. In general, patients are placed on 75 mg of indomethacin for 4 days, followed by 30 days of naproxen for prophylaxis of HO. Those who have had excision of HO are placed on 10 days of indomethacin, followed by the same course of naproxen. Early passive pain-free ROM is encouraged to decrease the likelihood of developing adhesions in the case of labral refixation. Physical therapy is generally initiated on postoperative day 1 and consists of passive ROM, gentle isometrics, and stationary bicycling. Patients leave the hospital with a continuous passive motion machine and a pneumatic cryotherapy device.

If a capsular plication is performed, extension to neutral and external rotation to 30 degrees are protected for 6 weeks. These patients are placed in an orthosis to restrict external rotation and

Figure 26-10. Capsular repair to the indirect head of the rectus femoris in a right hip as viewed from the mid-anterior portal.

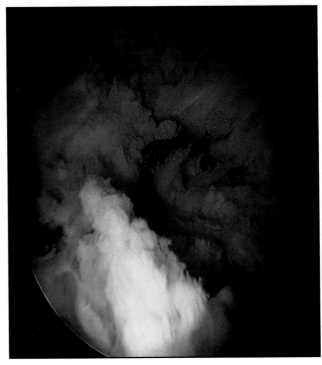

extension while outside of the home for 4 weeks. Patients are also placed in boots with a bolster to protect external rotation in the supine position when sleeping for the first 4 weeks.

Patients follow a structured progressive rehabilitation program, with emphasis on a functional criteria-based progression. Following revision surgery, patients may require a slightly slower progression, which will be determined by the patient's tolerance and muscular adaptations postoperatively. For the first 6 weeks postoperatively, the goal is to restore ROM (within the parameters of the specific procedure) and restore the ability to complete activities of daily living. Weeks 6 through 12 focus on restoring strength and eradicating patterns of compensatory dysfunction because there is often a prolonged period of neuromuscular dysfunction in the setting of a revision surgery. If the patient demonstrates adequate strength and stability at 12 weeks postoperatively, graduated progression toward recreational/sports activities may be initiated with the introduction of a running program.

Potential Complications

The general complications associated with hip arthroscopy hold true in the setting of revision hip arthroscopy. These include infection (most frequently limited to superficial wound infection), transient neuropraxia (including lateral femoral cutaneous, peroneal, and pudendal nerve), iatrogenic chondral and labral injuries, HO, and development of adhesions. Less likely complications include fluid extravasation and deep venous thrombosis.

Top Technical Pearls for the Procedure

1. Accurate diagnosis of the pain-generating structures preoperatively is of the utmost importance in maximizing the chance for a successful outcome from revision surgery.

2. Preoperative planning, including the use of CT scans to delineate areas of residual impingement, is imperative.

3. Careful management of the soft tissue structures, especially the capsule, is essential.

4. Recognize the strengths and limitations of the arthroscopic procedure because some complex deformities are better suited for an open approach.

5. Patient expectations must be managed appropriately in terms of recovery and outcomes and must be discussed at length prior to revision surgery.

References

1. Philippon MJ, Schenker ML, Briggs KK, Kuppersmith DA, Maxwell RB, Stubbs AJ. Revision hip arthroscopy. *Am J Sports Med.* 2007;35(11):1918-1921.
2. Heyworth BE, Shindle MK, Voos JE, Rudzki JR, Kelly BT. Radiologic and intraoperative findings in revision hip arthroscopy. *Arthroscopy.* 2007;23(12):1295-1302.
3. Aprato A, Jayasekera N, Villar RN. Revisions hip arthroscopic surgery: outcome at three years. *Knee Surg Sports Traumatol Arthrosc.* 2014;22(4):932-937.
4. Domb BG, Stake CE, Lindner D, El-Bitar Y, Jackson TJ. Revision hip preservation surgery with hip arthroscopy: clinical outcomes. *Arthroscopy.* 2014;30(5):581-587.
5. Larson CM, Giveans MR, Samuelson KM, Stone RM, Bedi A. Arthroscopic hip revision surgery for residual femoroacetabular impingement (FAI): surgical outcomes compared with a matched cohort after primary arthroscopic FAI correction. *Am J Sports Med.* 2014;42(8):1785-1790.
6. Ricciardi BF, Fields K, Kelly BT, Ranawat AS, Coleman SH, Sink EL. Causes and risk factors for revision hip preservation surgery. *Am J Sports Med.* 2014;42(11):2627-2633.
7. Bogunovic L, Gottlieb M, Pashos G, Baca G, Clohisy JC. Why do hip arthroscopy procedures fail? *Clin Orthop Relat Res.* 2013;471(8):2523-2529.
8. McCormick F, Slikker W III, Harris JD, et al. Evidence of capsular defect following hip arthroscopy. *Knee Surg Sports Traumatol Arthrosc.* 2014;22(4):902-905.
9. Fabricant PD, Bedi A, De La Torre K, Kelly BT. Clinical outcomes after arthroscopic psoas lengthening: the effect of femoral version. *Arthroscopy.* 2012;28(7):965-971.
10. Byrd JW. Hip arthroscopy utilizing the supine position. *Arthroscopy.* 1994;10(3):275-280.
11. Robertson WJ, Kelly BT. The safe zone for hip arthroscopy: a cadaveric assessment of central, peripheral, and lateral compartment portal placement. *Arthroscopy.* 2008;24(9):1019-1026.

Please see videos on the accompanying website at
www.ArthroscopicTechniques.com

Financial Disclosures

Dr. Geoffrey D. Abrams has no financial or proprietary interest in the materials presented herein.

Dr. William Brian Acker II has no financial or proprietary interest in the materials presented herein.

Dr. Eduardo Acosta-Rodriguez has no financial or proprietary interest in the materials presented herein.

Dr. Marco Acuna-Tovar has no financial or proprietary interest in the materials presented herein.

Dr. Asheesh Bedi is a consultant for Arthrex, Inc and owns stock in A3 Surgical.

Dr. J. W. Thomas Byrd is a consultant for and has received research support from Smith & Nephew, is a consultant for and owns stock in A3 Surgical, and receives royalties from Springer.

Dr. Emily Cha has no financial or proprietary interest in the materials presented herein.

Dr. John J. Christoforetti has no financial or proprietary interest in the materials presented herein.

Dr. Ryan M. Degen has no financial or proprietary interest in the materials presented herein.

Dr. Michael Dienst is a consultant for Karl Storz GmbH.

Dr. Benjamin G. Domb has no financial or proprietary interest in the materials presented herein.

Dr. Michael B. Gerhardt has no financial or proprietary interest in the materials presented herein.

Dr. Jonathan A. Godin has no financial or proprietary interest in the materials presented herein.

Dr. Carlos A. Guanche has no financial or proprietary interest in the materials presented herein.

Dr. Joshua D. Harris has no financial or proprietary interest in the materials presented herein.

Dr. Munif Ahmad Hatem has no financial or proprietary interest in the materials presented herein.

Dr. Elizabeth A. Howse has no financial or proprietary interest in the materials presented herein.

Dr. Víctor M. Ilizaliturri Jr is a consultant for ConMed.

Dr. Pedro Joachin-Hernandez has no financial or proprietary interest in the materials presented herein.

Dr. Brandon Johnson has no financial or proprietary interest in the materials presented herein.

Dr. Nicholas Johnson has no financial or proprietary interest in the materials presented herein.

Dr. Michael R. Karns has no financial or proprietary interest in the materials presented herein.

Dr. Bryan T. Kelly is a consultant for and shareholder in A3 Surgical and a consultant for Arthrex.

Dr. Scott R. Kling has no financial or proprietary interest in the materials presented herein.

Mr. Andrew W. Kuhn has no financial or proprietary interest in the materials presented herein.

Dr. Matthias Kusma is a consultant for Karl Storz GmbH.

Dr. Christopher M. Larson is a consultant for Smith & Nephew Endoscopy and owns stock in A3 Surgical.

Dr. G. Peter Maiers II has no financial or proprietary interest in the materials presented herein.

Dr. Matthew Mantell has no financial or proprietary interest in the materials presented herein.

Dr. Hal D. Martin has no financial or proprietary interest in the materials presented herein.

Dr. Richard C. Mather III has no financial or proprietary interest in the materials presented herein.

Dr. Lance Maynard has no financial or proprietary interest in the materials presented herein.

Dr. Jeffrey J. Nepple is a consultant for Smith & Nephew.

Dr. Shane J. Nho has no financial or proprietary interest in the materials presented herein.

Dr. Eilish O'Sullivan has no financial or proprietary interest in the materials presented herein.

Dr. Ian J. Palmer has no financial or proprietary interest in the materials presented herein.

Dr. Sunny H. Patel has no financial or proprietary interest in the materials presented herein.

Dr. Marc J. Philippon receives royalties from Smith & Nephew, Linvatec, Bledsoe, DonJoy, and Arthrosurface; is a paid consultant for Smith & Nephew and MIS; and owns stock or stock options in Smith & Nephew, Arthrosurface, HIPCO, and MIS.

Dr. James R. Ross has no financial or proprietary interest in the materials presented herein.

Dr. Marc R. Safran has no financial or proprietary interest in the materials presented herein.

Dr. Michael J. Salata is a paid consultant for Smith & Nephew.

Dr. John P. Salvo has no financial or proprietary interest in the materials presented herein.

Dr. Joshua D. Sampson has no financial or proprietary interest in the materials presented herein.

Dr. Thomas G. Sampson is a consultant for ConMed Linvatec.

Dr. Chris Stake has no financial or proprietary interest in the materials presented herein.

Ms. Rebecca M. Stone has no financial or proprietary interest in the materials presented herein.

Dr. Allston J. Stubbs is a consultant for Smith & Nephew, owns stock in Johnson & Johnson, and has received research support from Bauerfeind.

Dr. Eric P. Tannenbaum has no financial or proprietary interest in the materials presented herein.

Dr. Fotios Paul Tjoumakaris has no financial or proprietary interest in the materials presented herein.

Dr. Christiano A. C. Trindade has not disclosed any relevant financial relationships.

Dr. William Kelton Vasileff has no financial or proprietary interest in the materials presented herein.

Dr. Patrick Vavken has no financial or proprietary interest in the materials presented herein.

Dr. Andrew B. Wolff is a consultant for Stryker and Arthrex.

Dr. Thomas H. Wuerz has no financial or proprietary interest in the materials presented herein.

Dr. Yi-Meng Yen is a consultant for Smith & Nephew Endoscopy and Orthopaedatrics.

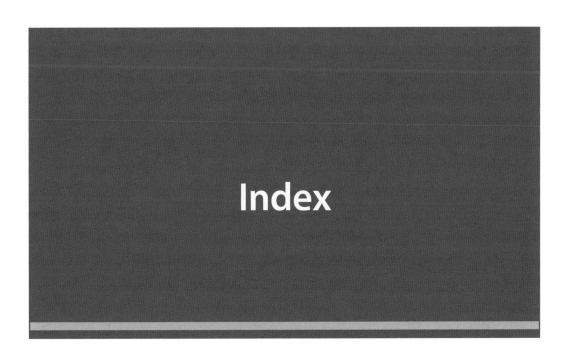

Index